Treatment of Severe Personality Disorders

RESOLUTION OF AGGRESSION AND RECOVERY OF EROTICISM

Treatment of Severe Personality Disorders

RESOLUTION OF AGGRESSION AND RECOVERY OF EROTICISM

Otto F. Kernberg, M.D.

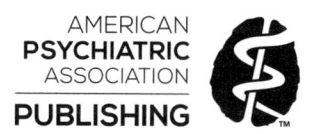

AMERICAN
PSYCHIATRIC
ASSOCIATION
PUBLISHING

Note: The author has worked to ensure that all information in this book is accurate at the time of publication and consistent with general psychiatric and medical standards, and that information concerning drug dosages, schedules, and routes of administration is accurate at the time of publication and consistent with standards set by the U.S. Food and Drug Administration and the general medical community. As medical research and practice continue to advance, however, therapeutic standards may change. Moreover, specific situations may require a specific therapeutic response not included in this book. For these reasons and because human and mechanical errors sometimes occur, we recommend that readers follow the advice of physicians directly involved in their care or the care of a member of their family.

Books published by American Psychiatric Association Publishing represent the findings, conclusions, and views of the individual authors and do not necessarily represent the policies and opinions of American Psychiatric Association Publishing or the American Psychiatric Association.

Copyright © 2018 American Psychiatric Association Publishing

ALL RIGHTS RESERVED
First Edition
Manufactured in the United States of America on acid-free paper
22 21 20 19 18   5 4 3 2 1

American Psychiatric Association Publishing
800 Maine Ave., SW, Suite 900
Washington, DC 20024
www.appi.org

Library of Congress Cataloging-in-Publication Data
Names: Kernberg, Otto F., 1928– author. | American Psychiatric
   Association Publishing, issuing body.
Title: Treatment of severe personality disorders : resolution of aggression
   and recovery of eroticism / Otto F. Kernberg.
Description: Washington, DC: American Psychiatric Association
   Publishing, [2018] | Includes bibliographical references and index.
Identifiers: LCCN 2017043849 (print) | LCCN 2017044627 (ebook) |
   ISBN 9781615371884 (ebook) | ISBN 9781615371433 (pbk. : alk. paper)
Subjects: | MESH: Personality Disorders—therapy | Psychotherapy—
   methods | Transference (Psychology)
Classification: LCC RC480 (ebook) | LCC RC480 (print) | NLM WM 190 |
   DDC
616.89/14—dc23
LC record available at https://lccn.loc.gov/2017043849

British Library Cataloguing in Publication Data
A CIP record is available from the British Library.

*To Kay,
with all my love*

Contents

Introduction xi
Acknowledgments xvii

PART I
Personality Disorders

1 What Is Personality? 3

2 Overview and Critique of the Classification of Personality Disorders Proposed for DSM-5 19

3 Neurobiological Correlates of Object Relations Theory 31

PART II
Spectrum of Psychoanalytic Psychotherapies

4 The Basic Components of Psychoanalytic Technique and Derived Psychoanalytic Psychotherapies 49

5 Interpretation in Borderline Pathology
A CLINICAL ILLUSTRATION.................. 73

6 The Spectrum of Psychoanalytic Techniques ... 81

7 New Developments in Transference-Focused Psychotherapy........................ 105

8 A New Formulation of Supportive Psychodynamic Psychotherapy 131

PART III
Narcissistic Pathology

9 An Overview of the Treatment of Severe Narcissistic Pathology 153

10 Narcissistic Defenses in the Distortion of Free Association and Their Underlying Anxieties ... 181

11 The Differential Diagnosis of Antisocial Behavior
A CLINICAL APPROACH..................... 197

PART IV
Erotism in the Transference

12 Erotic Transference and Countertransference in Patients With Severe Personality Disorders
PART I: THE EVALUATION OF SEXUAL PATHOLOGY..... 215

13 Erotic Transference and Countertransference in Patients With Severe Personality Disorders
PART II: THERAPEUTIC DEVELOPMENTS 235

PART V
Denial of Reality, Mourning, and the Training of Psychotherapists

14 The Denial of Reality 251

15 The Long-Term Effects of the Mourning Process 265

16 A Proposal for Innovation in Psychoanalytic Education 273

Index **285**

Introduction

This book presents an overview of my recent work regarding the neurobiological and psychodynamic determinants of the structure, development, and functioning of normal personality and personality disorders. It updates the findings of the Personality Disorders Institute of the Weill Cornell Medical College Department of Psychiatry that were derived from the empirical research and clinical investigation of severe personality disorders, and the related experience of the effectiveness of transference-focused psychotherapy (TFP), a specific psychodynamic treatment for these disorders developed at our institute. In this book, I focus particularly on an essential group of techniques common to all psychoanalytically derived treatments and clarify the corresponding differential features of various psychodynamic treatment approaches. Parts I and II of this book present this material.

Part III of this book is dedicated to an updated review of severe narcissistic psychopathology, and in Part IV, I review the psychopathology of eroticism and the problems in the love life of patients with severe personality disorders. In the last section, Part V, I examine general existential issues related to the management of the challenges of life tasks experienced by these patients, the effects of the capacity for mourning processes, and lastly, some essential preconditions in the education of psychodynamic psychotherapists to carry out the challenging and complex psychotherapeutic work in this field.

What follows is a capsule summary of the context of all the chapters of this book.

Part I of this book, "Personality Disorders," deals with the concept of personality disorders. Chapter 1 explores a contemporary concept of personality that does justice to both the genetic and constitutional determinants of personality functioning as expressed in the vicissitudes of the organization of the central nervous system, and the derived influence of intrapsychic developments that constitute a second level of structural determinants of personality functioning. In short, this chapter represents an effort to integrate genetic and neurobiological influences with psychodynamic and environmental influences on the organization and functioning of the personality.

Chapter 2 examines the present classification of personality disorders by the American Psychiatric Association. In the process, it discusses the consequences of the various viewpoints that, in their mutual confrontations, have influenced the way in which both the traditional classification of DSM-III and DSM-IV have come about, and the impact of new knowledge on the new classification of DSM-5. This latter proposal does greater justice to our current understanding of personality structure while illustrating the conflicts between scientific and political considerations that have hindered the classification of personality disorders in the past.

Chapter 3 illustrates in some detail how our present knowledge of neurobiological structures and neurotransmitters meshes with the psychodynamic determinants of organization of psychic experience. In the process, the complex interaction between neurobiological and psychodynamic features that determine psychological organization is spelled out.

Jointly, these three chapters provide an updated review of what we know about personality functioning, the relationship between personality and personality disorders, and the developmental aspects of the constitution of severe personality disorders.

Part II of this book, "Spectrum of Psychoanalytic Psychotherapies," deals with psychodynamic psychotherapies and the contemporary developments and controversies in this field. Chapter 4 describes four essential psychoanalytic techniques that are considered the common basis for standard psychoanalysis as well as for all derived psychoanalytic psychotherapies. They are *interpretation, transference analysis, technical neutrality,* and *countertransference utilization.*

Chapter 5 illustrates how the key technique of interpretation is applied in the TFP of severe personality disorders, demonstrating with a clinical case the fact that, in contrast to older assumptions, patients with severe personality disorder are able to benefit from interpretation as an essential technical tool.

Chapter 6 conveys the full spectrum of psychodynamic techniques that constitute the application of the basic techniques outlined in Chapter 4. In essence, the combination of Chapter 4 and Chapter 6 reflects a complete technical psychotherapeutic armamentarium that is common to psychoanalysis and all psychoanalytic psychotherapies.

Chapter 7 is a brief summary of TFP, the specific psychodynamic psychotherapy for the treatment of severe personality disorders developed by the Personality Disorders Institute, and updates this treatment with the latest clinical and research findings. This chapter also describes the four essential psychoanalytic techniques—interpretation, transference analysis, technical neutrality, and countertransference utilization—that are considered the common basis for standard psychoanalysis as well as for all derived psychoanalytic psychotherapies.

Chapter 8, the final chapter of this section, summarizes a contemporary supportive psychodynamic psychotherapy, thus completing the entire spectrum ranging from psychoanalysis, on one end, to supportive psychotherapy, on the other.

Part III of this book, "Narcissistic Pathology," deals with severe narcissistic pathology, its diagnosis, prognosis, and treatment. Chapter 9 presents an overview of the clinical syndromes and the corresponding treatment approaches of narcissistic personality disorder. It reflects the rapid development, in recent years, of clinical and research findings that have clarified a wide spectrum of degrees of severity and differences of clinical manifestations of a common, particular organization that is specific to narcissistic personality disorder, and the differential prognostic criteria and therapeutic techniques that this complexity implies.

Chapter 10 describes the particular distortions of verbal communication in the therapeutic interaction with narcissistic patients. These distortions are reflected in the efforts to carry out free association by narcissistic patients undergoing psychotherapeutic treatment.

Chapter 11 focuses more sharply on the differential diagnosis of antisocial behavior as the most important indicator of potential limitation of psychotherapeutic treatment of patients with narcissistic pathology. This chapter also clarifies the still controversial nature of the relationship between narcissistic pathology in a broad sense, and the specific antisocial personality disorder, the most severe form of pathological narcissism. This differential diagnosis should be of great practical interest to all mental health providers working with narcissistic psychopathology.

Part IV of this book, "Erotism in the Transference," deals with the diagnosis and treatment of sexual pathology, and explores the vicissitudes of the love life of people with severe personality disorders. Chapter 12 explores the diagnostic process of evaluating difficulties in the love life and sexual functioning of people with personality disorders, and correspondent countertransference developments in the therapist. This chapter also examines typical sexual conflicts at the level of neurotic personality disorganization of less severe personality disorders.

Chapter 13 specifically explores erotic transference and countertransference in patients with borderline personality organization. This chapter reflects an effort to present a comprehensive view of the different symptoms and interpersonal problems derived from serious sexual inhibitions and limitations these patients present in their capacity to commit to intimate relationships. It deals, in short, with a major, still largely unexplored, complication of personality disorders and technical approaches to the respective treatment.

Part V of this book, "Denial of Reality, Mourning, and the Training of Psychotherapists," reflects a focus on particular problems that have emerged as important consequences of severe personality disorders. Chapter 14 focuses on the denial of reality as an important existential problem of patients with severe personality disorders, the importance of clinical alertness to blind self-destructiveness, and the need to clarify and deal with the consequences of denial of reality. This issue has emerged as a major challenge in long-term psychotherapeutic treatment of these patients, and the resolution of the denial of reality may open major new life experiences and success.

Chapter 15 is a reflection on the effects of normal mourning processes as part of dealing with the reality of life and focuses on the fact that mourning processes constitute a permanent aspect of personality functioning rather than a temporary consequence of severe object loss or having to deal with death. This chapter also stresses that mourning is a counterpoint to the denial of reality and constitutes a potential enrichment of emotional life.

Chapter 16 deals with the concept of an ideal learning institution in which psychodynamic psychotherapy could be taught and developed, using psychoanalytic institutions as an example of what might characterize such an institution. It is an implicit critique of present-day psychoanalytic education as well as a description of what might be an optimal way to develop and teach psychodynamic psychotherapy as a task of psychoanalytic institutes.

In conclusion, this book attempts to present an integrated update of our knowledge of personality disorders, their neurobiological and psychodynamic determinants, and a specific psychodynamic psychotherapy geared to resolve the nuclear psychopathology of these conditions, namely, the syndrome of identity diffusion and its influence on the capacity for emotional well-being and gratifying relationships with significant others. Two specific aspects of severe personality disorders are explored here in sharp focus: the nature of narcissistic pathology and its

Introduction

treatment, and the traditionally neglected, crucial importance of exploration and treatment of the impoverishment of the love life of patients with severe personality disorders, particularly those with significant narcissistic pathology. It is hoped that this book will be helpful to all clinicians working to help these patients.

Acknowledgments

In recent years, Drs. Betty Joseph and André Green, whose departure signifies a great loss for contemporary psychoanalytic thinking, have profoundly influenced my explorations in psychoanalytic theory and technique. Other European colleagues whose work has been inspiring have included, in Great Britain, Dr. Anne-Marie Sandler and the late Dr. Joseph Sandler, and Dr. Ronald Britton. In Germany, Dr. Peter Buchheim, Dr. Horst Kächele, the late Dr. Irmhild Kothe-Meyer, and Drs. Rainer Krause, Ernst Lürssen, Gerhard Roth, Almuth Sellschopp, and Peter Zagermann have influenced my thinking regarding the boundaries between contemporary psychiatric and psychotherapeutic endeavors, on the one hand, and psychoanalytic thinking, on the other. Similar influences and interactions have involved Drs. Anna Maria Nicolò and Paolo Migone in Italy and Dr. Miguel Angel Gonzalez Torres in Spain. In the United States, I am grateful for the many scientific and personal exchanges with the late Dr. Martin Bergmann, Dr. Harold Blum, Dr. Robert Michels, the late Dr. Robert Wallerstein, Dr. Robert Tyson, and Dr. Robert Pyles. My thinking on psychoanalytic education has been profoundly influenced by Drs. Cláudio Eizirik and Elias Mallet da Rocha Barros in Brazil, by Drs. Sara Zac de Filc and Dr. Isidoro Berenstein in Argentina, and by Dr. César Garza Guerrero in Mexico.

This book would not have been possible to develop without the intense collaborative work with my friends and colleagues at the Personality Disorders Institute of the Weill Cornell Medical College. I warmly thank the senior members of this Institute—in particular, Drs. Eve Caligor, Monica Carsky, Diana Diamond, Eric Fertuck, Catherine Haran, Kenneth Levy, Michael Stone, Mallay Occhiogrosso, Barry Stern and Frank Yeomans. Ms. Jill Delaney, another senior member of our group, deserves my special gratitude for her careful, critical editing of all the chapters in this book. Our research collaboration with Drs. Mark Lenzenweger, Michael Posner, David Silbersweig and B.J. Casey, in the United States, and the vigorous collaboration of our specialized adolescent personality disorders group that includes Dr. Alan Weiner in New York, Drs. Lina Normandin and Karin Ensink in Canada, and Drs. Marion Braun, Werner Köpp, and Maya Krischer in Germany have stimulated the development of our joint endeavors regarding psychotherapeutic methods and research. Similar stimulating and creative contributions have originated from Drs. Peter Buchheim, Susanna Hörtz, Mathias Lohmer, Manfred Lütz, Philipp Martius, Almuth Sellschopp, and Agnes Schneider-Heine in Germany; from Drs. Stephan Doering, Melitta Fischer-Kern, Peter Schuster, Anna Buchheim, and George Brownstone in Austria; and from Dr. Gerhard Dammann in Switzerland.

Above all, I wish to express my profound appreciation to Dr. John Clarkin, Co-Director of the Personality Disorders Institute of the Weill Cornell Medical College, and the mastermind in the transformation of our theoretical and clinical hypotheses into workable research designs. He has been able to achieve the successful development of our research efforts in the middle of the administrative challenges related to the professional and financial infrastructure of our work. In this regard, I wish to express my profound gratitude and appreciation to Mr. Alvin Dworman and Mr. and Mrs. Michael Tusiani for their confidence and generous support of our work with severe personality disorders. Their interest and understanding have been essential stimulating factors in our research and educational functions. All of this would not have been as fruitful as it has been without the consistent, concerned, effective, and inspiring leadership support by Dr. Jack Barchas, Professor and Chairman of the Department of Psychiatry of the Weill Cornell Medical College.

I also wish to thank warmly Ms. Janie Blumenthal, who diligently typed and organized the various chapters of this book, and express my heartfelt gratitude to my personal secretary and longstanding former administrative secretary of the Personality Disorders Institute, Ms. Louise Taitt, who has been supporting my work and protecting my time over the years, permitting me to invest consistently in the production of this book as well as all the previous ones. And, last but not least, I want to thank my wife, Dr. Catherine Haran, who in her double function as senior clinician and researcher of the Personality Disorders Institute, and loving provider of unfailing emotional support under all conditions of professional institutional weather, has helped me to achieve this task. This book is dedicated to her as an expression of my profound love and gratitude.

PART I

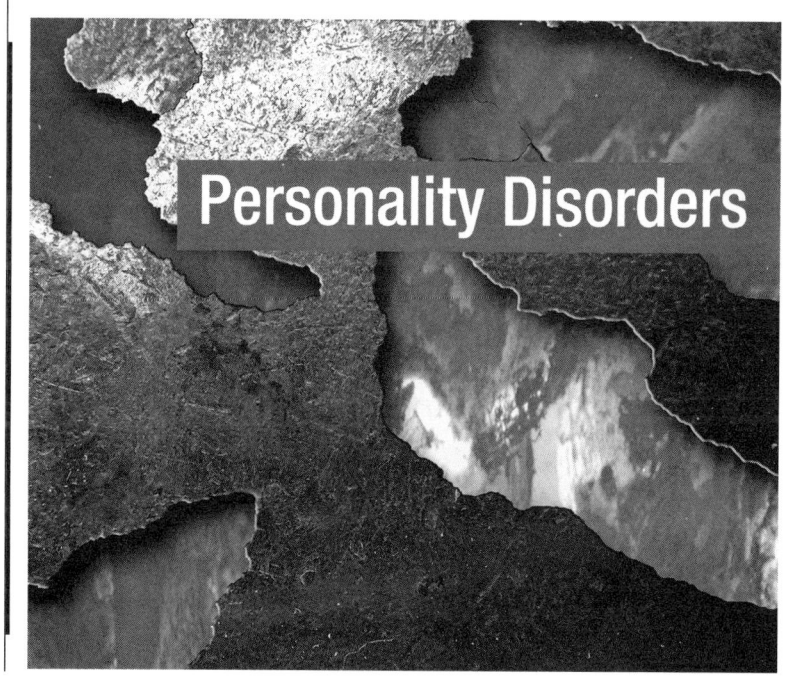

Personality Disorders

CHAPTER 1

What Is Personality?

The concept of *personality*, in my view (Kernberg and Caligor 2005; Posner et al. 2003), refers to the dynamic integration of the totality of a person's subjective experience and behavior patterns—including both conscious, concrete and habitual behaviors and experiences of self and of the surrounding world; conscious, explicit psychic thinking and habitual desires and fears; unconscious behavior patterns, experiences, and views; and intentional states. Personality is a dynamic integration insofar as it implies an organized, integrated association of multiple traits and experiences that influence one another, the final outcome of the coordination of multiple dispositions. In this regard, it represents a much more complex and sophisticated entity than simply the sum of all its component features.

Personality derives from the human organism's capacity to experience subjective states that reflect the internal condition of the body as well as the perception of the external environment within which this body functions. It includes discrete psychic functions such as affects, perception, cognition, instrumental as well as declarative memory, and various levels of self-reflective functions, from relatively simple mirror-

---

This chapter was originally published as Kernberg OF: "What Is Personality?" *Journal of Personality Disorders* 30(2):145–156, 2016. Copyright © 2016 Guilford Publications. Adapted with permission.

ing of perceived and intended motor movements and perceived sensory experiences, to complex self-reflective evaluation of cognitive and affective states.

The combined scientific advances in genetic determination of neurotransmitters that activate and regulate various affective states, the observation of interacting relationships between baby and caregiver from birth on, and the observation of psychological functioning throughout early development and into adulthood are gradually facilitating an integrated view of the determinants of the personality. The study of brain structures related to affect activation and control, and of instrumental and declarative development of memory and cognitive capacities, combined with the psychodynamic study of the intrapsychic relationship between behaviors, motivational states, fantasy, and perception of psychosocial reality, is providing a broader context for our understanding. The study of the sociology of small groups and the psychological influence of educational and cultural mores, and the study of specific types of organic and personality pathology, jointly permit, I believe, establishment of a general frame of reference for the dominant features of the personality and their harmonious or disharmonious functioning in health and illness.

Personality researchers and experts would probably all agree that personality is codetermined by genetic and constitutional dispositions as they interact with the individual's environment, particularly psychosocial features, during psychological development. Nonetheless, there remain enormous differences among the relevant fields regarding the key determinants of the personality, their mutual influences, and assessment (Konner 2010; Widiger and Mullins-Sweatt 2005). I believe that the main obstacle to progress in this general area of human knowledge is the temptation for reductionism in the development of theoretical frames that then influence the development of corresponding approaches and instruments to the study of personality.

For example, the psychoanalytic studies of personality constellations in the clinical practice of psychoanalytic investigation have permitted the description of major personality disorders such as the narcissistic personality disorders (Akhtar 1992) and have provided major advances into the description of the constellation of features characterizing the entire field of personality disorders. At the same time, however, the neglect of neurobiological determinants of motivational systems and intentional states, and of the environmental determinants of personality features, has made any efforts to construct a satisfactory, purely psychoanalytically informed theory of personality and personality disorders clearly inadequate. By the same token, reducing personality studies to the descriptive mapping of personality traits and factor analysis of clusters of epidemiologically predominant characterological traits neglects deeper structures of organization of behavior, and would seem to be equally inadequate (Kernberg and Caligor 2012b). This is reflected in the problematic efforts to relate such a trait psychology to specific neurobiological structures and functions, without considering the complexity of the internal psychological organization of behavior that gives the same traits a completely different meaning in the context of different underlying structural dynamics. A simplistic model of traits determined by neurobiological features reflecting specific genetic determinants seems as inadequate as a simplistic psychodynamic model based on unconscious conflict constellations. The same criticism, I believe, could be directed at other theoretical approaches regarding personality that neglect the complexity of the neurobiological and intrapsychic structures involved, such as a simplistic model of normal or pathological psychosocial adaptation.

What follows is an effort to approach the organizational structure of the personality from multiple viewpoints that corresponds to the collaborative work of the Personality Disorders Institute at Weill Cornell Medical College over the past 30 years. The main findings of this group, with respect to identity and identity disturbances (disorders of the self), have now been incorporated in the classification of personality disorders of DSM-5 (American Psychiatric Association 2013). The foregoing is not intended to be an all-inclusive understanding of personality formation, but, rather, an approach that attempts to do justice to the various fundamental scientific developments now available for our evolving understanding of this field.

The Components of the Personality

Our fundamental proposal considers personality as an umbrella organization that includes a small number of major component systems: temperament, object relations, character, identity, ethical value systems, and cognitive capability (intelligence).

TEMPERAMENT

I consider temperament as the fundamental constitutive structure of the personality, represented by the general psychological reactivity of the individual, particularly psychomotor, cognitive, and affective reactivity (Kernberg 1992; Panksepp 1998). Affective reactivity is the fundamental aspect of a person's psychic operation, constituting the primary motivational system, relating the individual to the environment in terms of positive, rewarding or negative, aversive affect states reflected, particularly, in peak affect state activation. Neurobiological affective systems are activated in response to organismic requirements that trigger alternative or combined activation of some of these systems. I am referring, particularly, to the attachment-separation panic system, the fight-flight system, the play-bonding system, the erotic system, the feeding system, and the agentic panic system (Panksepp 1998; Wright and Panksepp 2012). Each of these systems' response to organismic needs of the individual is constituted by a combined activation of specific brain structures and neurotransmitters, particularly specific neuropeptide and neuroamine affective neurotransmitters, the serotonergic, dopaminergic, and noradrenergic systems.

Of central relevance in early development is the attachment-separation panic system. It motivates the baby's search for mother's breast and mother's bodily contact and represents the prototype of the establishment of relations with significant others ("object relations"). This system determines the establishment of internalized representations of these interactions with mother in the form of dyadic, affective memory units constituted by representations of self and representations of the "object," within the context of a dominant positive or negative primary affect.

CHARACTER AND EGO IDENTITY

These internalized affective memory traces constitute the building blocks of internal representation of relationships with significant others (Kernberg 1976). The repetitive activation of both extremely pleasurable and extremely unpleasurable, and potentially traumatic, affective experiences determines the primary motivation toward or away from an object. Within contemporary attachment theory, these motivational structures constitute internal models of behavior. Within psychoanalytic theory, these primary "ideal" and "all bad" internalized object relations will become organized around mutually dissociated major segments of either "idealized" or feared (persecutory) earliest experiences. Out of these internalized representations of relations with significant others—internal models of behavior—will derive habitual behavior patterns that, in their dynamic integration, eventually will constitute *character*. Thus, character is the dynamically integrated structure of habitual behavior patterns. At the same time, in the gradual consolidation of all the integrated representations of self, surrounded, so to speak, by an integrated set of representations of significant others, *ego identity*—or rather, self-identity—crystallizes as the overall integrated view of oneself and the nature of one's habitual relations with significant others.

In summary, so far, all these processes might be subsumed under the statement that temperament reflects the motivation for activation of interpersonal behavior, and the resulting internalized object relations will determine the development of character and identity: character as the *objective*, individualized integration of habitual behavior patterns, and identity as the *subjective* correspondent of character. Identity and character are mutually complementary expressions of the organization of psychic life.

Character traits, the behavioral expression of the internal models of behavior derived from internalized self and object representation units, express the reflection of past experience on present, mostly automatized functioning modes of reaction. These traits depend in varying degrees on temperamental predispositions that influence past affective gratification or frustration of the person's own needs and desires in the context of adaptive relations with significant others. In addition, character traits may represent protective reactions against the expression of deeper needs felt to be risky or unacceptable in the interpersonal field. In other words, character traits may serve a defensive purpose, sometimes directed against opposite impulses to the behavior expressed in the character trait.

For example, habitual timidity may be an expression of a defensive reaction against projected aggressive trends, the projection onto others of intense negative affective experiences that are considered too risky to express in the environment. But timidity, to stay with this example, may also express a defensive reaction against exhibitionistic impulses expressing erotic wishes that, equally, cannot be tolerated consciously. In general terms, character traits may serve defensive purposes against intolerable primitive aggressive and erotic impulses linked to early infantile and childhood experiences that can no longer be freely expressed in later developmental stages of the personality (Kernberg and Caligor 2005).

Defensive character traits are characterized by their rigidity—that is, by their habitual activation, whether they are adaptively indicated at a certain point or not—leading to rigidification of the personality, which is characteristic in many personality disorders. They may signal inhibition within certain areas of affective expression, typically of a sexual or aggressive origin, or else, in a paradoxical mode, reactions against feared instinctual impulses may lead to exaggerated *counterphobic* behaviors. In short, defensive character traits may be inhibitory, exaggerated, or "reaction formations," and, particularly in the case of severe personality disorder, a combination of inhibitory and reactive formations that conveys a chaotic nature to the character structure, which is typical for these disorders. As mentioned earlier, some traits may reflect nonconflictual, dominant temperamentally based dispositions, particularly introversion or extraversion. Character traits may reflect vicissitudes of the major neurotransmitters that influence the activation of primary affective systems, such as the accentuation of intensity of negative affects derived from decrease in the functioning of the serotonergic system, and genetically determined hyperreactivity of the amygdala to aversive perceptions.

To this point, I have related character traits to the behavioral activation of internalized models of behavior represented by dyadic units of self and object representations under the dominance of certain affects, particularly peak affect states. However, significant learning, of course, gradually occurs more and more under conditions of low affect states, when direct perception and cognitive elaboration of the perceived environment permit cognitive learning relatively uninfluenced by the expression of organismic needs reflected in affect activation. Character formation, in other words, does not depend exclusively on peak affect states. Basic affective states, however, correspond to basic motivational tendencies that, in turn, are ultimately activated by the basic neurobiological systems geared to express the instinctual needs related to attachment, feeding, self-protection, peer bonding, and sexuality.

So far, I have referred to dyadic relations between self and object representations. It needs to be added at this point that from the beginning of life and gradually in a more articulated way, triadic internalized object relations complicate the original dyadic structures and determine more complex mechanisms of identity formation. As a child learns to accept and understand the relationship between the caretaking person and other significant adults and siblings in his or her psychosocial environment, the child begins to evaluate interactions between significant others and to relate them, by projection, to his or her own experiences in dyadic relations. Internalized dyadic relations now become influenced by the awareness of dyadic relations in the individual's immediate environment, usually the relationship of the parents.

In other words, triangulations emerge, leading to the significant conflicts around infantile aggression, sexuality, and dependency described in psychoanalytic developmental theory, and are of interest here because such triadic relations contribute to more realistic assessment of the self and of significant others in the interpersonal and internalized world of object relations. These developments foster the emergence of idealized, as opposed to realistic, representations of self, modeled by parental demands and prohibitions, praise, and criticism. A "moralistic" assessment of one's self—with dismantling of primitive illusions of one's own absolute goodness, power, and righteousness and a gradual internalization of expectations, demands, and prohibitions—evolves that creates tension between one's desired sense of self and the realistically perceived one. The psychological structuralization of this tension represents the origin of the *superego* in psychoanalytic theory (Jacobson 1964).

NORMAL IDENTITY AND IDENTITY DIFFUSION

As previously mentioned, the *subjective* aspect of the dynamic organization of character is the development of identity. A major developmental process extends from the first 2–3 years of life to crucial developments during late childhood and then again in adolescence. I am referring to the gradual integration of the representations of the self into a durable self-concept, and the gradual integration of multiple representations of significant others as whole, separate objects. This developmental process facilitates the capacity for awareness, concern, and empathy for others. An early stage of development in which rewarding, pleasurable peak affect states and their corresponding internalized object relationships are completely separated, dissociated, or split off from negative, aversive peak affect states with early caretakers leads to the consolidation of two separate segments of psychic experience, one an ideal or idealized view of intrapsychic and external reality, and the other a frightening, threatening, potentially destructive, and catastrophic world of experience. This latter segment of psychic experience, by means of projective mechanisms, is mostly projected outside and expressed as a diffuse panic, eventually originating the construction of a fantastic, primitive, persecutory external world.

These two segments of psychic experience originally represent the parallel buildup of idealized and persecutory dyadic units, linked to the separate channeling and corresponding cognitive-affective memory built up from the respective self representation–object representation units. Later, primitive psychological mechanisms of protection against overwhelming fears may lead to the defensive maintenance of this split organization, resulting in a character structure that relies upon the primitive defenses of splitting, projective identification, denial, primitive idealization, devaluation, and omnipotent control, as described by Melanie Klein (1946/1952, 1957) and her school. These primitive defensive operations can be observed clinically in the interpersonal behaviors of patients with severe personality disorders; under certain experimental situations, such as completely unstructured small and large study groups; and under extremely traumatic social circumstances.

Under normal circumstances, however, when the strong predominance of positive experiences permits the development of basic trust in a loving and reliable world of object relations, this experience and the gradual predominance of a low affect activation learning environment facilitate the linking between positive and negative, idealized and persecutory representations of self and others. The predominance of positive experiences permits the absorption, integration, and mentalization of the negative segment of experience. Usually between the third and the fifth or sixth year of life, an integrated view of self is consolidated in the context of a more realistic, integrated view of significant others: this constitutes normal identity (Kernberg and Caligor 2012a).

The failure of this process constitutes the syndrome of *identity diffusion*. Here a *permanent* splitting of the idealized and persecutory realm of experience is established, interfering with the integration of the concept of the self and of significant others. The syndrome of identity diffusion is reflected clinically in a patient's incapacity to convey to an observer a coherent, integrated description of self and significant others in his or her life (Kernberg and Caligor 2012a). This incapacity is reflected psychopathologically in chaotic behavior patterns, severe feelings of insecurity, rapidly fluctuating self-assessments and degrees of self-regard, and uncertainty about one's major interests and commitments. By the same token, these patients present great difficulties in commitment to work or profession, and in commitment to intimate mature relations in which sex and love need not be split off from each other. These patients have unstable and chaotic interpersonal relationships with significant others because of a severe lack of capacity to assess others in depth and rapid internal shifts of perception of self and others.

It is this structurally fixated lack of integration of the self and of the representations of significant others that represents the main etiological features of character traits of the various prototypes of severe personality disorders. We have designated these patients as presenting *borderline personality organization*. In contrast, *neurotic personality organization* refers to those personality disorders that, although still presenting significant rigid, defensive, pathological character traits, do *not* present the syndrome of identity diffusion. This type of personality organization, therefore, represents a less severe level of personality disorder.

From this general perspective, the proposal in the DSM-5 classification of personality disorders of *identity pathology* as the central criterion of severity of personality disorders, defined by the combination of lack of integration of the self and of the self's willful self-determination, and by abnormal relations with others characterized by a lack of capacity for empathy and intimacy, clearly corresponds to the syndrome of identity diffusion (Kernberg and Caligor 2012a).

AN INTEGRATED SYSTEM OF ETHICAL VALUES (SUPEREGO)

Having explored the constituent components of the personality represented by temperament, character formation, and identity, I now return to the establishment of an internalized "moral" structure as reflected by a commitment to ethical values and to universally accepted ethical principles of relationships with significant others and in social life in general. Such value systems and ethical commitments are in contrast to, and transcend, the practical requirements of direct interactions with the surrounding human society. This component of the personality corresponds roughly to the Freudian *superego*. By the same token, the Freudian *id*, or *dynamic unconscious*, corresponds to the totality of primitive aggressive, sexual, and dependent longings and their corresponding desired and feared primitive object relations that cannot be accepted in consciousness as ego identity consolidates. Active rejection of such intolerable desires and fears tends to eliminate them from consciousness by means of repression and other advanced defensive operations that depend on the very establishment of ego identity. The Freudian *ego,* from the viewpoint of the organization of the personality, is centered on the functions of identity—that is, it is constituted by an integrated self and its surrounding world of internalized, integrated object representations. In other words, the self and its internal world of object relations govern, in the end, the organization of character traits that permit the harmonious activation of effective, intimate, empathic, and stable relations with significant others.

The superego is a complex structure, the pathology of which is an important indicator of the severity—and the psychotherapeutic prognosis—of personality disorders. From the point of view of the corresponding internalization of ethical value systems, the work of Edith Jacobson (1964), it seems to me, has clarified the developmental stages of the establishment of this segment of the personality. What follows is a brief summary of her overall conclusions.

The earliest precursor of the superego, in Jacobson's (1964) proposal, is the internalization of the earliest prohibitions in the parent–child interactions, signaled by mother's clear and parental "no!," which is usually a response to the baby's behavior that may constitute an active danger for him or her (at least in mother's view). The fantastic distortions of such early prohibitions under the activation of negative peak affect states belonging to the *persecutory* segment of early experience derive from the combination of projective mechanisms and external frustrations. The prohibitions are amplified in terms of the baby's misunderstanding and misinterpretations of them under the effects of such projective mechanisms. The internalization of this first, negative layer of internalized prohibitions stimulates primitive, implicitly life-threatening fantasied dangers and punishments, mostly centering around threatened abandonment under the effect of the activation of the attachment-separation panic system. The internalization of these prohibitions implies an acceptance of them as a protective mechanism against greater threats of abandonment and even annihilation. Obviously, under conditions of severe traumatic circumstances, physical abuse, sexual abuse, or chronic witnessing of physical or sexual abuse, such an early negative internalized sense of basic threats to survival may become much more dominant than would be the case under ordinary circumstances.

This first, most primitive level of internalized prohibitions begins to influence both positive and negative segments of early experience, and is gradually followed by a second level of experiences, under the activation of positive peak affect states and, in part, under conditions of low affect activation, reflecting the environmental demands for "good" behavior. The expression of appreciation of the child's behavior—its stimulation, rewards, and gratitude on the part of the parental objects—fosters behaviors that the baby comes to see as ideal in terms of the rewards associated with them. This layer constitutes the early *ego ideal*. It is constituted both by the internalization of the demanding and rewarding aspects of the ideally perceived images of the significant others and as a result of the development of more realistic "ideal" self representations under conditions of the gradual toning down and integration of the idealized and persecutory segments of the self.

The buildup of the ego ideal as an internalized structure reinforces a sense of security, inner goodness, and warm connection with significant others. This structure gradually tends to neutralize the most primitive, persecutory segment of experiences within the superego. Throughout the second and third year of life, a process of integration between the most primitive persecutory and the secondary idealized level of realistic and fantasied, desired, and feared demands and prohibitions takes place. This neutralization of negative experiences tends to reduce projective processes and facilitates the internalization of yet a third level of demands and prohibitions. This is what Freud described as the *advanced oedipal state of development,* which is consolidated approximately between the fourth and sixth year of life (Freud 1923/1961).

This third, more realistic level of internalized demands and prohibitions already contains many expectations derived from the family, reflecting the cultural expectations of the immediate social environment and their specific ethnic, social, national, religious, or racial traditions and biases. By the beginning of the school years (the *latency years* in traditional psychoanalytic theory), sufficient integration of these levels of internalized value systems, under the dominance of the third, more realistic and complex one, has taken place to permit the child to enter a socially shared value system. This system regulates behavior in terms of justice and concern for others as well as responsibility for one's own behavior.

Throughout the years leading to adolescence, a gradual process of depersonification, abstraction, and individualization of the superego takes place. In other words, an abstraction/general integration of value systems is no longer linked concretely to demands or prohibitions from any particular parental image (Jacobson 1964). Now, both deep, unconscious dispositions from the early childhood years—as well as later preconscious and conscious identifications with value systems acquired at home, school, and one's social group—characterize the pubescent child. Finally, in early adolescence, with the activation of intense sexual strivings that reactivate, deepen, and expand sexual impulses, fantasies, fears, and desires from early childhood, and the impact of the development of secondary sexual characteristics, a profound transformation takes place. Now infantile prohibitions against sexuality and aggression have to be somewhat modified to conform with the more adult demands of intimate relationships under the combined impact of instinctual desires, efforts to harmonize them with the adolescent's identity and character formation, and the conscious and unconscious value systems reflected by the developed, integrated superego. In short, the development of an internalized set of ethical principles derives from particular aspects of internalized object relations, namely, those in which different levels of a broad spectrum of demands and prohibitions initiate the child's identification with the moral and ethical values of his or her home and social environment.

Under pathological circumstances, different levels of severity of personality disorders may affect the integration of this internalized system of ethical values and, in turn, influence the development of different levels of psychopathology. Identity diffusion may become fixed under the dominance of severe aggressive impulses, whether derived from genetically determined, temperamentally established predominance of negative affects and lack of cognitive control and contextualization of affects, or severely pathological attachment experiences, or a traumatic early infancy and childhood. The lack of identity integration negatively influences the integration of the different layers of the superego system. The first, persecutory superego level becomes excessively dominant by aggressive internalized object relations; the relative weakness of the ego ideal level interferes with the integration of these two levels and brings about a persistent dominance of the first, persecutory superego level. The establishment of the third, higher level of ethical values suffers as well, a consequence of excessive projection of the negative earlier superego features. Clinically, this predisposes the person to the activation of ego-syntonic aggressive antisocial behavior.

In fact, the development of antisocial behavior is the most important complication of the most severe level of borderline personality organization and signifies a poor prognosis for psychotherapeutic treatments. It causes damage to the capacity for relationships with others and to the normal modulation of affective expression of one's own emotional needs. In contrast, under conditions when normal identity development proceeds adequately, this positively influences superego integration. Under circumstances when normal superego integration takes place, but with a strong induction of excessive guilt feelings over instinctual impulses, the early superego level may "contaminate" the ego ideal with the development of sadistic demands for perfection. Under these circumstances, the prohibitions against infantile sexuality during the development of the third level of superego development may appear as excessively prohibitive, even violent, so that an integrated but sadistic superego may inhibit sexual, aggressive, and dependent impulses, leading to a defensive character structure that characterizes the higher level of personality disorders (neurotic personality organization).

One may summarize, in a simplified way, the dominant etiological features of personality disorders at different levels of severity in stating that at the level of borderline personality organization, conflicts (whatever their origin) around aggressive impulses predominate. At a higher level of development, with the establishment of normal identity, conflicts around infantile sexuality and dependency are predominant in the pathology of neurotic personality organization (Kernberg and Caligor 2012a). Obviously, this is a very general statement that includes a broad spectrum of variations in terms of individual history and development.

INTELLIGENCE

The final major component of the personality is the cognitive potential of the individual, *intelligence,* particularly expressed in the achieved level of abstraction. It is generally agreed that intelligence level is dependent both on genetic disposition and on early experiences. The stimulation of cognitive processes and linguistic development, and the explicit attention to a child's motivations, thought processes, and fantasy development, exert a fundamental influence on the development of cognitive ability. In general, a high cognitive potential facilitates an ever more realistic and subtle perception of the environment and the capacity to respond adequately to cognitive cues. The genetically determined development of the prefrontal and preorbital cortex, the anterior cortical midline structures, and the linguistic brain centers powerfully influences effortful control and participates in modulating affective response (Silbersweig et al. 2007).

In that regard, cognitive control may mitigate the effects of a severely traumatic environment, although under severely pathological circumstances, intelligence even may amplify trauma by the development of complex distorted cognitive interpretations of a threatening environment. Conversely, cognitive systems of rationalization of pathological character traits may powerfully reinforce faulty adaptive strategies that may be encountered in severe personality disorders. In clinical practice, we find patients with very high intelligence and patients with very low intelligence at all levels of severity of personality disorders. Intelligence has a positive prognostic implication for the indication of psychotherapeutic treatments and, of course, for the general level of social adaptation in terms of educational development and level of work or profession.

From the viewpoint of both the development of the normal personality and the etiology of personality disorders, we may distinguish two general organizational levels of psychic life: first, a neurobiological level of development that determines the organization of basic neurobiological structures that find expression in psychological life, particularly the development of perception and memory, the activation of consciousness, and, fundamentally, the development of affect systems that protect homeostasis and become the primary motivator of object relations. To this basic level of psychic development has to be added a second level of organization at a purely symbolic, intrapsychic level, which is best formulated in terms of the gradual building up of an internal world centered around personal identity and the realistic perception and investment in a world of significant others. This internal world organizes the satisfactory expression of basic instinctual needs, autonomy, and self-affirmation, and, by the same token, gratifying and effective relations with the surrounding social world. This includes sexual and romantic intimacy, friendship and commitments, and effectiveness and gratification in work and personal creativity. The limitations in this development represented by personality disorders are now within the realm of our understanding regarding etiology, mechanisms of interactions and organization, and the potential for treatment, as well as the present limitations of our therapeutic endeavors. Further progress in all these areas requires the attention to these two systems, the neurobiological and the intrapsychic, and their mutual influences in normality, pathology, and treatment.

References

Akhtar S: Broken Structures: Severe Personality Disorders and Their Treatment. Northvale, NJ, Jason Aronson, 1992

American Psychiatric Association: Diagnostic and Statistical Manual of Mental Disorders, 5th Edition. Arlington, VA, American Psychiatric Association, 2013

Freud S: The ego and the id (1923), in Standard Edition of the Complete Psychological Works of Sigmund Freud, Vol 19.Translated and edited by Strachey J. London, Hogarth Press, 1961, pp 12–66

Jacobson E: The Self and the Object World. New York, International Universities Press, 1964

Kernberg OF: Object Relations Theory and Clinical Psychoanalysis. New York, Jason Aronson, 1976

Kernberg OF: Aggression in Personality Disorders and Perversion. New Haven, CT, Yale University Press, 1992

Kernberg OF, Caligor E: A psychoanalytic theory of personality disorders, in Major Theories of Personality Disorders, 2nd Edition. Edited by Clarkin JF, Lenzenweger MF. New York, Guilford, 2005, pp 114–156

Kernberg OF, Caligor E: Identity: recent findings and clinical implications, in The Inseparable Nature of Love and Aggression: Clinical and Theoretical Perspectives. Washington, DC, American Psychiatric Publishing, 2012a, pp 3–30

Kernberg OF, Caligor E: Overview and critique of the classification of personality disorders proposed for DSM-V. Swiss Archives of Neurology and Psychiatry 163(7):234–238, 2012b

Klein M: Notes on some schizoid mechanisms (1946), in Developments in Psycho-Analysis. Edited by Riviere J. London, Hogarth Press, 1952, pp 292–320

Klein M: Envy and Gratitude. New York, Basic Books, 1957

Konner M: The Evolution of Childhood: Relationships, Emotions, Mind. Cambridge, MA, The Belknap Press of Harvard University Press, 2010

Panksepp J: Affective Neuroscience: The Foundations of Human and Animal Emotions. New York, Oxford University Press, 1998

Posner MI, Rothbart MK, Vizueta N, et al: An approach to the psychobiology of personality disorders. Dev Psychopathol 15(4):1093–1106, 2003 14984139

Silbersweig D, Clarkin JF, Goldstein M, et al: Failure of frontolimbic inhibitory function in the context of negative emotion in borderline personality disorder. Am J Psychiatry 164(12):1832–1841, 2007 18056238

Widiger TA, Mullins-Sweatt SN: Categorical and dimensional models of personality disorders, in The American Psychiatric Publishing Textbook of Personality Disorders. Edited by Oldham JM, Skodol AE, Bender DS. Washington, DC, American Psychiatric Publishing, 2005, pp 35–56

Wright JS, Panksepp J: An evolutionary framework to understand foraging, wanting, and desire: the neuropsychology of the SEEKING System. Neuropsychoanalysis 14(10):5–39, 2012

CHAPTER 2

Overview and Critique of the Classification of Personality Disorders Proposed for DSM-5

Background

The Work Group on Personality and Personality Disorders for DSM-5 (American Psychiatric Association 2013) began their work making several assumptions. First, the DSM-IV classification (American Psychiatric Association 1994) had proved unsatisfactory because of the high comorbidity among the various personality disorders and because the most frequent diagnostic conclusion, in clinical practice, was personality disorder not otherwise specified (NOS). Second, within the work group there would continue to be a long-standing dynamic tension between, on the one hand, empirical researchers interested in developing classification systems for the personality characteristics of normal populations and, on the other, clinicians who were concerned about developing a classification system that would do justice to the personality disorder constellations found in clinical settings.

Many factor analysis studies of large samples have demonstrated the consistent findings of the "five-factor system" in describing the major dimensions that determine the differential profile of personality structures within a normal population. These five dimensions are openness, conscientiousness, extraversion, agreeableness, and neuroticism. Clinical psychiatry and psychology, in contrast, have consistently found certain predominant constellations of pathological personality traits that could be translated into differential categories of personality disorders, although mixed features of several of them might combine in certain patients. These clinical categories have differential prognostic and therapeutic implications. In short, competing dimensional and categorical systems of classification constituted a significant dynamic within the committees/work groups involved in DSM-III, -IV, and -5 (American Psychiatric Association 1980, 1994, 2013).

DSM-IV was a purely categorical system, and the 10 categories of personality disorders it described represented well-differentiated entities, each of them characterized by a certain number of traits, which, in turn, signified that any diagnosis might be achieved by a particular combination of such respective traits. The underlying heterogeneity of at least some of these disorders was illustrated by the fact that different combinations of the traits representing one category could determine the same diagnostic presence in another.

The DSM-5 personality and personality disorders work group operated under strong instructions from the overall leadership of DSM-5 to shift from the categorical system of DSM-IV into a dimensional system (Kupfer et al. 2002). In addition to the dissatisfaction with the DSM-IV categorical classification system, other fundamental considerations also played a role. First, the search for a new classification system should link concrete behavioral traits with assumed underlying neurobiological dispositions and functions, and with the possibility of developing neurobiological and genetic markers to determine the disposition to a specific personality disorder (Donaldson and Young 2008). In this regard, this effort corresponded to a major emphasis on *translational research,* relating psychopathology to neurobiological functioning and to pathology in the neurobiological realm. Second, and less explicit but present as an underlying ideological influence, this orientation reflected a long, ongoing struggle between the neurobiological and psychodynamic disciplines, and the growing strength of neurobiological psychiatry in reducing the influence of clinical psychodynamic concepts and findings on the personality disorders classification system, bringing it in line with the dramatic growth in knowledge about the genetic and neurobiological basis of major domains of clinical psychiatry (Krueger et al. 2011; Skodol et al. 2011).

A Major Compromise Solution

The dynamic tension between researchers interested in empirical studies of normal populations, whose aim was to relate these findings to the predominant prototypes of personality disorders, and clinical psychiatry researchers, who were trying to preserve what they saw as their confirmed experience of the validity of major categories described in DSM-IV, evolved in the direction of a compromise. This compromise included an important, major new development: the agreement on a common basic factor of *all* personality disorders, a factor that represented a major criterion for the assessment of the severity of any personality disorder, namely, the integration or lack of integration of the *self* (i.e., the degree of normality or pathology in the relations of the individual with others) (Bender et al. 2011). Here, what might be called the common-sense observation that patients with personality disorders have difficulty in their comprehension and management of themselves and of their relationship with significant others was recognized for the first time as a basic characteristic of personality disorders. The fact that this dimension could be explicated, operationalized, and clinically evaluated in terms of the degree of its disturbance satisfied both empirical dimensionalists and, particularly, psychodynamic psychotherapists, who for over 40 years have observed, described, and used this dimension in their assessment and therapeutic approaches to patients with personality disorders (Kernberg 1975, 1980).

With regard to the differentiation of major personality prototypes, the struggle between the clinical experience of those interested in maintaining the categories of the DSM-IV system and the researchers who wished to relate the five-factor model to clinical prototypes of pathological personality structures led to a compromise. Of the 10 DSM-IV personality prototypes, those retained would be the prototypes that could evince significant empirical research carried out in recent years in support of their maintenance and that were clinically important from the viewpoint of their frequency in clinical practice (Skodol et al. 2011). This led, first, to maintaining the schizotypal, antisocial, borderline, avoidant, and obsessive-compulsive personality disorders—five of the original 10 categories.

This decision, which in itself already involved significant tensions and disagreements within the work group, evolved toward a minor crisis of a sort because narcissistic personality disorder has been the subject of abundant recent empirical studies and is of high prevalence in clinical practice and yet was slated to be excluded! In all fairness, it may be said that this attempted exclusion manifested the antipsychodynamic bias prevalent in the work group, because the clinical description, the study of the psychopathology, and empirical research on the features of this disorder had been carried out mostly by psychodynamically oriented researchers and clinicians (Russ et al. 2008). In fact, narcissistic personality disorder was reinstated and became a sixth category within the proposed DSM-5 nomenclature (Ronningstam 2011).

The Excluded Categories

The work group decided that the excluded DSM-IV personality disorders—paranoid, schizoid, histrionic, and dependent personality disorders, and the personality disorders from the appendix of DSM-IV (i.e., the depressive and the negativistic personality disorders, as well as the category of personality disorder NOS)—would now be subsumed under the diagnosis of a "trait-specified personality disorder." This in practice would mean that the clinician would have the option of diagnosing a personality disorder on the basis of the pathology of self and relationships with others, and tailoring the description of the personality disorder to fit the specific patient, by using the specific features included by the corresponding pathological traits (Skodol et al. 2011).

Needless to say, serious questions may be raised by excluding personality disorders that have a long history of significant clinical observations and specific therapeutic interventions, such as paranoid personality disorder and histrionic personality disorder, the latter corresponding to a broad spectrum of pathology described in psychodynamic literature, ranging from the hysterical to the histrionic or infantile personality disorders, and depressive personality disorder, which has a prognostically favorable implication for psychodynamic psychotherapies. Also, the fact that no major research has been carried out in recent years regarding paranoid personality disorder seems a problematic reason for eliminating it. In any case, from the viewpoint of the psychodynamically oriented proponents of a categorical nomenclature, the reinstatement of narcissistic personality disorder represented a significant positive development, corresponding to clinical reality. Clinicians may feel that histrionic personality disorder can still be considered a less severe form of borderline personality disorder, and that schizoid personality disorder is a less severe form of the schizotypal one, and may refer to them in their practice in that context.

For the neurobiologically oriented, and those preferring the dimensional trait system, the influence of the five-factor model seems to be relatively assured by the relationship of the factors of conscientiousness, extraversion, agreeableness, and neuroticism, respectively, to obsessive-compulsive personality, avoidant personality (reflecting detachment, as the polar opposite of extraversion), antisocial personality as an expression of antagonism (the polar opposite of agreeableness), and borderline personality disorder as the expression of neuroticism, in the sense of negative affectivity, reflecting emotional dysregulation and lability. Insofar as conscientiousness is considered the polar opposite of disinhibition, reflected by impulsivity, it would indicate another relationship between personality disorders and the five-factor model (Widiger 2011). It should also be pointed out that the factor of openness—reflecting, in fact, openness to unusual, idiosyncratic, bizarre ideas—that would seem to be related to schizotypal personality disorder raised sufficient methodological and conceptual questions for it to be discarded. A new factor, "psychoticism," was considered as representing the factorial personality dimension reflected in the schizotypal personality disorders. In short, with the exception of narcissistic personality disorder, the five-factor model, either by direct representation of these factors in the clinical picture or by means of their expression by their polar opposite, thus could be related to basic domains of personality underlying the personality disorders included in DSM-5.

The Overall Alternative Model

In summary, the alternative model for DSM-5 personality disorders includes two fundamental assessments: 1) the Level of Personality Functioning Scale, including the assessment of self and of interpersonal functioning; and 2) the diagnostic criteria for the six selected specific categories of personality disorders.

The assessment of degrees of pathology of the experience of self includes the following components:

1. *Identity:* the experience of oneself as unique, with clear boundaries between self and others; self-esteem and accuracy of self-appraisal; capacity for, and ability to regulate the range of emotional experience.
2. *Self-direction:* the pursuit of coherent and meaningful short-term and life goals; utilization of constructive and prosocial internal standards of behavior; ability to self-reflect productively.

The assessment of interpersonal functioning includes

1. *Empathy:* comprehension and application of others' experiences and motivations; tolerance of different perspectives; understanding of the effects of own behavior on others;

2. *Intimacy:* depth and duration of positive connection with others; desire and capacity for closeness; mutuality of regard reflected in interpersonal behavior.

In short, the components central to a personality functioning continuum are identity, self-direction, empathy, and intimacy, and the corresponding scale differentiates five levels of impairment, ranging from little or no impairment (healthy functioning) to extreme impairment.

The diagnostic criteria for six specific personality disorders types—antisocial, avoidant, borderline, narcissistic, obsessive-compulsive, and schizotypal—are defined by the level of personality functioning reflected by the self (the A criteria) and by the corresponding specific pathological personality traits (the B criteria). In addition, all discarded categories, those in the appendix of DSM-IV, and personality disorders NOS will now be classified as personality disorders with specific predominance of certain constellations of traits, and the personality disorder NOS no longer will be required.

Some Critical Reflections

From my viewpoint, the major innovative contribution and strength of these decisions resides in the belated recognition of the essential nature of the experience of the self and of relationships with significant others in the assessment of normality or degree of pathology of the personality. The concept of an integrated self—in contrast to severe lack of integration that characterizes what, in psychoanalytic literature, Erik Erikson introduced many years back as the concept of *identity diffusion*—is the central issue in the evaluation of a personality disorder. Identity is a fundamental structure of the personality that defines, more than anything else, the nature and degree of severity of personality disorders. The criteria of identity and self-direction now proposed reflect that aspect of the self accurately. The relationship with others, as DSM-5 has recognized, intimately relates to the degree of integration of the self and reflects, I would add, the integration of the representations of significant others implicit in the actual capability of empathy and intimacy as now defined in the alternative DSM-5 model.

It is remarkable that the essential characteristics of personality disorders are described in terms of predominantly subjective experiences, a very important aspect in the evaluation of the personality, which complements the analysis of the actual interpersonal and social functioning.

The research on attachment has provided the objective evidence for the intimate connections among the earliest relations with significant others, the buildup of internal models of those relationships as reciprocal, and dyadic constellations of self and object representations, and psychoanalytic theory has provided an explanatory theory of how these early intrapsychic structures become integrated, respectively, into an integrated concept of self and of significant others (Kernberg 2006).

The maintenance of the six major diagnostic categories of personality disorders, albeit within an effort to link them to a predominantly trait-oriented psychology (with an expectation of direct, linear relationships to neurobiological functioning and to underlying genetic predispositions), does indeed reflect clinically predominant categories of personality disorders, and the decision to retain these categories seems justifiable. The elimination of the other four categories from DSM-IV, however, raises questions. That there has not been empirical research in recent years regarding these other personality types does not seem to be reason enough to eliminate them if they are clinically relevant and, therefore, important in the general differential diagnostic and therapeutic approach to personality disorders. Paranoid personality disorder, for example, would be easily recognized by most clinicians and has been described in the psychiatric literature of many countries. But even if their diagnostic utilization in clinical practice is less frequent than the disorders that have been retained, the wisdom of including only the most frequent conditions while discarding less frequent yet clinically discriminant conditions is questionable. Would we exclude relatively rare types of illness in other medical fields just because of the rarity of cases in which the diagnosis has been established?

Another issue with the excluded personality disorders is that some represent milder forms of underlying pathologies, the elimination of which does not quite do justice to the spectrum of certain related personality disorders. Thus, as mentioned previously, histrionic personality disorder may represent a less severe form of borderline personality disorder but presents a different prognosis and indication for therapeutic management. The same may be stated regarding schizoid personality disorder, reasonably considered a less severe form of schizotypal personality disorder, with important implications regarding genetic predisposition to schizophrenia in the latter, but less likely so in the former. Here we touch upon an area explored by neither the DSM-IV nor the DSM-5 work group: the dimensional aspect of relationships between groups of personality disorders such as schizoid and schizotypal, or histrionic and borderline, and the unacknowledged relationship between narcissistic and antisocial personality disorder, the latter an extremely severe form of pathological narcissism that presents the symptoms of a narcissistic personality as an important aspect of its features. What I am suggesting here is that there exists a dimensional aspect of relationships between various personality disorders that, by itself, justifies a classification of personality disorders that combines categorical and dimensional features (Kernberg and Caligor 2005). From this very general viewpoint, the adoption in DSM-5 of such a combined, "hybrid" model seems appropriate.

The effort to link the five-factor model as representative of descriptive studies of large normal populations with the prototypes of clinically observed personality disorders may be questioned from the standpoint of the particular structure of an individual personality disorder: regardless of their neurobiological or psychosocial dispositions, the nature of personality disorders may reflect an organization of constellations of personality traits that may not have any psychopathological relevance regarding the statistically predominant constellations of traits of normal populations (the five-factor system). The assumed relationship between the five-factor system and the nature of the retained personality disorders seems rather forced, with the factor of openness not relevant at all, and the need to establish a new factor, psychoticism, in order to find a possible connection with schizotypal personality disorder seemingly well illustrating this point.

The Double Layer of Neurobiological and Subjective Intrapsychic Structures

The most important critique, in my view, of the conceptual underpinning of the alternative model for DSM-5 personality disorders relates to the underlying assumption that a trait psychology, in contrast to a categorical one, may permit a direct relationship between concrete personality traits and underlying neurobiological mechanisms. There are, of course, underlying neurobiological mechanisms related to all psychological functioning: subjectivity and intentionality, as we know by now, are clearly dependent on complex structural arrangements of the central nervous system, and there are concrete linkages between the functioning of different areas of the brain and subjective and behavioral aspects of human psychology. The function of neurotransmitters such as oxytocin in activating the attachment system and being influential in the passionate aspects of erotic life illustrates one such relationship: that the orientation of the self with regard to its immediate psychological environment and its influence on affect control relate to functions of the medial prefrontal cortex and the anterior part of the cingulum has been clearly established. In our own research on borderline personality disorder, we have found that the hyperactivity of the amygdala, combined with a primary inhibition of the prefrontal and preorbital cortex, differentiates these patients from normal control subjects. There is abundant literature that has confirmed these findings (Silbersweig et al. 2007).

We have also learned, however, that the central nervous system operates not through the isolated activation of particular structures or neurotransmitters, but through the integrated activation of multiple structures. For example, emotional dysregulation depends on a complex interaction between the activation of limbic areas (the hippocampus and amygdala), cortical areas (particularly the prefrontal and preorbital cortex and the anterior cingular region), and even broader areas (including insula and aspects of the parietal, temporal, and occipital cortices). We also have evidence that certain key psychological functions derive, in turn, from the organization of underlying psychological structures such as the very concept of the self, which are derived from the integration of centers of self-reflection that provide information about the location of the body in space and time, the information from the linguistic self, the status of the historical self, and the assessment of the perception of self by others. In other words, although all these psychological functions derive from a neurobiological basis, they in turn become organized at a psychological level. The study of subjective intentionality of behavior, I believe, has to consider two levels of organismic organization: a basic neurobiological one and a derived, secondary, symbolic or psychological one that, as recent research also has shown, in turn may influence the functioning of the underlying neurobiological structures.

This conceptualization of the double layer of neuropsychological organization raises serious questions about the organization of our nomenclature of personality disorders in terms of the linear concept of interaction of isolated multiple traits, which are practically considered as almost equivalent in their functionality. This problem is clearly reflected in the main dimension rightly proposed for personality disorders—namely the integration of the self, which is reflected by identity and self-direction on the one hand and the capacity for empathy and intimacy on the other.

Conclusion

My view is that the classification of personality disorders in the alternative DSM-5 model represents a significant improvement over DSM-IV, by adding as central criteria the severity of pathology of the self and of relations with others, incorporating, in this regard, the findings and clinical contributions from psychoanalytic object relations theory. The decision to maintain 6 of the 10 categories of DSM-IV is wise and will permit continuity in the research regarding those respective areas. The elimination of the other four categories seems to me questionable but perhaps may be compensated in practice by signaling the constellation of the corresponding, predominant traits in those personality disorders that also fulfill criterion A (regarding identity) but cannot be classified within the six categories that remain. The main problem with the new classification lies not, it seems to me, in the decisions regarding its shape, to the point at which it has been agreed upon until now, but in the untouched conceptual and methodological problem of dealing with the disposition to personality disorders stemming from two interrelated levels of organization of the mind: a basic neurobiological level and a symbolic or psychological level (Kernberg 2012). The achievement of such integration implies tasks for future research.

References

American Psychiatric Association: Diagnostic and Statistical Manual of Mental Disorders, 3rd Edition. Washington, DC, American Psychiatric Association, 1980

American Psychiatric Association: Diagnostic and Statistical Manual of Mental Disorders, 4th Edition. Washington, DC, American Psychiatric Association, 1994

American Psychiatric Association: Diagnostic and Statistical Manual of Mental Disorders, 5th Edition. Arlington, VA, American Psychiatric Association, 2013

Bender DS, Morey LC, Skodol AE: Toward a model for assessing level of personality functioning in DSM-5, part I: a review of theory and methods. J Pers Assess 93(4):332–346, 2011 22804672

Donaldson ZR, Young LJ: Oxytocin, vasopressin, and the neurogenetics of sociality. Science 322(5903):900–904, 2008 18988842

Kernberg OF: Borderline Conditions and Pathological Narcissism. New York, Jason Aronson, 1975

Kernberg OF: Internal World and External Reality: Object Relations Theory Applied. New York, Jason Aronson, 1980

Kernberg OF: Identity: recent findings and clinical implications. Psychoanal Q 75(4):969–1004, 2006 17094369

Kernberg OF: Commentaries: the seeking system and Freud's dual-drive theory today. Neuropsychoanalysis 14(1):47–49, 2012

Kernberg OF, Caligor E: A psychoanalytic theory of personality disorders, in Major Theories of Personality Disorders, 2nd Edition. Edited by Clarkin JF, Lenzenweger MF. New York, Guilford, 2005, pp 114–156.

Krueger RF, Eaton NR, Derringer J, et al: Personality in DSM-5: helping delineate personality disorder content and framing the metastructure. J Pers Assess 93(4):325–331, 2011 22804671

Kupfer DJ, First MB, Regier DE (eds): A Research Agenda for DSM-V. Washington, DC, American Psychiatric Association, 2002

Ronningstam E: Narcissistic personality disorder in DSM-V—in support of retaining a significant diagnosis. J Pers Disord 25(2):248–259, 2011 21466253

Russ E, Shedler J, Bradley R, et al: Refining the construct of narcissistic personality disorder: diagnostic criteria and subtypes. Am J Psychiatry 165(11):1473–1481, 2008 18708489

Silbersweig D, Clarkin JF, Goldstein M, et al: Failure of frontolimbic inhibitory function in the context of negative emotion in borderline personality disorder. Am J Psychiatry 164(12):1832–1841, 2007 18056238

Skodol AE, Bender DS, Morey LC, et al: Personality disorder types proposed for DSM-5. J Pers Disord 25(2):136–169, 2011 21466247

Widiger TA: The DSM-5 dimensional model of personality disorder: rationale and empirical support. J Pers Disord 25(2):222–234, 2011 21466251

CHAPTER 3

Neurobiological Correlates of Object Relations Theory

What follows is an overview of present neurobiological understanding of early development that is relevant for the assumptions of contemporary psychoanalytic object relations theory. I shall review briefly some major areas of neurobiological investigation that jointly provide a neurobiological background and a foundation for the analysis of early development of internalized object relations. The relevant areas of neurobiological development include the activation of affective systems, the differentiation of self from others, the development of a theory of mind and of empathy, the evolution of the self-structure, and the development of processes of mentalization.

This chapter was originally published as Kernberg OF: "Neurobiological Correlates of Object Relations Theory: The Relationship Between Neurobiological and Psychodynamic Development." *International Forum of Psychoanalysis* 24(1):38–46, 2015. Copyright © 2015 Routledge/Francis & Taylor. Adapted with permission.

Neurobiological Foundations

THE CONCEPT OF PERSONALITY

In Chapter 1, I described the formation and components of personality and personality pathology. To repeat, the basic components of personality organization include temperament, character, identity, value systems, and intelligence (Kernberg 2016).

Temperament is the genetically determined, constitutionally given reactivity of the organism in terms of affective, cognitive, and behavioral responses to environmental stimulation. Affective responsivity is the essential aspect of temperament, observable from birth on. Affects are considered as primary motivators of behavior and may be grouped as systems that involve various basic affects in different combinations (Diamond and Blatt 2007; Krause 2012). The basic affective systems are attachment, eroticism, fight-flight, play-bonding, separation-panic, and seeking (Wright and Panksepp 2012). Specific search for stimulus gratification is based on the activation of a series of corresponding affect-determining neurotransmitter activity. Affects now are considered as complex neurobiological systems that bridge the boundary between physiological and mental experience, signaling to the organism its internal, desirable, or undesirable subjective state, while simultaneously signaling to the infant's mothering object the affective state of the infant. In short, affects have a subjective and a communicative function in addition to their direct behavioral manifestations, neurovegetative discharge, and cognitive framing. Cognitive framing is an essential aspect of affect activation and conveys information regarding the stimulus impinging on the organism in terms of "Where is it?" "Is it good or bad for me?" and/or "What shall I do about it?"

From a psychoanalytic point of view, affects as primary motivational systems raise the question regarding the extent to which drives are constituted by the integration of corresponding positive ("libidinal") or negative ("aggressive") affects, and the extent to which affects are the expression of these assumed underlying corresponding drives. In any case, affects initiate the interactions between self and other, and the internalization of these interactions, in the form of affective memory, determines internalized models of behavior (in attachment terminology) or internalized object relations (in object relations theory language).

DEVELOPMENT AND INTEGRATION OF AFFECTIVE SYSTEMS

There is now clear evidence of the very early emergence of major primary affects, which make their appearance in the first few weeks and months of life. The neurobiological structures and neurotransmitter systems are in place at the time of birth. These primary affects include joyfulness, rage, surprise, fear, disgust, sadness, and sensual excitement (related to bodily surfaces, which becomes the basis of the capacity for sexual excitement). Each of these is characterized by specific neurotransmitters activated by organismic disequilibrium of homeostatic balance, and rewarding or aversive environmental stimuli.

Affects are grouped into the systems referred to previously—particularly, attachment, fight-flight, play-bonding, separation-panic, eroticism, and seeking. Seeking is a basic nonspecific motivation for stimulus gratification that may attach itself to any of the other affective systems mentioned and provides a basic explanation regarding why, under particular conditions of gratification or stimulation, there may be a tendency toward excessive activation of aversive or affiliative affective systems (Wright and Panksepp 2012).

The brain structures that control affect expression are centered in various levels of the limbic system (Roth and Dicke 2006). The hypothalamus controls homeostatic bodily systems and is involved in the activation of both positive and negative affects in terms of the regulation of temperature, hunger, thirst, fight-flight reactions, and sexual excitement. A general classification of affective systems into affiliative and aversive ones reflects the motivational tendency of movement toward the affiliative gratifying stimuli and situations and away from aversive situations and stimuli. The nucleus accumbens and the tectum are involved in activation of positive affects, and the amygdala is involved in the activation of negative affects: the lateral amygdala is related to fear, and the central amygdala is related to rage. Sexual stimulation is activated at the ventral septal area, the ventral area of the stria terminalis, and the preoptic area of the hypothalamus.

It needs to be stressed that positive affect–activating and negative affect–activating brain structures are separate from each other and that at a basic level of affect activation a complete separation of positive and negative affect evolves. The integration of positive and negative affects—both in terms of the cognitive framing of an actual situation in which such affects are activated and in terms of a mutual modulation of such combined affect states itself—only occurs at a higher level of limbic structures and functions that involve limbic and cortical interaction, particularly the prefrontal and preorbital cortex and the anterior cingulum. In that general area, affect activation integrates the presently determined affect, the corresponding declarative or semantic memory input from sensorial-thalamic information, and affective memory input derived partly from hypothalamic sources and mostly from the affective memory storage entered in the hippocampus. The hippocampus represents the structure involved in the registration and preservation of affective memory. It is only at the higher level, at the prefrontal and preorbital cortex–anterior cingulate junction, that positive and negative affect systems can be integrated into a total affective-cognitive frame (Roth and Dicke 2006).

ORIGIN OF THE SELF: SELF-REFLECTION AND INTEGRATION

The subjective experience of the self involves the activation of several independent brain structures signaling the various components of the self-concept that are brought into play simultaneously (Zikles 2006). These brain structures include the left and right temporoparietal junction, the superior temporal sulcus, the medial prefrontal cortex, and the paracingulate cortex. In addition, a broader network involving the bilateral temporal cortex, the precuneus, and the amygdala is also activated. The perception of others, in interaction with self, involves the dorsolateral prefrontal cortex, the posterior parietal cortex, and the temporo-occipital cortex. This broad spectrum of involvement of various brain structures in the activation of the full experience of self–other interaction reflects, in terms of the total subjective self experience, the following functions of the "embodied self."

The embodied self includes the availability of the contribution of consistent subjective background information and the actual consciousness of the self experience. The background information includes the ownership of one's own body (derived from information provided by the thalamocortical system) and the internal affective state. This state involves information from the hypothalamic and midbrain structures—that is, the amygdala, the nucleus accumbens, the periaqueductal gray, and the tegmentum. In addition, background information involves the location of self in space (given by the superior and inferior colliculi), the authorship and control of one's own actions provided by the mirror system (Gallese and Goldman 1998), and, finally, cognitive development involving the "theory of mind"—that is, the capacity to differentiate clearly one's own fantasy (wishes and fears) and realistic perceptions from the realistic perceptions of another person's thinking activity (Förstl 2012). Against all this background information, several functions imply actual consciousness of the self: the perception of the present environment and the identification of social reality; cognitive functions involving thinking, imagining, and remembering; and the affective system reflecting present motivation.

In short, the psychological permanence of the concept of the self corresponds to a neurobiological potential that flickers on momentarily when we evoke our self experience. In terms of the integration of varying experiences of self under different circumstances, it needs to be repeated that only the prefrontal cortex–anterior cingulate system can integrate positive and negative affective self experience, and that this integration cannot occur at the level of the hypothalamus, the amygdala, or the hippocampus, where positive and negative affective systems run separately.

In terms of the developmental stages of integration of the self, one may define an early proto-self, which is determined by bodily homeostasis; the core self, which involves conscious placement of oneself in space and time; and the mature, stable self-concept, which includes autobiographical memory, anticipation, the linguistic self, the mental self, and the social self. The central neurobiological structure involved in this integration is the junction of the ventromedial prefrontal cortex (vmPFC) and the anterior cingulate cortex (ACC). The vmPFC/ACC carries out a central function in the neurobiological integration of all the components of the self.

EARLY DEVELOPMENT OF DIFFERENTIATION OF SELF AND OTHER

There is general agreement about and broad confirmation of the capacity for an early cognitive differentiation between self and other, including the now classical evidence of such differentiation that emerges during the first 6–8 weeks of life (Gergely and Unoka 2011; Roth 2009). Infants, at that point, show different reactions to animate faces and inanimate patterns and are able to differentiate their mother's voice from other voices. They present a smiling response to "not me" interactional experiences and have a capacity for multimodal transfer—that is, to visually identify an object that differs from another in terms of its shape previously experienced while holding that object in their mouth. Infants also are able to follow movement and size of visual stimuli. These early indications of the capacity to differentiate experience originating in the self from external experience develops dramatically during the first 6 months and up to the first 18 months of life.

At 6 months, there is a further discrimination of facial expression of others as representing emotions. Between 6 months and 2 years, there develops a capacity to understand the action of others as indicating desire. Between 12 and 14 months, gaze perception is understood as indicating interest, and between 12 and 18 months, there is evidence of attribution of mental states to others, mostly as *equivalency*. This means that throughout all these functions, there is an early attribution of mental states to others that, under peak affect states, is overshadowed by attribution to others of the same emotion the infant experiences. By the third to fourth year, there develops the capacity to attribute complex beliefs to others, and somewhere between the end of the third and the beginning of the fourth year, there appears the capacity to attribute false beliefs to others (in contrast to the child's realistic knowledge of the present situation) (Förstl 2012).

The capacity to understand others is strongly dependent on Gallese's mirror neuron systems (Gallese and Goldman 1998)—that is, the internal replication at a neuronal level of actions, perceptions, and emotions of others. This replication determines the development of social cognition, as do actual interpersonal interactions. The role of emotional recognition is powerfully reinforced by language. Between 18 months and 3 years, the development of the verbal self contributes to differentiating clearly between "I" and "you." Between 24 and 36 months, the potential for negativism develops, but so also does the capacity for integration of good and bad images of mother, indicating the achievement of *object constancy*—that is, the integration of positive and negative affective relations. Between 3 and 5 years, finally, a full development of a private self evolves, and all these systems in the development of understanding of self and others contribute to strengthening the capability of a theory of mind (Gemelli 2008; Newen and Vogeley 2012).

EMPATHY AND COMPASSION

The capacity for empathy has to be differentiated from the capacity for theory of mind. Empathy involves feeling what the other is feeling, knowing what the other is feeling, and, particularly, empathy for pain in another. Empathy involves the activation of several brain structures: the anterior portion of the insula, the vmPFC, the ACC, the lateral prefrontal cortex, and the cerebellum. The lateral prefrontal cortex is central to empathic assessment of others. In addition, the anterior portion of the insula has a significant function in general recognition of social situations.

Empathy seems to be dependent on various brain functions—first of all, *contagion*. From the first few weeks of life, by mechanisms as yet unknown, a contagion of feelings among infants can be observed that may not involve mirror systems at all, but, rather, constitute an ancient phylogenetic subcortical system. In addition, the *gating function*, by which affects related to attachment, play bonding, and erotic stimulation (i.e., all positive, affiliative affective systems) determine intense attention to the other, may play a role in the activation of empathy. Finally, empathy is strongly influenced by the mirror neuron systems: first the cortical (primordial) mirror systems are involved, but later, widely distributed mirror functions involving the insula and the parietal and temporal cortex contribute to a general *cognitive-emotional recognition system*.

There is empirical evidence for the early development of the capacity for empathy (Bråten 2011; Richter 2012). The observation of infants between 12 and 14 months in the presence of another infant who shows indication of negative affective reactions or suffering permits the classification of infants' reactions into four types: 1) helping infants, who try to go to the aid of another who seems to suffer; 2) affected but not helping infants, who are concerned but who do not intervene; 3) confused infants, who do not respond but who in some way resound with the suffering other; and 4) indifferent infants, who also show a reaction of non-self-recognition in the mirror.

In general, empathy appears to originate in affective processes but gradually becomes enriched with cognitive development (Roth and Dicke 2006; Zikles 2006). At first, structures with affective activation are involved such as the brain stem regions, periaqueductal gray, amygdala, striatum, septal region, hypothalamus, and autonomic nervous system. Gradually, structures underlying cognitive processes become more and more involved, including the paralimbic region, cingulate cortex, insula, and orbitofrontal region. In short, the capacity of empathy has genetic roots, but it is intimately related to affective development and the differentiation between self and other.

Psychoanalytic Object Relations Theory

BASIC DEVELOPMENTAL CONCEPTS

In all its major variations, psychoanalytic object relations theory corresponds to a dominant contemporary development of psychoanalytic theory and technique. It proposes the internalization of significant relations between self and others as fundamental building blocks of the mind (Kernberg 2004). The internalization of such significant relations in the form of dyadic units of self and object representations, linked by the affect in which they are experienced, constitutes the basic infrastructures of the mind. Consolidation and gradual integration of these dyadic units into more complex, supraordinate structures lead to the development of the tripartite structure of ego, super ego, and id. In other words, the basic mental structures proposed by psychoanalytic object relations theory would really be constituted by various degrees of integration of component internalized dyadic and subsequent triadic object relations structures. This theory was first formulated by Fairbairn (1954) and Melanie Klein (1946/1952), and, in different ways, was also proposed by Edith Jacobson (1964) and Margaret Mahler and colleagues (1975) within ego psychology. In still different ways, this development also was conceived by various authors of the culturalist and relational psychoanalytic approach (Kernberg 2011). These basic internalized self–object representational dyads are conceived as embedded in peak affect states, both positive and negative, determining, respectively, "all good" and "all bad," and "idealized" and "persecuting," mental structures. It was the effort to objectify, in behavioral terms, these assumed intrapsychic structures that led Bowlby and Ainsworthy to develop contemporary attachment theory as the behavioral correspondence of the internalized object relations set up under the influence of the early mother–infant relationship (Diamond and Blatt 2007).

Psychoanalytic object relations theory implies two basic levels of development. First, under the dominance of peak affect states, a dual psychic structure is built up. On the one hand, a psychic structure constituted by idealized self representations relating to an idealized other (infant and mother) develops under the influence of strong positive, affiliative affective states; on the other, an opposite dyadic set of relationships develops under the dominance of strongly negative, aversive, painful affects, constituted by a frustrating or aggressive representation of the other related to a frustrated, enraged or suffering self representation (Kernberg 2004). This concept of the internalization of all good and, completely separately, all bad internalized object relations leads to an intrapsychic structure characterized by primitive dissociative or "splitting" mechanisms. In addition to primitive dissociation or splitting itself, there develop derived psychological mechanisms of projective identification, primitive idealization and devaluation, omnipotence and omnipotent control, and denial.

In contrast to these early developments under conditions of peak affect states, early development under conditions of relatively low affect states would evolve under the control of available cognitive functions, the instinctive (seeking system) impulses to learn about reality, and lead to early concepts and understanding of animate and inanimate reality that would develop in parallel with the splitting system of emotional experiences. At the early stage being described, there would not yet exist an integrated sense of self or the capacity of an integrated view of significant others. The representations of significant others would be split or dissociated similarly to those of the self, according to the corresponding idealized or persecutory peak affect states. In this regard, the term *persecutory* refers to the attribution of the state of pain or rage, or of "badness" in general, to the correspondent intentionality attributed to the significant other within such a negative or aversive state. However, under low affect states the more realistic representations of external reality are being built up to be integrated with the development of internalized object relations at the next, or second, stage of development.

At the second stage of development, gradually emerging over the first 3 years of life, the progressive development of realistic cognitive comprehension of the surrounding world and, particularly, the predominance of good over bad experiences facilitate the gradual integration of emotionally opposite conditions (i.e., the tolerance of the simultaneous awareness of both good and bad experiences). This development of tolerance of ambivalence, of combined positive and negative emotional relations with the same external objects, gradually leads to an integrated sense of self and significant others or, put another way, to normal ego identity. This second stage of development corresponds to the "depressive position" within Kleinian theoretical formulations. It signals the development of normal psychological functioning, or moderate pathology at a neurotic level of organization. In contrast, the development of character pathology at a borderline level of personality organization corresponds to Klein's "paranoid-schizoid position." Borderline personality organization, a severe level of personality disorder, is characterized, in fact, by lack of identity integration or the syndrome of identity diffusion, the permanence of predominant primitive defensive operation centering around splitting, and certain limitations in reality testing in terms of deficits in the subtle aspects of interpersonal functioning.

Psychoanalytic object relations theory proposes that the shift from borderline personality organization to neurotic and normal personality organization also corresponds to a shift from the predominance of primitive defensive operations to advanced defensive operations centering on repression and its related mechanisms, including a higher level of projection, negation, intellectualization, and reaction formations. This advanced level of development is reflected in a clear delimitation of a repressed, dynamic unconscious, or *id*, constituted by unacceptable internalized dyadic relationships reflecting intolerable primitive aggression and aspects of infantile sexuality. The *ego* now includes the integrated, conscious self-concept, and the representations of significant others, together with the development of sublimatory functions reflected in adaptive expression of affective, emotional needs regarding sexuality, dependency, autonomy, and aggressive self-affirmation. Internalized object relations that include ethically derived demands and prohibitions transmitted in the early interactions of the infant and child with his or her psychosocial environment, particularly the parents, are integrated into the *superego*. Layers of internalized prohibitions constitute this latter structure and idealized demands, significantly transformed into a personified, abstracted, and individualized system of personal morality (Kernberg 2004, 2012a).

The basic assumption of object relations theory regarding its relation to underlying neurobiological structures is that the dyadic units of internalized object relations reflect the availability of differentiation of self from others from the first few months of life on, and that representations of self and other become intimately related under the effect of peak affect states. It is assumed that such units of self and object representations are internalized as affective memory. The integration of the self and object representations from split or "partial" to "total" or whole representations would depend on the predominance of positive relationships and the corresponding positive segment of psychic experience. Otherwise, this integration would be threatened by the predominance of the negative segment of internalized object relations. In this case, to prevent a catastrophic "flooding" of mental experience by such a negative view of all reality, a defensive fixation at the early stage of primitive dissociation or splitting takes place, determining the syndrome of identity diffusion.

Primitive mental mechanisms of splitting and their derivatives would be based on biological, subcortical limbic developments of separate positive and negative affective systems, and their potential integration would be based on a cortical level of processing of emotional experience originally sharply dissociated (Roth 2009). In more general terms, the intrapsychic structures represented by object relations theory reflect a second, intrapsychic level of organismic organization, based upon a primary, neurobiological one (O. Kernberg, "The Unresolved Problem of the Classification of Personality Disorders," unpublished manuscript, July 2014) The review of present-day knowledge regarding early neurobiological development indeed strengthens the theoretical assumptions of psychoanalytic object relations theory and may provide a neurobiological basis reinforcing the developmental assumptions of personality organization (Gemelli 2008). The fact that positive and negative affects are strictly separated at lower limbic levels and can only be integrated at the level of the prefrontal and preorbital cortex and anterior cingulate level of elaboration of affective-cognitive experience reinforces the basic tenets of psychoanalytic object relations theory.

MENTALIZATION RECONSIDERED

Mentalization refers to the realistic interpretation of behavior of the self and others in terms of intentional mental states (beliefs, desires, fears) and the ability to reflect on such experienced mental states. Mentalization is a consequence of the gradual development of the cognitive differentiation of self and other, cognitive contextualization of affective states, the development of a theory of mind, empathy, and the very integration of the self (Kernberg 2012b). On the basis of what has been said so far, it is possible to differentiate two phases in the process of mentalization: an early phase, in which understanding of a present affect state develops in terms of an immediate object relationship, and a later phase, in which the understanding of this immediate object relationship may be related to the background of self experience and the background of the experience of others within the present social context. In other words, to be able to reflect on the meaning of a present interaction is not the same as to be able to modify that meaning under the impact of memory of related affective interactions that occurred under very different and opposite conditions to the present interaction. This second function, contextualizing the immediate present in the light of the reflected past, is severely disturbed under conditions of identity diffusion. The predominance of nonintegrated "persecutory" over "idealized" segments of experience predisposes the individual to a negatively distorted interpretation of present interpersonal interactions, reinforced by the activation of primitive defensive operations of splitting, projective identification, denial, omnipotent control, and devaluation, potentially determining vicious cycles of pathological interactions that reconfirm split-off negative mental experiences.

BORDERLINE PERSONALITY DISORDER: A PARADIGMATIC PERSONALITY DISORDER UNDER CONDITIONS OF BORDERLINE PERSONALITY ORGANIZATION

Neurobiological Features

There is evidence of genetic predisposition to borderline personality disorder, reflected in substantive family aggregation and genetically determined reduction in serotonin transporter gene functions. Patients with borderline personality disorder also show a deficit of the attentional control network, with hypoactivity in the prefrontal regions and abnormalities in the ACC, vmPFC, midbrain, and ventral striatum. We see a decreased function of cortical and subcortical midline brain structures, as well as "reflexive" versus "reflective" reactivity to emotional, particularly negative, stimuli, and evidence of hyperactivity of the amygdala, indicating augmentation of negative affectivity. In short, these patients evince neurobiological deficits and alterations in brain structures that clearly affect the normal integration of positive and negative segments of affective experience (O. Kernberg, "The Unresolved Problem of the Classification of Personality Disorders," unpublished manuscript, July 2014; Siever and Weinstein 2014; Sokol and Gunderson 2008).

Severe Childhood Trauma

Patients with borderline personality disorder show evidence of severe childhood trauma and sexual abuse, problematic parenting, predominance of hostile object relations beginning in early childhood, insecure attachment styles, and a limited capacity for symbolization or reflection (Koenigsberg et al. 2007). In short, severe childhood trauma represents another major etiological factor predisposing to dysfunction by the predominance of the segment of negative emotional experiences.

Relation of Neurobiological Features to Severe Childhood Trauma

How do all these features relate to each other? Genetic disposition to heightened temperamental negative affect reactivity is reinforced by severe childhood trauma. The decreased processes of self-regulation related to low executive function and low effortful control (derived from the combination of constitutionally low functioning prefrontal and preorbital control centers); the dominance of negative affects; and the failure of positive social reinforcement—all contribute to a predominance of negative reactivity that powerfully leads to lack of behavioral control and impulsivity (Sokol and Gunderson 2008).

The heightened rejection sensitivity derived from dominance of negative affective interactions, reflexive stimuli processing under conditions of an inadequate reflective function, the lack of mentalization related to the predominance of splitting mechanisms—all come together in contributing to these patients' impulsivity, aggression, affective dysregulation, abnormal interpersonal patterns, and chaotic self experience (Koenigsberg et al. 2007).

CONTRIBUTION OF OBJECT RELATIONS THEORY TO THE UNDERSTANDING AND TREATMENT OF BORDERLINE PERSONALITY DISORDER

The predominance of negative, persecutory segments of experience precludes the integration of normal identity. Dyadic units of self and other representations embedded in the context of peak negative or positive affect will retain the emotional valence in which they were experienced. When negative experiences overwhelm the positive, the borderline structure is maintained and reinforced through splitting and projective mechanisms. This becomes a self-perpetuating process wherein all negative affects take on an equivalence with archaic primitive experiences, leading to the apprehension of self–other interactions as binary between a victim and a persecutor. And finally, consistent efforts to reverse the persecutory relationship—that is, to become the victimizer rather than being the victim—in order to maintain an idealized dominant power position contribute further to reinforce and maintain the severely distorted bad relationships with significant others.

The predominance of primitive defensive operations, geared to maintain an idealized state, prevents the resolution of this split structure and perpetuates the cycle by defensively maintaining the segmentation of positive and negative experiences of self and other. Projective identification maintains the attribution of aggression to others. The reliance on omnipotent control translates into efforts of coercion and reinforces conflicts with others; the mechanism of devaluation leads to the destruction of potentially good relations, and the lack of affective integration maintains the primitivity of negative affects and fosters impulsivity to deal with unavoidable negative experiences (Kernberg 2012a).

TRANSFERENCE-FOCUSED PSYCHOTHERAPY AS A TREATMENT FOR BORDERLINE PERSONALITY ORGANIZATION

The general assumption that patients with borderline personality organization present with a predominance of the aggressive, persecutory segment of early experience (whatever its origin) that prevents identity integration leads us to propose a treatment geared to achieve identity integration and thus increase cognitive control. A stable sense of self would facilitate a more nuanced understanding and appreciation of others and would thus normalize social life and foster tolerance of ambivalence. This would in turn lead to affect modulation and reduction of impulsivity (Kernberg et al. 2008). With these assumptions, the strategy of transference-focused psychotherapy consists of clarifying the object relations activated in the treatment situation (the transference) at each affectively dominant point, regarding both positive and negative experiences. We attempt to facilitate the patient's tolerance and awareness of conflicting mental states. By means of clarification and, ultimately, interpretation of dissociated mental states, we foster mentalization. In treatment, the activation of such split-off object relations tends to produce "role reversals" in the transference. In other words, the interchanging of roles of self and object in the patient's experience of his or her relationship with the therapist permits the patient gradually to accept his or her unconscious identification with both victim and persecutor and, at the same time, to understand that his or her idealizations also have an unrealistic quality that represents a protective function against the opposite, negative segment of this experience (Clarkin et al. 2006).

The therapist, maintaining technical neutrality while protecting the therapeutic frame, permits a gradual introduction of a "three-person psychology." In other words, the therapist's specific function is that of an "excluded" outsider or third who helps the patient to diagnose the split-off idealized and persecutory states and gradually link them together, pointing to their distorting effects regarding the reality of the therapeutic interaction. In this context, the interpretation of primitive defenses and of the metaphorical significance of activated object relations in the transference permits the gradual tolerance of such primitive, split object relations, and their eventual elaboration into an integrated sense of self. At the same time, interpretations facilitate an integrated sense of the significant other; the achievement, in Kleinian terms, of the depressive position; and the expansion of analysis of the patient's corresponding problems in work and profession, love and sex, social life, and creativity as they surface in the transference.

In short, an object relations approach deals directly with the character structure of borderline personality disorder rather than focusing in a restricted way on particular symptoms of these patients. Clarification of the object relations implications of affect activation in the therapeutic hours increases cognitive control and permits the patient to overcome the splitting between persecutory and idealized relations. The mentalization of primitive affective states is commensurate with an interpretive approach to the primitive object relations activated in the transference. Integration of complex affective systems—involving aggression, sexuality, dependency, and autonomy—may be achieved in the study of the personal meanings at work in the activation of the patients' affect states.

In recent developments of this treatment, major attention has been given to the normalization of pathological consequences of insecure attachment. We would add that *all* primitive affective systems are involved in significant distortions of early experiences of these patients—not only the attachment system but also the play-bonding system and particularly the patient's erotic affective system. Important aspects of exploration of the transference in transference-focused psychotherapy involve disturbances of the capacity to integrate tenderness and eroticism, and a main focus of therapy is on developing normal object relations in depth, including the development of normal sexuality and its integration with love, and the capacity for commitment, effectiveness, and enjoyment in work and profession.

Conclusion

In consonance with what I suggested in earlier chapters, I would stress that there are two levels of personality development and personality integration—a neurobiological one and an intrapsychic/existential one—that influence each other and are influenced by the psychosocial environment. This is relevant for the analysis of personality structure, development, and pathology. The direct treatment of the personality *structure* of borderline personality organization is the ultimate objective of transference-focused psychotherapy.

References

Bråten S: Intersubjektive partizipation: bewegungen des virtuellen anderen bei säuglingen und erwachsenen. Psyche (Stuttg) 65(9/10):832–861, 2011

Clarkin JF, Yeomans FE, Kernberg OF: Psychotherapy for Borderline Personality: Focusing on Object Relations. Washington, DC, American Psychiatric Publishing, 2006

Diamond D, Blatt SJ: Introduction, in Attachment and Sexuality. Edited by Diamond D, Blatt SJ, Lichtenberg JD. New York, Analytic Press, 2007, pp 1–26

Fairbairn WRD: An Object-Relations Theory of the Personality. New York, Basic Books, 1954

Förstl H: Theory of Mind. Heidelberg, Germany, Springer, 2012

Gallese V, Goldman A: Mirror neurons and the simulation theory of mind-reading. Trends Cogn Sci 2(12):493–501, 1998 21227300

Gemelli RJ: Normal child and adolescent development, in American Psychiatric Publishing Textbook of Psychiatry. Edited by Hales RE, Yudofsky SC, Gabbard GO. Washington, DC, American Psychiatric Publishing, 2008, pp 245–300

Gergely G, Unoka Z: Attachment and mentalization in humans: the development of the affective self, in Mind to Mind: Infant Research, Neuroscience, and Psychoanalysis. Edited by Jurist EL, Slade A, Bergner S. New York, Other Press, 2011, pp 50–87

Jacobson E: The Self and the Object World. New York, International Universities Press, 1964

Kernberg O: Psychoanalytic object relations theories, in Contemporary Controversies in Psychoanalytic Theory, Techniques, and Their Applications. New Haven, CT, Yale University Press, 2004, pp 26–47

Kernberg OF: Divergent contemporary trends in psychoanalytic theory. Psychoanal Rev 98(5):633–664, 2011 22026541

Kernberg OF: Identity: recent findings and clinical implications, in The Inseparable Nature of Love and Aggression: Clinical and Theoretical Perspectives. Washington, DC, American Psychiatric Publishing, 2012a, pp 3–30

Kernberg OF: Mentalization, mindfulness, insight, empathy, and interpretation, in The Inseparable Nature of Love and Aggression: Clinical and Theoretical Perspectives. Washington, DC, American Psychiatric Publishing, 2012b, pp 57–79

Kernberg OF: What is personality? J Pers Disord 30(2):145–156, 2016 27027422

Kernberg OF, Yeomans FE, Clarkin JF, et al: Transference focused psychotherapy: overview and update. Int J Psychoanal 89(3):601–620, 2008 18558958

Klein M: Notes on some schizoid mechanisms (1946), in Developments in Psycho-Analysis. Edited by Riviere J. London, Hogarth Press, 1952, pp 292–320

Koenigsberg HW, Prohovnik I, Lee H, et al: Neural correlates of the processing of negative and positive social scenes in borderline personality disorder. Biol Psychiatry 61:104S, 2007

Krause R: Allgemeine PsychosomatischeBehandlungs—und Krankheitslehre. Stuttgart, Germany, Kohlhammer, 2012, pp 177–234

Mahler M, Pine F, Bergman A: The Psychological Birth of the Human Infant. New York, Basic Books, 1975

Newen A, Vogeley K: Menschlicher selbstbewusstsein und die fähigkeit zur zuschreibung von einstellungen, in Theory of Mind. Edited by Förstl H. Heidelberg, Germany, Springer, 2012, pp 161–180

Richter A: Empathie: wie können klinische erfahrungen und neurowissenschaften in beziehung gesetzt werden? in Psychotherapie und Neurowissenschaften. Edited by Böker H, Seifritz E. Bern, Switzerland, Huber, 2012, pp 181–200

Roth G: Aus Sicht des Gehirns. Frankfurt am Main, Germany, Suhrkamp, 2009

Roth G, Dicke U: Funktionelle neuroanatomic des limbischen systems, in Neurobiologie Psychischer Störungen. Edited by Förstl J, Hautzinger M, Roth G. Heidelberg, Germany, Springer, 2006, pp 1–74

Siever LJ, Weinstein LN: Neurobiology of personality disorders: implications for psychoanalysis. Paper presented to the New York Psychoanalytic Society, February 2014

Sokol AE, Gunderson JG: Personality disorders, in The American Psychiatric Publishing Textbook of Psychiatry. Edited by Hales RE, Yudofsky SC, Gabbard GO. Washington, DC, American Psychiatric Publishing, 2008, pp 821–859

Wright JS, Panksepp J: An evolutionary framework to understand foraging, wanting, and desire: the neuropsychology of the SEEKING System. Neuropsychoanalysis 14(10):5–39, 2012

Zikles K: Architektonik und funktionelle neuroanatomic der hirnrinde des menschen, in Neurobiologie Psychischer Störungen. Edited by Förstl H, Hautzinger M, Roth G. Heidelberg, Germany, Springer, 2006, pp 77–140

PART II

Spectrum of Psychoanalytic Psychotherapies

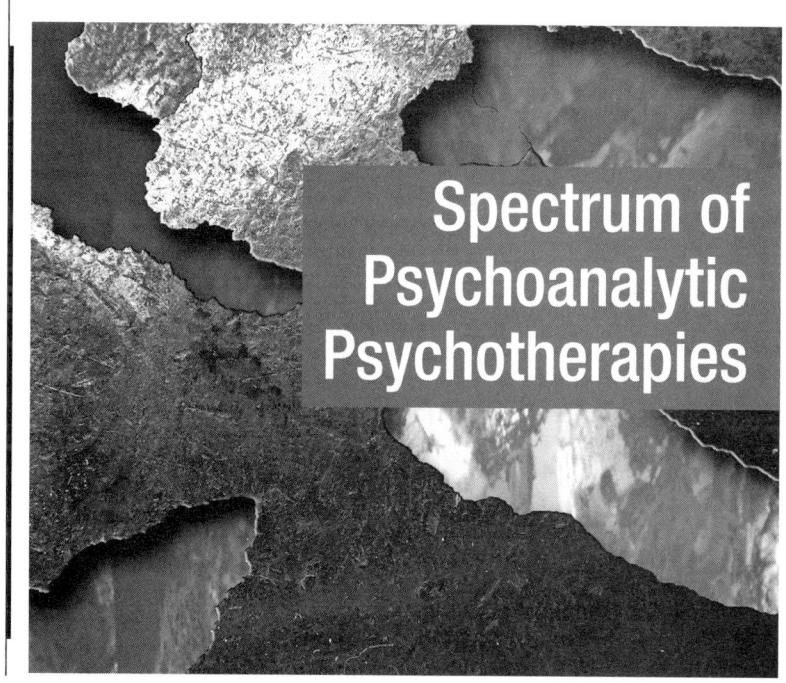

CHAPTER 4

The Basic Components of Psychoanalytic Technique and Derived Psychoanalytic Psychotherapies

What follows is an effort to describe the essential components of standard psychoanalytic technique, which are recognizable to most psychoanalytic practitioners, as well as a comprehensive delineation of techniques that derive from traditional psychoanalysis, yet can be broadly applied when psychoanalysis is not the treatment of choice. In fact, I propose that various psychoanalytic psychotherapies may be defined and differentiated in terms of specific modifications in one or several of these basic techniques. I attempt to provide contemporary definitions of these techniques that incorporate historical transformations in some of their underlying theoretical conceptualizations. Where contradictory models of these basic techniques have evolved as an expression of alternative psychoanalytic schools, I attempt to include these modifications of the corresponding techniques.

This effort derives from the work of the Personality Disorders Institute at Weill Cornell Medical College to develop a specific psychoanalytic psychotherapy for severe personality disorders, notably transference-focused psychotherapy (TFP). We have tried to spell out the differences between standard psychoanalysis and TFP and to relate this specific psychotherapy to other psychoanalytic psychotherapies such as supportive psychotherapy based on ego psychological principles, the German depth psychology–based psychoanalytic psychotherapy, mentalization-based therapy (MBT), and the rather nonspecific psychodynamic psychotherapy, which is practiced widely without a very sharp differential definition. In other words, this is an effort not only to describe the essential techniques of psychoanalysis, necessary and probably sufficient to qualify as such, but also to propose a frame that facilitates the differentiation of psychoanalysis proper from derived psychotherapies and the differences of these psychotherapies from one another within the context of this frame. In this chapter, I also discuss the application of these different techniques to comparative empirical studies of the relationships between process and outcome of psychoanalytic psychotherapies and standard psychoanalysis.

This effort should not be misinterpreted as a reductionist simplification of the richness and complexity of psychoanalytic technique. It is hoped that in elaborating this frame, the opposition to such reductionism should become clear.

Development of Classical Psychoanalytic Technique in the Context of Contemporary Object Relations Theory: A Capsule Overview

In general terms, the classical psychoanalytic theory of the nature of psychopathology treated by means of psychoanalytic technique proposes that the corresponding symptomatology is the result of unconscious conflicts between drive-derived impulses or wishes and defensive operations directed against them. Symptoms, in general, are compromise formations between impulse and defense. Repressed or dissociated libidinal and/or aggressive impulses, on the one side, and defense mechanisms originating from the tripartite structure of the mind, particularly from ego and superego, on the other, constitute the mutually opposed forces of these conflicts. While impulses derive mostly from the unconscious dynamics of the id, there are also id-derived defensive operations, namely repetition compulsion. The task of psychoanalytic treatment is to gradually reduce these defenses by means of the interpretive interventions of the psychoanalyst, thus facilitating the gradual emergence, in the conscious ego, of previously repressed or dissociated impulses, now to be explored by the conscious ego. This leads to conflict resolution, replacement of repression, and other defensive operations by sublimatory processes, and by a general harmonious integration of previously rejected unconscious impulses into adaptive psychic functions (Kernberg 2009).

During psychoanalytic treatment, transference developments come to reflect both the principal manifestations of the defensive operations and the gradual emergence of the repressed unconscious impulses, so that transference interpretation becomes the dominant feature of contemporary psychoanalytic technique. The interpretation of the transference requires a position of the analyst outside the conflict that is being enacted in the treatment situation—that is, the position of technical neutrality. One correlate of transference development, originally seen as an obstacle, but now seen as an important, often crucial, source of information to the analyst, is the development of countertransference. Its utilization as part of transference analysis has become an important aspect of psychoanalytic technique.

This (simplified) version of the classical psychoanalytic approach has been modified significantly but not replaced by contemporary psychoanalytic object relations theory. The essential tenet of object relations theory, shared by different theoretical schools using this approach within different technical and theoretical frames, is the assumption of the internalization, from birth on, of the relationship between the infant and the significant other, already highlighted in the classical discovery of the affective attachment system and enriched by the more recent knowledge of the crucial importance of the earliest mother–infant relationship in health and illness.

The basic assumption of psychoanalytic object relations theory is that the expression of instinctual drives or primary affect systems occurs in the context of the infant's affect activations that motivate interactional relations between infant and mother, and the infant's corresponding internalizations of the respective affective memory structures. These relationships are internalized first in the form of dyadic units of self and object representations within the frame of a dominant affect, and later in the form of triadic relationships that complicate the organization of the dyadic ones. Eventually they constitute the building blocks of the tripartite intrapsychic structure. The internalization of dyadic relationships occurs first in the context of a sharp division between positive and negative, idealized and persecutory relationships under the impact of corresponding positive and negative peak affect states. This is an early, originally neurobiologically based, developmental situation within which gradually primitive defensive operations, centering around splitting and projective identification, dominate. This early stage is followed by a stage of integration of positive and negative relationships, the development of tolerance of ambivalence, and the consolidation of an integrated self and integrated concepts of significant others. As this occurs, splitting and related primitive defenses tend to be replaced by repression and other related advanced defensive mechanisms, in the context of unconscious conflicts that now evolve as interstructural conflict. This developmental pathway is the essential contribution of contemporary object relations theory (Kernberg 2005).

What I wish to stress here is the essential change in the psychoanalytic theory of technique under the influence of object relations theory, in the sense that the conflict between impulse and defense is conceived no longer as a conflict between a "pure" impulse, on the one hand, and an "impersonal" defensive operation, on the other; rather, both impulse and defense are considered to be constituted by an internalized object relation of an impulsive or, respectively, a defensive nature. The implication is that the struggle between impulse and defense becomes a struggle between contradictory, conflictual internalized object relations, with significant implications for the analysis of the transference.

Now the transference is conceptualized as an *enactment*, not only of a regressed aspect of the self under the impact of a certain impulse or the defenses against it, but also of a defensive or impulsive relationship of self with object representations, with role distributions between self and object played out in the transference. The activation of opposite or contradictory internalized relationships between self and other play out the conflict between impulse and defense in the transference.

For example, a patient with subservient agreeableness, a reaction formation against profound rebellious hostility, would be considered not simply to be activating a defense mechanism—a reaction formation against a repressed drive derivative (i.e., aggression)—but to be presenting a defensive object relationship between a submissive self representation and a dominant, protective but demanding object representation. Thus, the superficial friendliness evident in the transference would suggest a surface dyad that defends against its opposite, the enraged opposition to a threatening authority. The unconscious conflict is between affectively opposite internalized object relations that enact the conflict between drive and defense in the transference. These considerations are relevant for the definitions of basic techniques that follow. Thus, object relations theory suggests a redefinition of basic transference developments to reflect the activation of internalized dyadic units embedded in an affective valence.

Different theoretical psychoanalytic schools may highlight different consequences of these complex developments, but what interests us here is the implicit highlighting of the basic technical therapeutic interventions that constitute indispensable instruments of transference analysis as the essential clarification of impulse—defense developments. I am referring to the following four technical aspects: 1) interpretation, 2) transference analysis, 3) technical neutrality, and 4) countertransference utilization. I propose that these four aspects jointly determine the very essence of psychoanalytic technique and that all other aspects of psychoanalytic technique really constitute specific applications or derivatives, depending on subject matters, complications, or developmental stages in the psychoanalytic treatment regarding how these four basic techniques are applied.

The combined application of these four basic techniques may be focused on different areas of the psychoanalytic treatment, which in turn imply particular technical approaches that are an important part of the total repertoire of techniques. This includes the analysis of the vicissitudes of free associations (to be discussed later in this chapter); the analysis of character, dreams, acting out, and separation anxiety and termination; the analysis of repetition compulsion and negative therapeutic reaction; and the analysis of specific defensive operations, and even countertransference complications during the treatment. So, while the focus of application may vary depending on the patient's dynamics, the basic four techniques remain at the heart of the psychoanalytic endeavor.

Preconditions for Psychoanalytic Work

I am referring here to the nature of the expectations regarding the work to be carried out by the psychoanalyst and by the patient. Other than the usual contractual arrangements such as time, frequency, and financial responsibility, the patient is expected to be capable of free associations. The instruction for free association is an essential precondition for psychoanalytic work, and difficulties or defensive interference with free association may become a major area of psychoanalytic intervention with some patients or, in some circumstances, with many. In practice, this very important requirement and the analysis of the related disturbances in verbal communication are frequently neglected, and it has been a major contribution of French analysis to point to this issue. Free association is a technical requirement that is common to many types of psychoanalytic psychotherapy (Hoffer 2006; Kris 1982, 1992).

The expectation for the analyst to intervene with "evenly suspended attention" is a complementary precondition for psychoanalytic work. This requirement—or, rather, the possibility of its achievement—has been questioned in terms of the unavoidable influences on the analyst, not only those due to countertransference but also those related to the limitations derived from his or her theoretical orientation. In this regard, I believe, with some reservation, that Bion's (1967) proposal to intervene "without memory or desire" is a relevant, important contemporary contribution to the analyst's specific task (Aguayo and Malin 2013). Bion's recommendation to attempt to start each session without preconceived ideas or theories of what is happening with this patient, or the wish for a significant change in the patient to be achieved, seems eminently reasonable. The unconscious conflicts that are presently relevant and emotionally dominant should emerge in the session itself, thereby activating aspects of the analyst's memory of previous knowledge about the patient, guiding any intentional approach to this patient that now may become relevant.

Bion's recommendation, however, is part of a paradox. It presupposes an analyst who is knowledgeable about the patient's background history and unconscious conflicts as they have been played out in the treatment and in external reality. This leads to an unavoidable internal conflict between his knowledge and his total openness to the unknown. To the contrary, ignoring the patient's "real" life outside the treatment situation, and past transferential developments, would impoverish the analyst's ability to contextualize new elements emerging in the present session. I believe this paradox needs to be tolerated and worked through by the analyst. This is a precondition for technical neutrality. In any case, I assume that the combination of evenly suspended attention on the part of the analyst, and the patient's effort to follow the rule of free associations are essential *preconditions* for psychoanalytic work, and not part of the actual technical interventions.

Definition and Analysis of the Four Basic Components of Psychoanalytic Technique

In explicating the basic four techniques, I have taken into consideration the corresponding definitions of several major dictionaries of psychoanalytic terms and concepts, including the *Dictionnaire International de la Psychanalyse*, edited by Alain de Mijolla (2002); *The New Dictionary of Kleinian Thought*, edited by Elizabeth Bott Spillius et al. (2011); *Psychoanalytic Terms and Concepts*, edited by Elizabeth Auchincloss and Eslee Samberg (2012); *Comprehensive Dictionary of Psychoanalysis*, by Salman Akhtar (2009); *The Language of Psychoanalysis*, by J. Laplanche and J.-B.

Pontalis (1988); *The Edinburgh International Encyclopaedia of Psychoanalysis,* edited by R.M. Skelton et al. (2006); *A Dictionary of Kleinian Thought,* by R.M. Hinshelwood (1991); the 4th edition of *Handbuch Psychoanalytischer Grundbegriffe,* edited by Wolfgang Mertens (2014); *Los Fundamentos de la Técnica Psicoanalitica,* by R. Horacio Etchegoyen (1986); and *The First Dictionary of Psychoanalylsis,* by Richard Sterba (2013). It was surprising, but reassuring, to see that there was tremendous overlap and complementarity among the definitions found in these sources.

INTERPRETATION

Interpretation is the basic technique of psychoanalysis and the main instrument to help the patient become aware of the conflict between defense and impulse and between defensive and impulsive relationships—in short, to become aware of his or her unconscious conflicts. Interpretation is the verbal communication by the analyst of the hypothesis of an unconscious conflict that seems to have dominantly emerged in the patient's communication in the therapeutic encounter. This may be considered the basic common technical approach in all psychoanalytically based treatments. It includes stages of communications that go from conscious surface to unconscious depth, and from defense and the motivation for this defense, to the underlying impulse.

In general, interpretation of a defense or a defensive relationship initiates the interpretive process, followed by the interpretation of the context, or the impulsive relationship against which the defense was erected, and the analysis of the motivation for this defensive process. Interpretive interventions may be classified into 1) *clarification,* by which the analyst attempts to clarify what is consciously is going on in the patient's mind; 2) *confrontation,* by which the analyst tactfully brings into the patient's awareness nonverbal aspects of the patient's behavior (the silent introspective utilization of the analyst's countertransference—in addition to the information from clarification and confrontation—may help assess the affectively dominant theme in the session); and 3) *interpretation proper,* by which the analyst proposes a hypothesis of the unconscious meaning that relates all these aspects of the patient's communication with one another. This condensed hypothesis is interpretation in the "here and now," to be followed or completed with interpretation in the "there and then"—that is, the genetic aspects of interpretation that refer to the patient's past and link the unconscious aspects of the present with the unconscious aspects of the past.

Transference interpretation is the most important application of interpretive interventions in psychoanalytic treatment and probably the most specific therapeutic factor of this approach. It needs to be pointed out that interpretation takes a different form in the treatment of patients with a neurotic personality organization and normal identity, in which repression and related defensive operations dominate the defensive process and interpretations involve bringing repressed content to awareness, than it does in the treatment of patients with severe personality disorders. Patients with borderline personality organization present identity diffusion and predominance of splitting and related primitive defense mechanisms, in which interpretation concerns contents that may emerge in the patient's consciousness or preconscious awareness but remains separate from other, conflictually linked contents by these very mechanisms: splitting and/or denial, projective identification, primitive idealization, devaluation, and omnipotent control. Here interpretation reveals *not* previously unconscious contents, but the unconscious motivation that determines the fragmentation of conscious experience (Kernberg et al. 2008).

The possibility of including in the interpretation of conflict not only in the transference but in external reality as well, as also in the intrapsychic elaboration and transformation of unconscious aspects of the past (in other words, the elements of construction and reconstruction), indicates that interpretation may be considered a *process* rather than single isolated interventions by the analyst. Although affective dominance in the therapeutic hour should determine the selection of the material to be interpreted—Bion's "selected fact"—the appropriate depth of interpretation varies according to the predominant transference situation. Interpretations that are too superficial will lead nowhere, and interpretations that are too deep may be rejected or lead to a purely intellectualized acceptance. Interpretations at an appropriate level of depth should provide confirmatory evidence by opening the patient's mind to new, previously unavailable material.

In general, given the uncertainty about the level of interpretation that may be indicated at a certain point, it seems preferable to go "too deep" rather than to stay on the surface. The patient's reaction will indicate whether the level chosen was appropriate, and further interpretations at a more appropriate level will be facilitated. Different psychoanalytic schools may differ in the material and level of depth they would focus on, but not, as far as I am aware, in the concept of interpretation itself as a basic psychoanalytic technique. They may differ in the frequency of interpretive intervention and the scope of material incorporated in each, as well as in the degree of "saturation" versus "evocativeness" of interpretations. French psychoanalysis, for example, tends to use infrequent, evocative, "strategic," widely integrating interpretive interventions, whereas

Kleinian analysis is characterized by frequent, "tactical," sharply transference-focused interpretation (Kernberg 2011).

Recent developments in interpretive styles seem to reveal a potential divergence between what may be called the relational, the neo-Bionian, and a "mainstream" approach, the last-mentioned one constituted by contemporary Kleinian, ego psychological, and French approaches. Relational authors are particularly attentive to the objective contribution of the analyst's countertransference and personality to the transference/countertransference bind. The neo-Bionian approach pays particular attention to the "psychoanalytic field" as a general emotional ambience generated in the analytic session and the analyst's reverie in generating a correspondent narrative that becomes an essential aspect of the interpretations. And, finally, the mainstream approach maintains the emphasis on the patient's material as reflecting the unconscious past as the "total transference" expressed in the patient's verbal, nonverbal, and external reality features and the countertransference. This last approach strongly focuses on the unconscious elements of the preconscious here and now, with the assumption that the interpretation will bring about transformation in the underlying structural past conflicts.

In short, within the generally accepted definition of interpretation as a basic psychoanalytic instrument, there are variations in the level of depth of the interpretive process and in the privileging of particular elements of the analyst's various sources of information included in his or her interpretive work.

TRANSFERENCE ANALYSIS

As mentioned before, transference is at the center of the manifestation of the patient's unconscious conflicts in the treatment situation, a predominant defensive operation that functions as resistance in the clinical setting, as well as a fundamental source of information regarding the patient's unconscious conflicts. *Transference* may be defined as the unconscious repetition in the here and now of pathogenic conflicts from the past. The analysis of transference is the main source of specific change brought about by psychoanalytic treatment.

This statement has been partially questioned by psychoanalysts with a relational approach, who would put equal emphasis on the therapeutic function of the actual relationship between patient and analyst established during the analytic treatment, a viewpoint that dovetails with their view that transference is not exclusively the activation in the here and now of the patient's unconscious conflicts from the past, but is contributed to by the personality and the behavior of the analyst. In the view of relational analysts, in the same way as the patient's transference induces countertransference reactions in the analyst, the analyst's personality and countertransference reactions influence transference developments. In their view, transference is considered as jointly constructed, and the analyst's recognition of his or her contribution, which is often shared with the patient, leads to a collaboration in the understanding of the transference, which functions as an important therapeutic factor containing both interpretation and recognition of realistic aspects of the actual therapeutic relationship (Kernberg 2011).

Insofar as this relational approach also involves the potential for some communication of countertransference reactions—in contrast to their exclusive introspective analysis by the analyst as material to be included in transference interpretation—this also signals a potential departure from strictly classical definitions of the essential components in the processes of analytic technique. In this regard, then, the relational psychoanalytic approach modifies the concept of transference and the utilization of countertransference reactions to some extent as conceived in the classical psychoanalytic model. Without discussion of the pros and cons of the relational approach, this difference signals how a strict definition of the four basic techniques within the classical model permits the differentiation of more recent psychoanalytic models, and their correspondent techniques, from standard psychoanalytic technique proper.

The classical concept of transference analysis has been expanded significantly by the concept of the analysis of the total transference proposed by the Kleinian approach (Joseph 1985). It involves a systematic analysis of the transference implications of the patient's total verbal and nonverbal manifestations in the hours, the patient's direct and implicit communicative efforts to influence the analyst in a certain direction, and the consistent exploration of the transference implications of material from the patient's external life that he or she brings into the session. The inclusion of a systematic consideration of the patient's total functioning at the point of the activation of a predominant transference seems an important reinforcement of the centrality of transference interpretation and points to an important implicit consequence of transference interpretation, namely, the analysis of character. Defensive characterological patterns tend to become dominant transference resistances and, in this regard, lend themselves to systematic analysis leading to characterological modification. This is a significant effect of psychoanalytic treatment, one of its most powerful therapeutic consequences, which is surprisingly underemphasized in the psychoanalytic literature on technique.

The question has been raised as to what extent is transference analysis the exclusively effective form of interpretation. This would seem an unwarranted extension: many problems in the patient's life that may draw the analyst's attention because they are affectively dominant in the communications of the hour and apparently linked with the transference may, in fact, be invested predominantly in a present relationship with an external object. Also, the interpretation of the corresponding unconscious conflict focused on that relationship, because of the affective dominance at this point, is located there. Eventually, however, major pathogenic unconscious conflicts tend to be anchored in characterological defensive structures that will become transference resistances. Systematic analysis of the transference is, I believe, the essential but not exclusive focus of the analyst's interpretive activity. The Kleinian approach always has tended to maximize systematic transference analysis, but the trend has now evolved in ego psychological and relationist approaches as well, and even French analysis has increased this aspect of analytic work.

The nature of transference regression also has shifted in the conceptualization of primitive, early, archaic object relations–determined transferences, in contrast to later advanced oedipal transferences. Oedipal and preoedipal conflicts tend to be condensed in regressive transferences of severe personality disorders, with dominance of aggressive developments, in contrast with clearer differentiation of stage of development in less regressive transferences of neurotic personality organization, where we see mostly infantile sexual conflicts.

In patients with neurotic personality organization, transference-related material is expressed in the verbal communication of subjective experience. In contrast, in patients presenting borderline personality organization, subtle (or not so subtle) efforts to influence the analyst by means of projective identification and omnipotent control foster enactments and intense and shifting countertransferences that lead to a focus on the influence of the analytic field in the analytic situation. Severe acting out, of course, focuses the analytic attention on what is going on in the patient's external life situation. The relative importance of the various sources of transference expression and its interpretation varies with alternative characterological features of the patient.

In the light of contemporary object relations theory, the understanding of identificatory and projective aspects of transference developments in severe personality disorders has been clarified and enriched. In the case of neurotic personality organization, the predominant enactments in the transference/countertransference bind involve the patient's identification with an aspect of his or her infantile self while projecting the corresponding object representation onto the analyst. Reversals of this enactment, in which the patient identifies with the object representation while projecting the corresponding self representation onto the analyst, are less frequent. In contrast, in the case of severe psychopathology, such reversals are frequent, and the consistent alternating reversals of self and object representations are the rule, which gives an apparently chaotic character to the transference developments (Kernberg et al. 2008). In addition, other complications emerge in these cases. One is the reciprocal activation of the patient's grandiose self and his or her depreciated self representation as dominant object relations pathology in the transference developments of narcissistic pathology. Another complication is the regression to symbiotic relations, in which the patient cannot tolerate any differences of views and relatedness in the therapist, experiencing all triangulations as intolerable traumatic situations. The interpretation and working through of these primitive transference regressions may represent the dominant therapeutic feature of these cases.

TECHNICAL NEUTRALITY

The technique of technical neutrality tends to be misinterpreted as a recommendation for an analyst's distant, uninvolved attitude, a "mirror to the patient's presentations." In essence, technical neutrality simply refers to the analyst's not taking sides in the patient's activated internal conflicts, remaining equidistant, as Anna Freud put it, from the patient's id, ego, and superego, and from his or her external reality (A. Freud 1936/1966). Technical neutrality consists of an attitude of concerned objectivity. It implies a potential alliance with that part of the patient's ego in which he or she is able to carry out self-observation, however strong or weak that aspect of the patient's personality may be. Technical neutrality, in addition, implies the analyst's not attempting to influence the patient with his or her own value systems. Freud's early metaphor of the analyst as a "mirror" clearly was questioned by himself, and he protested against a view of analytic objectivity as "disgruntled indifference" (Laplanche and Pontalis 1988, pp. 271–272).

Technical neutrality also implies the concept of *abstinence*, in the sense that the analytic relationship should not be utilized for the gratification of libidinal or aggressive impulses of the patient or the analyst. In contrast, technical neutrality does not imply the concept of *anonymity*, a questionable development in psychoanalytic thinking in the 1950s and importantly related, in my view, to the development of authoritarian pressures within psychoanalytic education, and the institutionally fostered idealization of the training analyst, who should not show any usual personal human characteristic to the patient. This implicit fostering of an unanalyzable idealization of the analyst has been sharply criticized in recent years, particularly by the relational school.

Technical neutrality implies an attitude of the analyst "in role," a natural and sincere approach to the patient within general socially appropriate behavior, as part of which the analyst avoids all references or focus upon his or her own life interests or problems. The analyst cannot avoid that personal features emerge in the treatment situation and become the source of transference reactions. The patient's realistic reaction to realistic aspects of the analyst's behavior should not be considered a transference reaction. Not everything is transference! Maintaining the definition of *transference* as an inappropriate reaction to the reality presented by the analyst that reflects the activation of the unconscious conflicts of the patient should differentiate transference from other of the patient's realistic reactions to natural, as well as idiosyncratic, aspects of the treatment situation.

Technical neutrality refers to the analyst's actions but not to his or her internal emotional experiences. Countertransference reactions may shift from moment to moment or over an extended period, but the analyst has to attempt to intervene at points in which he or she has achieved or regained a position of technical neutrality and is no longer under the sway of his or her particular activated emotional reaction to the patient. To sum up, it is the analyst's behavior and interventions that should be carried out from a point of technical neutrality, not the analyst's emotional experience. That experience should be subject to countertransference analysis, our next subject.

There are forms of psychoanalytic psychotherapy in which technical neutrality clearly must be abandoned, namely, at points of severe acting out that threaten the survival of the treatment or the life of the patient. In standard psychoanalysis, the need to abandon the treatment frame is usually not indicated or necessary.

Within the relational approaches, self psychology has explicitly abandoned technical neutrality in so far as the analyst consciously adopts the position of the patient's self-object, in an effort to complement and normalize a deficient self-object relation from the past (Kernberg 2011). Further, the relational approach to occasionally communicate selected aspects of the countertransference to the patient also decreases technical neutrality, so that it seems fair to state that relational analysis moves in the direction of a modification of this aspect of standard analytic technique.

COUNTERTRANSFERENCE UTILIZATION

Countertransference is the analyst's total, moment-to-moment emotional reaction to the patient and to the specific material that the patient presents. The contemporary view of countertransference is that of a complex formation codetermined by the analyst's reaction to the patient's transference, the reality of the patient's life, the reality of the analyst's life, and specific transference dispositions activated in the analyst as a reaction to the patient and his or her material. Under ordinary circumstances, countertransference mostly is determined by the vicissitudes of the transference, and as such, the analyst's emotional reactions may fluctuate significantly within each session. In contrast to acute fluctuations of the countertransference, chronic distortions of the analyst's internal attitude toward the patient usually signify significant difficulties in the analyst's understanding of the transference. They usually indicate a stalemate in the analytic situation that the analyst may need to resolve through self-exploration or consultation. Serious characterological difficulties of the analyst may contribute to such chronic countertransference distortions, but frequently they relate to more limited difficulties in his or her understanding and are related to particular developments in the transference (Kernberg 2012).

Racker's classification of countertransference reactions is a very helpful indicator of the developments in the transference. In Racker's classification, there are two types of reaction: *concordant identification* in the countertransference—that is, the analyst's emotional identification with the patient's central subjective experience at this point—and *complementary identification* in the countertransference—that is, identification with the transference object of the patient projected onto the analyst, an identification with an internal object that the patient cannot tolerate. Concordant identification in the countertransference facilitates an increased empathy with the patient's subjective experience, and the analysis of complementary identification in the countertransference is an important instrument for the analysis of primitive defensive operations, particularly projective identification. The analyst's interpretive analysis of what has been projected into his or her subjective experience facilitates a full understanding of the dominant object relationship activated in the transference.

The technical utilization of countertransference requires analysts to first maintain themselves "in role" to protect themselves from countertransference acting out, while remaining open to a full exploration of their subjective countertransference experience. Full internal tolerance of countertransference reactions, including regressive fantasies about specific relations with the patient, may be followed by the analyst's internal exploration of the meanings of his or her reaction in terms of the present transference situation, and the motivation of the analyst's particular way of reacting to it, and thus prepare the road for transference analysis. In fact, as mentioned previously, the basic material for interpretive interventions is a combination of the analysis of the patient's verbal and nonverbal behavior, present references to his or her external reality, and the countertransference.

If countertransference reactions cannot be fully elaborated and controlled and are expressed or acted out in the sessions, and the patient indicates his or her awareness of that aspect of the analyst's behavior, the reality of that behavior should be acknowledged, but without any further analysis of the analyst's motivation determining that behavior. The point is to maintain an honest relationship with the patient, acknowledging the reality of perhaps questionable behavior of the analyst that the patient has become aware of, and not to consider that as part of the transference. It may, of course, determine the activation of particular transference reactions and developments.

As previously mentioned, relational psychoanalysts may decide to selectively communicate aspects of the countertransference to patients to signal the universality of such emotional reactions--in short, their own humanity. In this way, they may decrease the objectively regressive aspects of the psychoanalytic situation, in which a parental relationship is enacted with an analyst whose internal life the patient can never know, similar to the relationship the patient had with his or her parents. An anti-authoritarian intention, as well as the conviction that the actual therapeutic relationship has a significant therapeutic effect, underlies this approach. Again, I believe that this represents a variation from standard psychoanalytic technique that permits to differentiate techniques of different psychoanalytic approaches, illustrating the utilization of this outline.

Acting out of the countertransference must be differentiated from *enactment*, in which an emotional situation reflecting a transference development is enacted countertransferentially without a specific actual behavior of the psychoanalyst but is certainly present in his or her emotional experience in consonance with the emotional relationship that is implied in the transference development of the patient. Enactments may signal important transference/countertransference developments that should be differentiated from countertransference acting out.

So far, we have the overall outline of the basic techniques that, I suggest, essentially define psychoanalytic technique and that may be applied to the analysis of various developments in the analytic situation, such as the analysis of dreams, character analysis, the analysis of acting out, and repetition compulsion—all of which will culminate in transference analysis.

Differentiation of Psychoanalysis From Psychoanalytic Psychotherapies

Before comparing various derivatives of psychoanalysis proper, I need to clarify several points regarding the general treatment setting and the objectives of treatment. Regarding the treatment setting, one question relates to the frequency of sessions and another one to the use of the couch. I assume there exists a general agreement regarding the minimal frequency of psychoanalysis of three sessions per week, with different views regarding the essential or necessary nature of a higher frequency, of four or five weekly sessions. This is a controversial subject that requires empirical research. It is reasonable to assume that cases of significant narcissistic pathology require a higher frequency of sessions than cases in which this pathology is not a major issue.

Regarding psychoanalytic psychotherapies, TFP explicitly requires a minimum frequency of two sessions per week, with the rationale that a lesser frequency would not permit careful exploration of the patient's external life situation and of transference developments at the same time (Clarkin et al. 2006). It is reasonable to state that all other forms of psychoanalytic psychotherapy are less specific regarding frequency, although all of them, except supportive psychotherapy proper, would see a frequency of two sessions a week preferable to once-a-week sessions.

The use of the couch seems optimal for psychoanalysis, but it needs to be kept in mind that by itself, a strictly psychoanalytic technique with an appropriate psychoanalytic frequency is feasible in the psychoanalysis of patients who present various reasons for enormous resistance to use of the couch. There seems to be no good rationale for use of the couch for psychoanalytic psychotherapies that are usually carried out in a face-to-face position. In fact, TFP is strongly committed to a face-to-face treatment of patients with severe personality disorders, a setting that highlights the behavioral aspects of the transference as well as facilitates countertransference analysis in the case of patients with very restricted capacity for verbal expression. With such patients, it is often nonverbal communication that provides clues to the transference developments. In general, the more severe the psychopathology, the more the transferences are predominantly expressed in severely distorted characterological patterns, which emerge as powerful distortions in the interpersonal field with the therapist. Face-to-face settings permit opportunities for observing and interpreting these developments.

The assumed essential mechanism of change in psychoanalytic treatment—the dominant mediator of its effectiveness—is the achievement of insight into the unconscious conflicts that determined the patient's psychopathology and the use of this insight to elaborate such infancy- and childhood-derived unconscious conflicts into conscious and sublimatory solutions. Major changes in dominant transference developments are outstanding indicators of therapeutic improvement. The basic correspondent assumption of optimal effectiveness of psychoanalytic treatment involves a definite improvement in the overall personality functioning of the patient in the major areas of psychological realm, including work and profession, love and sex, social life, and creativity, and a corresponding increase in effectiveness and gratification with life. TFP, probably the most ambitious of the psychoanalytic psychotherapies, has similar goals for patients with borderline personality organization, a very severe character pathology that usually presents contraindications for psychoanalysis proper. Mentalization-based therapy expects significant symptomatic and interpersonal functioning improvement based upon its specific mediating mechanism of increase in mentalization, a point that requires further discussion (Bateman and Fonagy 2004). MBT proposes that interpretation is contraindicated in the treatment of severely regressed borderline patients. In contrast, TFP uses interpretation from the beginning of treatment. This difference requires further elaboration.

Mentalization refers to the capacity to realistically assess mental states in oneself and others as intentional, motivated wishes, feelings, and aspirations. In a sense, it corresponds to the concept of insight, with emphasis on the centrality of realistic self-assessment, assessment of others, and the capacity for self-reflection. There has been a broadening use of the concept of mentalization, so that it is difficult to differentiate it from the general psychoanalytic concept of insight. Insofar as MBT is a specific form of psychotherapy developed for the treatment of borderline personality disorder and severe personality disorders in general, it is focused on the distortions characterizing these patient's therapeutic interactions and helps them systematically to acquire more realistic assessments of their own and their therapist's emotional experiences and behavior in their interactions. MBT does not attempt to highlight and interpret these patients' dissociative or splitting processes that interfere with integration of the concept of self and the integration of the concept of significant others.

TFP, to the contrary, although starting out with clarifying the patient's emotional experiences and his or her interpretation of the patient's and the therapist's interaction, does not attempt to normalize these experiences by their reality-oriented clarification, but attempts to clarify and preserve the conscious awareness by the patient of extremely distorted, split self and object representations and then proceeds to clarify the function of the separation of the extremely *bad/feared* and *good/desired* relationships to maintain the split between idealized and persecutory segments of experience (Clarkin et al. 2006). In this regard, TFP also starts out with mentalization-focused interventions as an early clarifying stage of full interpretation of primitive internalized object relations in the transference. In other words, in TFP, mentalization would refer to the specific acquisition of realistic insight related to the faulty interpretation of self representations and the corresponding faulty interpretation of representations of significant others—in short, the achievement of insight by transforming identity diffusion into normal identity. TFP interprets primitive splitting and related defensive mechanisms to achieve realistic insight. In fact, we have empirical data showing that TFP, indeed, produces increased mentalization in borderline patients, leading to an increase in their capacity for realistic assessment of self and others as consequence of identity integration. Both MBT and TFP use mentalization as a specific clarification of the nature of the relationship activated in the transference, but for TFP this is only a preliminary step to the interpretation of primitive defensive operations and object relations. Thus, significant differences in the use of interpretation permit us to differentiate the technical approaches of these two psychoanalytic psychotherapies.

So far, I have not referred to the introduction of supportive techniques in various types of psychoanalytic psychotherapy (Kernberg 1999). The development in the 1960s and 1970s in the United States of insight-oriented or expressive psychotherapy coincided with the development of supportive modalities of psychotherapeutic treatment based on psychoanalytic understanding of psychopathology and the consideration of transference developments during treatments. The Psychotherapy Research Project of the Menninger Foundation relied on the classification of psychoanalytically derived treatments into standard psychoanalysis, expressive psychotherapy, and supportive psychotherapy. This classification was based on the technical criteria of the use of interpretation, transference analysis, and supportive measures, particularly cognitive and emotional support and guidance, selective reduction of transference regression by educational means, and direct environmental interventions, initially labeled (somewhat derogatorily) "manipulation." For practical purposes, psychodynamic psychotherapy as practiced in the United States is still characterized to a major extent by varying degrees of combination of interpretive and partial transference interpretive techniques, combined with direct guidance and reassurance, and generally re-educative efforts to strengthen adaptive compromises between impulse and defense.

The German *Tiefenpsychologisch fundierte Psychotherapie* (depth psychology–based psychoanalytic psychotherapy) utilizes a combination of interpretation—particularly of extratransferential manifestations of unconscious conflicts, partial clarification and reality-oriented reduction of the transference, and direct supportive and re-educative measures (Wöller and Kruse 2005). In comparing various types of psychoanalytically derived psychotherapy, the assessment of the extent to which supportive techniques are included in the technical repertoire is important in their differentiation.

Using the four technical instruments explored above and the extent to which supportive techniques are included in the treatment approach, we may now tentatively classify psychoanalysis and psychoanalytic psychotherapies as a set of related treatments that use these techniques to different degrees and with some differences in emphasis. This should facilitate the establishment of a matrix evaluating the relationship between these approaches, including frequency of sessions and setting, their indications and contraindications or limitations, and effectiveness. This chapter is intended as a tentative approach to clarifying a complex subject with clinical and research implications, a first step in the direction of an effort to facilitate the clarification of their mutual relationships and facilitate scientific research in this area.

All the approaches that constitute what may be called the "mainstream" of standard or classical psychoanalysis—the contemporary ego psychological approach, the contemporary Kleinian approach, the British Independent approach, and the French (non-Lacanian) approach—apply interpretation, transference analysis, technical neutrality, and countertransference analysis and are fully cognizant of and committed to these techniques as mutually necessary and complementary. Differences within these approaches relate to 1) the use of the "tactical" (Kleinian), in contrast to the "strategic" (French), approach regarding the frequency of transference interpretations, and the different emphasis on various contents and levels of unconscious conflicts interpreted among these orientations; 2) the focus on archaic in contrast to later oedipal developments, preoedipal in contrast to later oedipal conflicts; and 3) the focus on the expression of unconscious conflicts in linguistic characteristics (in the French approach).

The relational psychoanalytic approach uses the same four basic techniques, but with a variation derived from their conceptualization of transference (considered as determined in part by the analyst's personality and reactions) and with sharing with the patient the effects of the combined enactment of contributions to the transference by patient and analyst (Akhtar 2009; Auchincloss and Samberg 2012). A limited communication of countertransference reactions to the patient, an implication of this approach, also differentiates the relational school from classical psychoanalysis in terms of the four techniques considered. This approach somewhat reduces technical neutrality and may limit transference interpretation at the deepest levels of negative transference developments, particularly because relational analysts are concerned about the traumatic origin of patient's unconscious conflicts, in contrast to the primarily drive-determined origins of them. Self psychology, in turn, presents a major reduction in technical neutrality and transference analysis derived from the analyst's consciously assuming the role of a self-object for the patient, as part of the specific emphasis of this approach to help development and maturation of normal narcissism. Here, a significant limitation of transference analysis, particularly of negative transference analysis, may be a consequence (Kernberg 2011).

TFP is the psychotherapeutic approach closest to standard psychoanalysis. It applies the four basic techniques with significant emphasis on systematic analysis of the transference. A major difference with standard psychoanalysis is the occasional abandonment of technical neutrality to protect the frame and the continuity of the treatment, and to protect the patient from life-threatening self-destructive behavior. Departures from neutrality under these conditions usually involve limit setting to protect the patient's life, and the treatment itself, and the setting up of specific conditions under which the treatment can be continued. The severity of acting out of self-destructive, self-mutilating, or violently aggressive behaviors triggers such limit settings in selected individual cases. This significant deviation from technical neutrality is combined, however, with a systematic analysis, following such abandonment, of the reasons and related unconscious conflicts necessitating abandonment of technical neutrality, and its unconscious meanings for the patient, thus attempting to restore the position of technical neutrality. TFP relies heavily on countertransference analysis as an intrapsychic exploration by the therapist that is applied to the clarification and interpretation of transference developments.

Ego psychological expressive psychotherapy, which was developed in the United States in the 1960s and 1970s, explicitly uses interpretation, particularly of extratransferential developments, with limited transference analysis—particularly regarding the analysis of negative transference developments—and the therapeutic utilization of positive transference developments to strengthen the therapeutic alliance (Auchincloss and Samberg 2012; Kernberg 1999). In this context, this approach reduces the position of technical neutrality. Also, there is little emphasis on countertransference analysis. This expressive or insight-oriented psychotherapy may also be combined with supportive elements, and is quite prevalent in the practice of psychodynamic psychotherapy in the United States, in which cognitive and emotional support, selective reduction of negative transference developments, and direct environmental intervention are combined. A purely supportive psychotherapy, which uses supportive measures in addition to selective strengthening of adaptive compromise formations of impulse and defense, complements this set of expressive-supportive and supportive psychotherapies, in which a significant degree of reduction of technical neutrality and limited transference interpretation are matched with varying degrees of these supportive measures (Kernberg 1999). In Chapter 8 of this book, "A New Formulation of Supportive Psychodynamic Psychotherapy," I describe a supportive psychotherapy approach that is based on TFP principles.

German depth psychology–based psychoanalytic psychotherapy follows quite closely the principles of American ego psychological psychodynamic psychotherapies and was developed further in great technical detail in Germany. It has been enriched with theoretical and technical elements derived from the British psychoanalytic schools but limits interpretive approaches mostly to extratransferential material and combines partial transference interpretation with direct efforts to reduce negative transferences, strengthen the therapeutic alliance, and reinforce the patient's resources for more adaptive environmental functioning (Wöller and Kruse 2005).

MBT specifically focuses on increasing the patient's realistic awareness of his or her experience and reactions and the present motivations of the self and the therapist, rejecting explicitly interpretive interventions and avoiding transference analysis. It attempts to strengthen the realistic aspects of the patient–therapist relationship. In that MBT acknowledges that it may constitute the first stage of subsequent psychoanalytic psychotherapy, dealing in more depth with patients' transferences and unconscious conflicts, it does not place itself in contradiction to a psychoanalytic approach.

There is empirical evidence for the effectiveness of TFP, MBT, and psychoanalytic psychotherapy in a broad sense (mostly following the general approach signaled by the developments in American ego psychology). It remains an open question as to what are specific indications, contraindications, and limitations, and, very importantly, how these treatments expand the realm of therapeutic effectiveness of a general psychoanalytic approach. It also needs to be stressed that in the development of the techniques of these psychoanalytically based psychotherapies, ongoing developments in psychoanalysis proper have had fundamental importance in enriching the corresponding technique and increasing the sophistication of these approaches. Thus, for example, the contributions of the Kleinian school to the understanding of primitive object relations and primitive defensive operations have been of enormous importance in the psychotherapeutic treatment of severe personality disorders. Similarly, the understanding of the nature and the potential for utilization of countertransference reactions developed within psychoanalysis proper has significantly enriched psychoanalytic psychotherapy approaches.

While the main intention of this effort to develop a conceptual frame for the comparison of psychoanalytically based treatments has been geared to the facilitation of clinical practice and research in this area, a practical implication may also be the question of to what extent psychoanalytic institutes should be systematically engaged in training their candidates both in standard psychoanalysis and in a spectrum of psychoanalytic psychotherapies. The fear has been expressed that such training may lead to dilution of psychoanalytic techniques and eventually threaten the psychoanalytic enterprise. On the basis of our experience in teaching TFP in various psychoanalytic institutes, this fear seems unjustified. To the contrary, when psychoanalytic psychotherapy is more clearly differentiated from psychoanalysis proper, the very approach to psychoanalytic technique tends to become more precise and sharpened. Psychoanalysts may have a much better theoretical and clinical basis for developing expertise in various types of psychoanalytic psychotherapy than many mental health professionals who are attempting to learn psychoanalytic psychotherapy without a solid psychoanalytic basis. The present effort to differentiate psychoanalytic techniques and their mutual relationship may foster the eventual development of a comprehensive, standard text on psychoanalytic technique, something that is urgently needed for learning psychoanalysis as well as for scientifically developing its technique and applications further, and for empirical research on its process and effectiveness.

From a broader perspective of the development of a general synopsis of contemporary psychoanalytic technique, the present effort to define the four basic technical psychoanalytic instruments needs to be complemented with a comprehensive synthesis of all the other psychoanalytic technical instruments that are facilitated by the combined employment of these basic ones. This task will be attempted in further exploration of psychoanalytic techniques in Chapter 6 of this book, "The Spectrum of Psychoanalytic Techniques."

References

Aguayo J, Malin B: Wilfred Bion: Los Angeles Seminars and Supervision. London, Karnac, 2013

Akhtar S: Comprehensive Dictionary of Psychoanalysis. London, Karnac, 2009

Auchincloss EL, Samberg E: Psychoanalytic Terms and Concepts. New Haven, CT, Yale University Press, 2012

Bateman A, Fonagy P: Psychotherapy for Borderline Personality Disorder: Mentalization-Based Treatment. New York, Oxford University Press, 2004

Bion WR: Notes on memory and desire. Psychoanalytic Forum 2:272–273, 279–290, 1967

Clarkin JF, Yeomans FE, Kernberg OF: Psychotherapy for Borderline Personality: Focusing on Object Relations. Washington, DC, American Psychiatric Publishing, 2006

de Mijolla A: Dictionnaire International de la Psychanalyse. Paris, Calmann-Lévy, 2002

Etchegoyen RH: Los Fundamentos de la Técnica Psicoanalítica. Buenos Aires, Argentina, Amorrortu, 1986

Freud A: The ego and the mechanisms of defense (1936), in The Writings of Anna Freud, Vol 2. New York, International Universities Press, 1966, pp 3–176

Hinshelwood RD: A Dictionary of Kleinian Thought. London, Free Association Books, 1991

Hoffer A: What does the analyst want? Free association in relation to the analyst's activity, ambition, and technical innovation. Am J Psychoanal 66(1):1–23, 2006 16544200

Joseph B: Transference—the total situation. Int J Psychoanal 66:447–454, 1985

Kernberg OF: Psychoanalysis, psychoanalytic psychotherapy and supportive psychotherapy: contemporary controversies. Int J Psychoanal 80(Pt 6):1075–1091, 1999 10669960

Kernberg OF: Object relations theories and techniques, in Textbook of Psychoanalysis. Edited by Person ES, Cooper AM, Gabbard GO. Washington, DC, American Psychiatric Publishing, 2005, pp 201–216

Kernberg OF: Countertransference: recent developments and technical implications for the treatment of patients with severe personality disorders, in The Inseparable Nature of Love and Aggression: Clinical and Theoretical Perspectives. Washington, DC, American Psychiatric Publishing, 2012, pp 81–101

Kernberg OF: Psychoanalysis: Freud's theories and their contemporary development, in New Oxford Textbook of Psychiatry. Edited by Gelder MG, Andreasen NC, López-Ibor JJ Jr, et al. New York, Oxford University Press, 2009, pp 293–305

Kernberg OF: Divergent contemporary trends in psychoanalytic theory. Psychoanal Rev 98(5):633–664, 2011 22026541

Kernberg OF, Yeomans FE, Clarkin JF, et al: Transference focused psychotherapy: overview and update. Int J Psychoanal 89(3):601–620, 2008 18558958

Kris A: Free Association. New Haven, CT, Yale University Press, 1982

Kris A: Interpretation and the method of free association. Psychoanal Inq 12:208–224, 1992

Laplanche J, Pontalis J-B: The Language of Psychoanalysis. London, Karnac, 1988

Mertens W (ed): Handbuch Psychoanalytischer Grundbegriffe, 4th Edition. Stuttgart, Germany, Kohlhammer, 2014

Skelton RM, Burgoyne B, Grotstein J, et al (eds): The Edinburgh International Encyclopaedia of Psychoanalysis. Edinburgh, Scotland, Edinburgh University Press, 2006

Spillius EB, Milton J, Garvey P, et al: The New Dictionary of Kleinian Thought. New York, Routledge, 2011

Sterba R: The First Dictionary of Psychoanalysis. London, Karnac, 2013

Wöller W, Kruse J (eds): Tiefenpsychologisch fundierte Psychotherapie. Stuttgart, Germany, Schattauer, 2005

CHAPTER 5

Interpretation in Borderline Pathology

A Clinical Illustration

Interpretation is the basic technique of psychoanalysis. It is the main instrument with which to help the patient become aware of his or her unconscious conflicts. Interpretation is the verbal communication by the analyst of the hypothesis of an unconscious conflict that seems to have emerged in the patient's communication in the session.

Interpretation takes different forms depending on the personality organization of the patient. With neurotic patients, in whom the primary defensive operation is repression, interpretations involve bringing into consciousness originally unconscious, repressed content. With patients with borderline personality organization, interpretations focus on content that emerges in the patient's consciousness or preconscious awareness but remains separate from other, conflictually linked contents by means of splitting and/or denial, projective identification, primitive idealization, devaluation, and omnipotent control. Here interpretation reveals not previously unconscious contents, but the unconscious motivation that determines the fragmentation of conscious experience (Kernberg et al. 2008).

The following case material is from session five with a borderline patient in treatment with transference-focused psychotherapy. This material illustrates the interpretation of projective identification as part of the interpretation of a primitive object relationship activated in the transference, with rapid reversals of the projection of the correspondent self and object representations.

Background

The patient is a 25-year-old violinist who has been failing in her work commitments, drifting for the past 2 years, and involved in several sadomasochistic relations with men, and has had severe disruption of her entire social life because of her emotional instability, angry outbursts, and impulsive behavior. Her primary symptoms are chronic anxiety and depression.

She has two younger siblings. Her parents divorced when the patient was 11 years old, and her father never remarried. She has had an overly dependent and chronically conflictual relationship with her father and a distant relationship with her paternal grandmother, who took over major maternal functions after her mother left the home.

The Session

The verbatim transcript of the following segment evolved approximately 10 minutes after the start of the session. It is included here because of its relevance to what follows later in the session.

> PATIENT: Well, I was talking about my father.
> THERAPIST: Yes.
> PATIENT: Because I have to listen to him, and I don't like to.
> THERAPIST: Okay?
> PATIENT: I don't like to feel submissive. I don't like to feel . . . listening feels submissive sometimes. 'Cause he goes on and on, you know. So (*long pause*) . . . I'll probably put up some distance between he and I so I wouldn't have to listen. Or either I'd listen but I didn't really have to be there. I'm not sure . . . but . . . it's hard for me to listen (*chuckles*) when, um, a male starts talking.
> THERAPIST: Why? Because males are particularly prone to have you become submissive?
> PATIENT: Yes. Yes. Yes, yes, yes. Sure, I grew up as my father's wife. You know.
> THERAPIST: What do you mean?
> PATIENT: My mother left when I was 11. I was daddy's little helper. Even now, he tells me things that if she were home he would tell her. You know, that kind of stuff. So, I grew up, you know, wanting to

Interpretation in Borderline Pathology: A Clinical Illustration

please him. So, it's there, it's just there in the . . . and it does cause a lot of problems. And a lot of pain.

THERAPIST: What problems? Why is it painful?

PATIENT: 'Cause I shoot myself down. I don't talk about things and do things that make me happy, you know. I'm just conditioned this way. Makes me want to be like whatever boyfriends I have, makes me want to be like them, if I'm gonna have to listen to them anyway, I mean that's not the reason, but, it's just like that. That's just how I grew up.

THERAPIST: So, are you saying that because of that, with all your boyfriends you tend to be very submissive, is that what you're saying? Or resentful because you felt tempted to be submissive or they were trying to . . .

PATIENT: (*Interrupts*) Certainly, yes. Yes.

THERAPIST: Yeah, which?

PATIENT: All of it! I mean I felt . . .

THERAPIST: (*Interrupts*) You were tempted to be submissive, they were trying to exploit that, and before you knew it, you were in a mess being exploited by your boyfriends. Is that what you're saying?

PATIENT: Well, it feels like a mess. It may not appear to be a mess because most of my boyfriends have been quite faithful and loyal. They haven't been (*clears throat*) . . . otherwise . . . . But the mess I find myself in is I feel lost. I don't like it that I can't talk well today.

What follows is the verbatim transcription of the second half of this session. It illustrates the interpretation of the alternative projection of a superior acting object and a corresponding humiliated self onto the therapist.

THERAPIST: So perhaps when you left disappointed last session, you left not only disappointed, but . . .

PATIENT: It wasn't last session. It was the session before, wasn't it?

THERAPIST: Okay.

PATIENT: I think.

THERAPIST: (*Continues*) In any case, when you left that session, first you felt not only disappointed but also put down.

PATIENT: Yeah, but I was also grateful that you pointed that out. I was also glad to know.

THERAPIST: Well, I'm aware that you are divided in your view of me. I have a sense that in part of you, you trust that I'm being straight with you and that I mean what I say. But another part of you sees me as one more of that series of males who are trying to take over the brainwashing. And if I became important and you felt like trying to please me it would be very humiliating to think that you try to please somebody who is controlling you, criticizing you, manipulating you, putting you down, not a very nice perspective.

PATIENT: So, what am I gonna do? It's always been that way. I mean that's why I'm here.

THERAPIST: That's right, so this is an opportunity for exploring that reaction and what it's all about.

PATIENT: I'm trying to. Don't you agree? Do you agree with me that it has something to do with my father?

THERAPIST: (*Interjects*) Yes.

PATIENT: (*Continues*) And how I was raised.

THERAPIST: Yes, I would be surprised if it wasn't . . .

PATIENT: (*Interjects*) Okay.

THERAPIST: (*Continues*) It makes sense. What I'm trying to stress here is how powerful that part of you that sees apparently all relations with men as a replica of the relationship with your father. And makes you try to get away, when you feel again threatened with being taken over and humiliated.

PATIENT: You know, I think I'm experiencing some of that in my relationship with Antonio. Um . . . he has moved to the West Coast, you know . . .

THERAPIST: He has left already?

PATIENT: Oh yeah. He left on Monday. When he asked me how I feel talking to him on the phone, there's a part of me that's so apprehensive. There's a part of me that likes to talk to him, but I told him I said I'm still very apprehensive, but I don't think it has so much to do with, um, whether things are gonna work out or not. It seems that I just feel that talking to him . . . I'm scared, and I feel sort of revved up (*chuckles*), like an engine, you know, I feel . . .

THERAPIST: Scared about what?

PATIENT: I'm just, um, I'm real scared about his approval. I know that, I can sense that. Wanting . . . not getting it. Getting disapproval, criticism, and, um, I'm scared to feel my feelings for him. I'm scared to feel how I really feel, so I stay defensive, you know?

THERAPIST: And what would happen if you accept your feelings about him? What are you scared of? That you might miss him more than he misses you? That it might seem as a serious loss and you might get depressed over that?

PATIENT: (*Pause*) Yeah. Yeah, and my feelings and my mind would be focused on him too much. That's happened before with other boyfriends.

THERAPIST: Too much in the sense that you would be focused on somebody whom you know, there would be no future in the relationship. Is that it?

PATIENT: No, because that's not true.

THERAPIST: Well, didn't you tell me that he said you shouldn't waste your time with him? Didn't you?

PATIENT: He said that. . . . Yes, I did tell you that he said that. But, he said something else other times later. Later this week. So, my best judgment about the whole thing is the sounds of marriage and children scares him, certainly, but he seems to warm up to that whole idea and starts talking about the future in some sort of plan type way, even had a dream and I called right when he was having the dream or something the other night, about going ahead,

Interpretation in Borderline Pathology: A Clinical Illustration

and telling me that yes, he would give me a kid. And he felt good about it.
THERAPIST: That's the dream? (*Pause*) That's a dream?
PATIENT: (*Laughing*) Yup, that's the dream.
THERAPIST: So, are you saying that because he dreamt that it makes it more likely to happen?
PATIENT: You tell me what it means.
THERAPIST: I beg your pardon?
PATIENT: Well, you tell me what it means.
THERAPIST: What the dream means? Well, it sounds to me from your attitude that at least the content of the dream reflects a wish of yours.
PATIENT: Yup, and maybe his.
THERAPIST: That's not clear to me.
PATIENT: He had the dream.
THERAPIST: Oh, I'm sorry, I misunderstood that. I thought you had the dream.
PATIENT: Ahhhhhhh!!! (*claps*)
THERAPIST: I misunderstood.
PATIENT: Good, so I'll stay suspicious of you because you still didn't understand. (*Chuckling*). I'm just kidding. I'm teasing. You misunderstood me, see! Why should I trust you? Why should I . . . you don't understand me anyway. I can spell it out, and you still don't get it. That's the way men are. That's the way my dad is. I can spell it out, write it in French, German, English, or Spanish . . . . Does he get it? Does he understand me? The nature of me? No. Why should I? How many diffe— I could go to 20 years of therapy, and learn how to express myself 20 different ways. I could wear 20 different outfits. Would he still understand me? No. Why not? 'Cause he has his thing about women. So, what am I to do?
THERAPIST: Because he has what?
PATIENT: A thing about women.
THERAPIST: What thing?
PATIENT: Women are either this or this. Who knows what his thing is. This is my father you know, not Antonio.
THERAPIST: I understand. You looked very happy when I said I had misunderstood.
PATIENT: 'Cause I'm right.
THERAPIST: Yes.
PATIENT: (*Laughing*) 'Cause I was right. Is it me? Is it me because I don't explain it well? Is it normal just because people don't understand each other the first time sometimes? Yes. I will let it slide, you know. I'll get over this and get back to my point, but . . . I do get upset about it. I have intense reactions about not being understood. I get mad like that. (*Snaps fingers*) (*Sighs*) Antonio had the dream. Two nights ago. I picked up the phone to call him, um, because he had tried to call a couple of nights before, and while I called he was having this dream and he wouldn't tell me about it. Anyway, I just sensed that, um, I can't…I'm having a hard time how I feel. I'm

having a hard time feeling how I feel about it. And it's . . . What do you want to say?

THERAPIST: I'm still mulling over your feeling happy because you were right and I was wrong. Um, it puts you in a position of superiority . . .

PATIENT: Ahh, yes!

THERAPIST: Right?

PATIENT: Yes.

THERAPIST: Well, I wonder whether you feel that if I'm right in what I'm saying. I may feel happy about it and feel superior to you, and one more reason to feel the danger here of being humiliated. So . . .

PATIENT: (*Interjects*) I can't follow you.

THERAPIST: (*Continues*) Do you follow me?

PATIENT: No, I have a hard time . . .

THERAPIST: Have a hard time following me?

PATIENT: I know what you're saying but I can't quite . . .

THERAPIST: Well, it creates a problem for you. If I'm right in what I'm telling you, you may perceive me as reacting the same way you do, feeling superior because I'm right, so I'm on top and you are down, and that's humiliating for you. If I'm wrong, you feel fine, you are on top, but by the same token there's nothing to be expected from me. So, you can't win.

PATIENT: I can't win?

THERAPIST: That's right.

PATIENT: Why can't I win because I can't expect anything?

THERAPIST: You can't win because if I'm right you feel humiliated. And if I'm wrong you feel disappointed. Do you follow me?

PATIENT: If you're wrong, I feel disappointed because you're my therapist and you're no good.

THERAPIST: Right. And if I'm right you feel humiliated because I know better than you and you feel put down.

PATIENT: Yeah, that one's very vague. The other one is the one that's more active.

THERAPIST: Yes.

PATIENT: I mean I know what you're saying . . .

THERAPIST: Okay, well, let's stop here.

The patient first experienced me as one more edition of her dominant father, resenting that she was expected to be submissive to me. I then misinterpreted her statement about the dream, which immediately triggered her sense of superiority over such a stupid man. The roles of a superior, dominant object and a humiliated self switched in the transference, and the patient felt disappointed with this incompetent therapist. I interpreted this role reversal and its implications for our relationship, and the patient immediately understood this interpretation.

Reference

Kernberg OF, Yeomans FE, Clarkin JF, et al: Transference focused psychotherapy: overview and update. Int J Psychoanal 89(3):601–620, 2008 18558958

Further Reading

Akhtar S: Comprehensive Dictionary of Psychoanalysis. London, Karnac, 2009
Auchincloss EL, Samberg E: Psychoanalytic Terms and Concepts. New Haven, CT, Yale University Press, 2012
Bion WR: Learning from experience, in Seven Servants: Four Works by Wilfred R. Bion. New York, Jason Aronson, 1977, p 73
de Mijolla A: Dictionnaire International de la Psychanalyse. Paris, Calmann-Lévy, 2002
Etchegoyen RH: Los Fundamentos de la Técnica Psicoanalítica. Buenos Aires, Argentina, Amorrortu, 1986
Hinshelwood RD: A Dictionary of Kleinian Thought. London, Free Association Books, 1991
Kernberg OF: Divergent contemporary trends in psychoanalytic theory. Psychoanal Rev 98(5):633–664, 2011 22026541
Laplanche J, Pontalis J-B: The Language of Psychoanalysis. London, Karnac, 1988
Mertens W (ed): Handbuch Psychoanalytischer Grundbegriffe, 4th Edition. Stuttgart, Germany, Kohlhammer, 2014
Skelton RM, Burgoyne B, Grotstein J, et al (eds): The Edinburgh International Encyclopaedia of Psychoanalysis. Edinburgh, Scotland, Edinburgh University Press, 2006
Spillius EB, Milton J, Garvey P, et al: The New Dictionary of Kleinian Thought. New York, Routledge, 2011
Sterba R: The First Dictionary of Psychoanalysis. London, Karnac, 2013

CHAPTER 6

The Spectrum of Psychoanalytic Techniques

In Chapter 4 of this book, "The Basic Components of Psychoanalytic Technique and Derivative Psychoanalytic Psychotherapies," I defined four basic aspects of psychoanalytic technique as the fundament for both standard psychoanalysis and derived psychoanalytic psychotherapies. These four basic components of psychoanalytic technique were *interpretation, transference analysis, technical neutrality,* and *countertransference utilization.*

I shall attempt to define and describe a full complement of psychoanalytic techniques that may be considered specific applications of the combined use of these four basic components of technique. The definitions that follow should facilitate the empirical assessment of their respective use in particular treatments, thus constituting a basic manualization of psychoanalytic modalities of treatment, geared both to clinical utilization and research endeavors. These descriptions are addressed to readers with practical experience in carrying out psychoanalytic psychotherapies as well as standard psychoanalysis. Thus, it is hoped that it is sufficiently clear without having to be illustrated by clinical vignettes. The risk is that these definitions may at first appear to be too schematized or abstract. However, the effort of a comprehensive enumeration of psychoanalytic techniques, including their mutual relationships, should facilitate the clarification of each of them. In each case, I shall attempt to define these techniques in their use as part of standard psychoanalytic treatment and then refer to their potential modifications in derived psychoanalytic psychotherapies.

Given the unfortunate fact that we do not have a universally recognized and agreed-upon dictionary of all psychoanalytic techniques or an integrated text of psychoanalytic technique that would be recognized by the different psychoanalytic schools, I have attempted to provide basic definitions that reflect common contemporary views of the respective concept by different psychoanalytic approaches, while spelling out significant differences in their conceptualization and utilization by alternative psychoanalytic models if such differentiations apply. Leading contemporary psychoanalytic dictionaries have provided the background for these definitions (Akhtar 2009; Auchincloss and Samberg 2012; de Mijolla 2002; Etchegoyen 1986; Hinshelwood 1991; Laplanche and Pontalis 1988; Mertens 2014; Skelton et al. 2006; Spillius et al. 2011).

Psychoanalytic technique is based on the availability of a psychotherapeutic relationship that involves work, including a particular attitude, on the part of both analyst and patient. On the part of the analyst, analytic listening involving "evenly suspended attention," and an implicit simultaneity of alertness to the content of the patient's free associations, verbal and nonverbal behavior, external reality, countertransference activation, and the implicit use of a particular theoretical view that is expressed in the intuitive application of knowledge and experience. On the part of the patient, the expectation or hope is that the patient will be able and willing to carry out free association and in the process express both emerging thoughts and emotional experiences activated in his or her mind, along with impediments, distortions, and difficulties emerging in the effort to free associate.

During this working situation, the analyst's focus (i.e., paying attention to what is affectively dominant in their interaction) will lead to specific areas that call for the application of features of psychoanalytic technique. These developments include the emergence of dominant defenses that frequently will present as transference resistances, repetitive characterological defenses that will lead to character analysis, the exploration of dreams, repetition compulsion, and a spectrum of transformations of emotional experiences into somatization or acting out. Acting out, in turn, will have to be differentiated from emotional enactment in the session, and the analytic work involved in an interpretive approach will lead to transformation or insight, resolution of repetition compulsion, or what we know as *working through*. Complications such as negative therapeutic reaction, treatment disruptions, and termination may require additional technical interventions. This list of the particular areas that will stimulate the focus of an interpretive approach also suggests the specific applications of the four basic components of general psychoanalytic technique, as we shall now examine in detail.

It should be emphasized that *affective dominance* emerges as the most important feature orienting the clinician to the simultaneous activation of the many aspects of the analyst–patient interaction. Affective dominance is referred to by different terms within different theoretical orientations but appears again and again as the point of departure of the analyst's orienting attention to the material of the session. What is affectively dominant may be derived from the patient's verbal or nonverbal communication, in one's countertransference, in a particular aspect of the analytic field, or in a blocking or an intrusive or bizarre perception, but it is where emotion seems to be concentrated at the moment.

Character Analysis

Character analysis refers to the exploration of the patient's dynamic organization as exhibited by his or her habitual behavior patterns, idiosyncratic reactive or inhibitory traits, and chaotic or fragmented repertoire of character traits. This approach practically coincides with the analysis of the patient's dominant defensive mechanisms and his or her mutual reinforcements (Kernberg 1993). In patients with neurotic personality organization, the "classic" cases for psychoanalytic treatment, defense mechanisms tend to emerge as blockings or distortions of free association. In fact, this is how the ego's mechanisms of defense were discovered and described. The analysis of defensive operations, their manifestations, their motivation, and the unconscious impulses against which they are directed may appear as specific contents of the analytic situation.

Defense analysis coincides with what used to be called *resistance analysis*—that is, the analysis of clinical manifestations of defense operations. Psychoanalytic technique has evolved to consider "resistances" not as forces to be overcome, but as defensive operations to be understood for their unconscious meanings, motivations, and functions (Busch 1996). Such exploration constitutes a central aspect of interpretive interventions. From the perspective of contemporary object relations theory, these defensive operations may be translated into unconscious, defensively activated object relations (dyadic self and object representations) in the transference, which are directed against opposite, and unconscious, impulsively dominated dyadic units of self and other representations. These defensive and impulsive object relations jointly represent the activation of the presently dominant unconscious conflict (Kernberg 2004).

In the case of severe personality disorders in which identity diffusion and predominance of primitive defensive operations center around splitting rather than repression, these defensive operations may become so dominant that they practically characterize patients' habitual behavior patterns and, in their overall mutual combinations, coincide with a primitive, severe character pathology. The analysis of these primitive defensive operations, particularly of paranoid-schizoid and depressive defenses, becomes part of the analysis of the patient's defensive character structure, and what may be called "character defenses" rapidly show as transference resistances. In the case of patients with neurotic personality organization, the fact that the prevalent constellation of higher levels of defensive operations also serves general defensive character patterns usually emerges only more gradually in the treatment. However, in the long run, the systematic analysis of ego defenses also comes to coincide with a systematic analysis of predominant characterological defenses.

The main point of this brief review is to stress that as a practical matter, defense analysis will become concentrated in the analysis of characterological defenses and thus the analysis of the patient's pathological character structure. This raises the question of when and how such predominant characterological patterns need to be explored. A contemporary consensus indicates that the analysis of the patient's habitual behavior as it acquires defensive functions in the treatment situation is indicated whenever it becomes *affectively dominant*. In some patients with severe character pathology, this may appear in the first session so that the treatment will start with analysis of a patient's characterological structure. In fact, this frequently is the case with severe narcissistic character pathology. In less severe cases involving a circumscribed pathology with specific symptoms relating to oedipal or preoedipal conflicts, these conflicts may dominate the transference situation without being reflected in a dominant character pathology. However, whenever defensive character traits are affectively dominant in the treatment situation, there is an indication for an interpretive approach.

The essential technique of character analysis has been well articulated by Wilhelm Reich (1933). However, given the idiosyncratic complications of Reich's personality and professional behavior, the term *character analysis* fell into some disrepute, and his early contributions have not been fully acknowledged. In contemporary psychoanalytic technique, the approach to character analysis may be summarized briefly as follows: 1) draw the patient's attention to a particular, predominant behavior that becomes central in one or several sessions; 2) raise the patient's interest in that particular behavior and ask him or her to associate regarding the implications of that behavior; 3) interpret the immediate transferential implications of the activation of that particular behavior; and 4) gradually interpret the defended-against, feared and/or desired relation under the impact of the respective aggressive or libidinal impulse that is being defended against.

Systematic analysis of the transference typically, and dominantly, involves character analysis. Its effect, under optimal circumstances, should bring about significant changes in the patient's experiences and/or behavior in his or her external life as well as in the analytic situation. In the case of patients with severe character pathology and identity diffusion, the predominance of primitive defenses centered on splitting mechanisms translates into severe dissociation between idealized and persecutory transference developments, and their analysis fosters characterological integration, progressing from a predominance of paranoid-schizoid to depressive transferences in advanced stages of the treatment.

Transference-focused psychotherapy (TFP), indicated for patients with borderline personality organization and the corresponding severe, primitive constellations of personality disorders, involves carrying out characterological analysis in the context of a severe potential for acting out of primitive defensive operations and corresponding object relationships in the sessions and in the patient's external life. It requires particular attention to the maintenance of the therapeutic frame, with temporary abandonment of technical neutrality, and the development of specific techniques to both limit acting out and restore technical neutrality (Yeomans et al. 2015). In these cases, the therapist's stress on immediate and external reality as a starting point of an interpretive approach is the counterpart to the limitations of free association as an ongoing work commitment on the part of the patient.

Characterological defenses may include defensive operations that not only reflect ego efforts to maintain characterological "armament" but also may reflect superego defenses and the enactment of profound guilt feelings, as well as the entire characterological structure of obsessive-compulsive, hysterical, masochistic, and narcissistic pathology.

In the application of TFP with neurotic personality organization, character analysis may be limited to a particular segment of the patient's habitual behavior and linked to the specific area of conflicts regarding which the patient entered into treatment. Here transference analysis is limited to the specific transference reflections of the dominant unconscious conflicts related to the patient's symptomatology in addition to the ever-relevant indication to analyze manifest negative transference in order to preserve a "workable therapeutic relationship."

This may be the point to refer to the problematic concept of the *therapeutic alliance*. This term refers to the alliance of the nonconflictual, "normal" part of the patient's ego with the work-related aspects of the psychoanalyst's interventions. There exists, undoubtedly, such a potential for collaborative work in patients with a well-integrated neurotic personality organization, signaling the patient's capacity to collaborate in the analytic work and to maintain a certain objectivity at points of activation of significant negative transference developments. That potential, which reflects in a deeper sense the availability of a secure positive transference disposition, should not, however, be artificially stimulated by the therapist's seductive behavior as that would counteract the nature of analytic work. In supportive psychotherapy, the effort to appeal to and strengthen the patient's wishes to be helped and his or her capacity for trusting the therapist may be part of the supportive repertoire, but it is not an aspect of psychoanalytic technique proper. In the case of severe personality disorders, the therapeutic alliance may be absent for extended periods of the treatment, and the patient's capacity to collaborate in the treatment situation depends on the systematic analysis and working through of the predominately negative transference.

Dream Analysis

Although dream analysis is no longer considered the exclusive "royal road to the unconscious," it continues to be an important source of information about unconscious processes and represents a focus of interpretation. Dream analysis also has acquired additional importance in the present time as renewed attention to the consistent psychic activity of daydreaming has gained attention under the heading of "waking dreaming" in Bion's formulation (Civitarese 2014; Ferro 2009). The neo-Bionian approach tends to treat free associations as equivalent to the manifest content of dreams—that is, it attempts to transform even patients' talking about aspects of their daily reality as if those aspects represented symbols of unconscious psychological processing. This development has led to a renewed emphasis on the value of dream analysis.

In its classical technical approach, dream analysis deals with the manifest content of dreams as surface material to be divided into meaningful partial segments, inviting the patient to associate to these segments of the dream with the expectation that latent content of each of these segments of the manifest dream would emerge. The interpretive integration of the latent meanings of the manifest segments, explored by means of the patient's free association and the analyst's corresponding "reverie," then would lead to the deeper unconscious meanings of the dream.

This general approach to the technique of dream analysis assumes that the manifest content of dreams is the product of unconscious elaboration, by means of "dream work," of the original, primarily wishful feeling fantasy expressed in dreams. The elaboration of unconscious dream thoughts involves exploring them as reflecting primary process thinking: logic that ignores the principle of contradiction, collapses time and space, tends to represent ideas visually, and uses condensation and displacement as the dream thoughts are undergoing secondary elaboration by the dream censorship, usually leading to a more rational or representational manifest dream narrative. Dream analysis, therefore, involves deconstructing the manifest content while considering all these distorting elaborations and considers the impact of day residue previous to the dream that may have stimulated unconscious infantile wishes. At the same time, it expresses these wishes in the context of the dominant transference situation. Contemporary stress on the stylistic and communicative aspects of dream narratives and Fairbairn's (1952) proposals that self and object representations may emerge in split forms and through multiple characters of the dream content add further complexity as well as informative value to dream analysis. Dream contents and other characteristics of dreams may point to specific meanings, such as in anxiety dreams reflecting the incapacity to control threatening unconscious impulses fully, examination dreams, dreams that provide gratification of immediate physiological needs frustrated in reality, and so on.

Important questions involve when and how dreams should be interpreted, to what extent they always or at times reflect an affectively dominant issue, to what extent dream analysis needs to be integrated in the analysis of the presently predominant transference, and so on. Chronically repetitive dreams very often deal with various aspects of an essential conflict of the patient and deserve particular attention, because their modifications in the course of treatment may reflect the transference modifications and elaboration of the corresponding conflict. In general, dreams should be interpreted when they seem affectively dominant in the sessions rather than systematically explored whenever they emerge. Dreams have a seductive quality, and their narrative may serve defensive purposes. Very confused dreams may, in fact, be closer to the possibility of their analytic understanding because they reflect a reduced secondary elaboration, whereas some very clear dreams with ordinarily unconscious content erroneously may convey the impression that repressions have been lifted. Undoubtedly, there also are good dreams, in which a significant conflict is being elaborated in an emotionally meaningful way, profoundly influencing the wake life of the dreamer.

Dream analysis depends on the patient's capacity to carry out free association and optimally is carried out in the context of standard psychoanalysis. In psychoanalytic psychotherapies, dream analysis also requires the patient's capacity for free association. In TFP with individuals with severe personality disorders, dreams in the early stages of the treatment tend to be explored in terms of their manifest content, linking the meanings of the manifest content to the presently predominant transference. In the middle stages of TFP treatment, partial analysis of the latent content of dreams may be attempted, and in advanced stages, full-fledged dream analysis may be carried out (Yeomans et al. 2015). Dream analysis is usually contraindicated in supportive psychotherapy, except in the utilization of manifest content in terms of the elaboration of the conscious conflict that is explored at that point.

It is rarely possible to elaborate and analyze fully a complex dream within one session. Sometimes the analysis might stretch over several sessions, because other issues may become affectively dominant during that time. Some patients use dream narratives to escape from a realistic examination of their lives. Narcissistic patients may eagerly "interpret" their own dreams in terms of their assumed knowledge and understanding of the meaning of particular contents, and the effect of such self-analysis in the countertransference reaction of the analyst is usually one of empty speculation.

An essential attitude of the patient that may indicate his or her capacity to participate in the analysis of dreams is an authentic curiosity about the unknown that may emerge in the patient's mind, in clear contrast to his or her competitive intellectualizing attitudes regarding dream analysis, or transference-related devaluation of dream contents.

Acting Out, Enactment, Repetition Compulsion, Working Through

ACTING OUT

In a strict sense, *acting out* refers to the behavioral expression of an unconscious conflict bypassing an emotional awareness of a conflict. A general tendency to expand the meaning of the concept to "bad" behavior does injustice to the technical implications of this concept, which requires transformation of the behavior into an emotional awareness of the corresponding conflict against which the patient is defending (Sandler et al. 1973).

Acting out may occur outside the sessions as well as in the session itself. Sometimes it takes unusual, subtle forms such as distortions in free association that lead to the use of language as action, which are intended to influence the analyst rather than to communicate emotional experience. *Accretion,* a super-condensation of meanings expressed in a brief, almost casual comment that tends to deny the emotional implications of the subject matter that has been evolving gradually in the patient's mind, is one such form of "mini-acting out." It may come to the analysts' awareness only by a sudden disruption of his or her understanding or a sudden loss of attention to what is going on in the session.

In severe personality disorders, such transformation of language into action, geared to control the therapeutic situation and directed against the possibility of cognitive communication with the therapist, may become a prevalent way of expressing transference developments, and the interpretation of this form of acting out practically coincides with systematic working through of transference resistances. In healthier patients with neurotic personality organization, acting out usually emerges more gradually, outside the analytic sessions, and reveals its affective dominance in the sessions by the analyst's careful attention to the "total transference" (Joseph 1985)—that is, the analyst's alertness to the expression of the dominant transference disposition in the session and simultaneously in the patient's external reality. Whereas attention to the transference in the patient's total emotional experience may alert the analyst to the subtler aspects of acting out, the obvious nature of persistent forms of emotionally charged behavior or acute crises in the patient's life situation usually becomes quite evident as an affectively dominant content of the sessions. Such material takes the highest priority for interpretive interventions.

There are, however, severe cases in which the nature of splitting operations is so effective that subtle but chronic forms of acting out, seriously affecting the patient's life in the long run, may remain undetected for a dangerously long time unless the therapist remains specifically alert to that potential in individual cases. Careful exploration of the patient's total life situation at the beginning of the treatment, and the alertness to his or her potential for the activation of severe, self-destructive acting out, may provide an important preventive therapeutic function (Kernberg 2016).

Long-standing experience has taught us that acting out is always intrinsically linked to the transference, even when it is expressed in behavior patterns that predate the treatment. The analyst's alertness to this new and now dominant function of "a long history" of acting out becomes an important requirement in the treatment of severe personality disorders.

Standard psychoanalytic technique does not require any technical modifications to deal with severe acting out potential and relies upon the systematic analysis of the unconscious meaning of acting out in the context of transference analysis from a position of technical neutrality. The activation of specific countertransference reactions to acting out—with the important implication of the patient's effort to unconsciously recreate a primitive object relationship or a particular defense against such a threatening object relationship—may provide important clues to the psychoanalytic understanding of the meanings expressed in this acting-out development. It may be utilized as part of the interpretive working through of acting out, its transformation into emotional experience to be explored during the sessions. In general, André Green's (1993) recommendation to systematically pay attention to acting out and to somatization as two major channels of defensive avoidance of emotional awareness of unconscious conflicts in the sessions becomes relevant. He recommends consistent work on transformation of acting out and somatization into emotional experience that enriches the available expression of the dominant transference and permits its exploration and working through.

In the case of borderline personality organization with indication for TFP, the prevalence of acting out that threatens the treatment or well-being of the patient requires certain steps before treatment can begin. First, a careful assessment of the total present life situation of the patient will expose potential activities such as suicidal behavior, severe violence, and antisocial behavior. Once potential threats have been identified, based on the patient's history, a discussion is indicated to agree on how these behaviors and impulses will be managed so that the treatment may proceed with a minimum of disruption. A "contract" will be negotiated (verbally) as to limits and responsibility for safety that the patient accepts. Lastly, the transference implications of the patient's reactions to the contract setting and restrictions of dangerous behavior must be interpreted from the beginning of treatment. The therapist should be prepared to explicitly grant the patient a second chance after breaking a contractual commitment, and such occurrence should be used to interpret the meaning of the patient's behavior as representing a destructive part of him or her that is perhaps triumphing over the therapist and risking continuation in the treatment (Yeomans et al. 2015).

Severe acting out may require the abandonment of technical neutrality, but in our experience the combination of limit setting and systematic interpretation of the necessity for such limits, the transference implication of the therapist's being pulled out of role, and the extent to which this situation reflects deeper transference dispositions constitutes an important technical modification of TFP that has permitted the expansion of this psychoanalytic psychotherapy to a broad segment of severe personality disorders.

Direct control of severe acting out in supportive psychotherapy requires the use of supportive techniques, such as the provision of information and advice giving and the use of external support, to facilitate and reinforce adaptive, protective behavior patterns that counteract the temptation and risk for the corresponding acting-out behavior (Rockland 1989). The exploration of the gratification derived from acting out and of the price paid for it, together with the suggestion of alternative ways to compensate for the loss of this gratification, constitutes important aspects of a supportive psychotherapeutic technique that is an alternative to the possibility of an analytic approach.

ENACTMENT

Enactment is a relatively recent enrichment of psychoanalytic technique highlighting that the activation of a certain transference disposition in the session and of its correspondent countertransference disposition in the analyst contributes to the development of a temporal modification of the analytic relationship under the effect of that specific transference/countertransference bind (Chused 1991). It is the "emotional enactment" of the unconscious conflict in the transference situation that powerfully influences the analyst's countertransference, often reinforced by what Joseph Sandler called the "role responsiveness" of the analyst, who may be particularly responsive to a particular transference activation (Sandler et al. 1973). For relational school analysts, it provides evidence for their important theoretical assumption that transference not only reflects the unconscious dispositions of the patient but also serves, in part, as a response to the countertransference dispositions of the analyst (Mitchell and Aron 1999).

In more general terms, the implication is that the countertransference influences the transference so that transference and countertransference constitute an interactional dyad that, naturally, is predominantly determined by the patient's transference. It leads, however, to a new experience of the patient determined not only by the analyst's interpretive attitude in the context of technical neutrality, but by the analyst's response to the transference, with his or her personality dispositions, and thus contributes potentially to a new therapeutic life experience in the context of transference development.

Within the Kleinian approach, enactment is conceptualized as the consequence of the activation of projective identification—an important primitive mechanism that tends to induce specific reactions in the analyst, which is unconsciously intended by the patient—that reflects the activation of a specific primitive object relationship of the patient (Spillius et al. 2011). Realistic features that the patient observes in the analyst's behavior facilitate the focus and the rationalization of projective identification, and the intensity of the corresponding countertransference reaction permits the analyst to experience by concordant or complementary identification in the countertransference the total transference activated in the psychoanalytic situation.

Enactment differs from acting out in that it is a very direct, intense expression of the dominant transference development, in contrast to the primarily defensive function against transference awareness in the case of acting out. Enactment in the analytic situation allows and facilitates transference interpretation and is practically a privileged aspect of systematic transference analysis, with the contribution of the self-analytic function of the analyst exploring his or her countertransference disposition at that point. Betty Joseph (1992) stressed the importance of the analyst's internal musing as to what the patient might be trying to achieve with his or her particular way of attempting to influence the analyst. Enactments allow a sharp focus on this issue.

For relational analysts, enactments may reflect a dissociated self state that needs to be integrated interpretively with the patient's dominant self experience. As mentioned previously, this interpretive process, influenced by the analyst's unconscious contribution to the transference/countertransference bind, contributes to a new object relation as an important therapeutic aspect of psychoanalytic treatment.

REPETITION COMPULSION

Repetition compulsion refers to the unconscious tendency to repeat past conflictual, particularly traumatic, painful experiences regardless of the pleasure principle, but it is also an effort to obtain general satisfaction of particular libidinal or aggressive needs. The compulsive nature of these behaviors is evident in their unremitting persistence despite analytic elaboration (Freud 1920/1955). It used to be described as a defense of the id, rather than a superego or ego defense. In fact, in the light of contemporary psychoanalytic experience, repetition compulsion appears to be linked more typically with significant activation of internal object relationships and the effort to repeat and overcome the unconscious conflicts linked to them.

In the case of severe traumatic experiences, repetition compulsion may involve an unconscious effort to gradually work through traumatic situations, and, in effect, a patient's working through of these repetitive experiences in the transference gradually may lead to their resolution. Very often, however, there are other important meanings expressed in repetition compulsion that must be considered in the correspondent interpretive approach. A frequent dynamic involves the unconscious reactivation of the relationship with a persecutory object of the past that is projected onto the therapist with the secret hope of turning a bad object into a good one despite one's consistent effort to destroy or undermine the present transferential relationship. Some sadomasochistic transferences evince such repetition compulsion as reactivation of past experienced traumatization or repeated sadistic assault and may reflect a combination of the projection onto the analyst of the sadistic object and, at the same time, an unconscious identification with that object in an effort to reverse the past relationship and transform the other into the victim. The unconscious envy of the analyst's not being controlled by such internal hostile forces as the patient is experiencing may be an important related dynamic, particularly in patients with narcissistic personality disorders.

The technical approach to repetition compulsion in standard psychoanalytic treatment is the ongoing reexamination of the behavior, exploring it as a pathological character pattern that reflects an internal pathological object relationship in terms of its different functions under different circumstances and within different moments of transference activation. Under optimal circumstances, such working through permits the resolution of repetition compulsion in consonance with the resolution of pathological character defenses expressed as transference resistances.

In the treatment of severely regressed patients with borderline personality organization by means of TFP, in some cases the impossibility of resolving repetition compulsion with the interpretive approach described may require the exploration of secondary gain possibly obtained by means of the repetition compulsion. Under such circumstances, limit setting to reduce the secondary gain may be indicated, followed by the analysis of the transference implications that necessitated the analyst to deviate from technical neutrality.

In supportive psychotherapeutic technique, the endless repetition of pathological behavior patterns requires a combination of informative and supportive induction of alternative or compensating behavior with adaptive function that reduces the pressure for carrying out the pathological repetitive behavior. A worst-case scenario is provided by patients in whom the repetition compulsion involving severe self-destructive, self-harming, and potentially life-threatening behavior expresses a narcissistic fantasy of being beyond the fear of pain or death, and in whom suicide may reflect an ultimate expression of the patient's omnipotence. Such developments may correspond to the most severe type of negative therapeutic reaction referred to later in this chapter.

WORKING THROUGH

Working through is an essential therapeutic process that implies joint work of analyst and patient on the activation and resolution of unconscious conflicts, particularly in the elaboration of intense transference resistances derived from the activation of pathological character patterns in the treatment situation. Working through acquires particular importance under conditions of repetition compulsion. Working through, under optimal conditions, also relates to the general work of mourning and refers to the elaboration of the depressive position, the patient's gradual capacity to resolve the dominance of primitive defensive operations centering around splitting and projective identification. It includes the development of the patient's capacity for self-observation and insight, conflict tolerance and elaboration of disillusionment about self and others, the gradual desensitization regarding potentially traumatic experiences and memories, and the assumption of autonomous growth. Working through implies, above all, the development of the capacity for insight—that is, the combination of cognitive and emotional understanding of unconscious conflict, concern over the effects of that conflict on the patient's life and the lives of others, the tolerance of guilt feelings and the strengthening of a sense of personal responsibility, and the wish to overcome the respective limitation to one's optimal functioning. Working through involves, in essence, a gradual resolution of transference regression as well as the regressive features of the patient's relationship to self and others in the present and in the reconstruction of his or her past.

Negative Therapeutic Reaction

Negative therapeutic reaction refers to the paradoxical reactions of patients in psychoanalysis and psychoanalytic psychotherapy expressed by worsening of the symptomatology or destructive transference regressions after becoming aware of the helpfulness of the analyst. Patients get worse after clearly having experienced something good coming their way. It typically involves any one of three potential developments in the psychoanalytic situation. First, it may be the expression of unconscious guilt; second, it may be the expression of unconscious envy of the analyst; and third, it may represent an unconscious identification within a primitive sadomasochistic relationship (see Chapter 9 of this book, "An Overview of the Treatment of Severe Narcissistic Pathology").

The first case, negative therapeutic reaction as an expression of unconscious guilt, frequently can be observed in cases of depressive-masochistic personality as an expression of profound guilt over being helped by the analyst. The patient harbors the unconscious conviction that he or she does not deserve to be helped or that to be helped implies an implicit injustice carried out regarding a third person, or regarding others who would be more deserving of such help. Unconsciously, the patient may fear that the analyst is not aware of the depth of the patient's unworthiness or the severity of the patient's unacknowledged aggression. The unconscious fear of the loss of the dependence on the analyst if the patient were to improve sometimes may be involved. Unconscious guilt over the good relationship with the analyst experienced as a forbidden oedipal triumph is another dynamic one may observe in this development.

The second possibility, negative therapeutic reaction from unconscious envy of the analyst, is a typical development in the psychoanalytic treatment of narcissistic pathology. Here, negative therapeutic reaction expresses the need to deny any dependency on the analyst and an effort to avoid the experienced inferiorization and humiliation perceived as part of the analyst's "triumphant" capability to help the patient. In a deep sense, the patient's unconscious envious reaction also expresses the intolerable experience of acknowledging the creativity of the analyst, who has been able to continue helping the patient despite the patient's resistances and negativity. This dynamic unconscious envy is by far the most frequent form of negative therapeutic reaction and replicates narcissistic patients' difficulties to learn from others as a major cause of their difficulty in learning and progression in work and studies.

The third type of negative therapeutic reaction is relatively rare. It is experienced by patients who have had a chronic, severely sadomasochistic relationship with a parental object and chronically traumatized patients who have developed the conviction that the only way in which a needed object expresses his or her interest in them is by sadistic attacks or mistreatment. The analyst's interest in the patient cannot be trusted unless it is motivated by rage or resentment. The conviction that only somebody who hates the patient is really interested in him or her tends to evolve hand in hand with severe self-destructiveness as well as a tendency to attack the analyst or therapist with chronic dangerous acting out. These usually are patients for whom psychoanalytic treatment proper is contraindicated but who may respond to TFP if strict control and limitation of self-destructive behavior, and at times careful supervision of the patient's life outside the sessions, become part of the conditions under which psychotherapy is undertaken. Here, the need to establish strict parameters around the treatment and abandonment of technical neutrality required by the need to protect the continuation of the treatment and the patient's life may color the essential nature of the transference. Consistent interpretation of the patient's needs to have the analyst control his or her life as a condition for survival, as well as a confirmation of the patient's fantasy of the therapist's sadism, needs to be carried out again and again as varying circumstances reactivate this transference in ever new forms.

The technical approach to negative therapeutic reaction consists in the interpretation of the respective underlying dynamic and, in the most severe type of negative therapeutic reaction, in the establishment of conditions and control that protect the stability of the treatment. Negative therapeutic reaction out of unconscious guilt is the easiest to detect and resolve analytically. Negative therapeutic reaction reflecting unconscious envy usually requires long-term working through and, in the analyst's countertransference, the tolerance of negative countertransference reactions within which the analyst may experience a sense of revengeful superiority over the patient who envies the life and capability of his or her therapist.

Somatization

Somatization is a broad spectrum of manifestations of physical symptoms related to psychological conflicts. It is important to differentiate the organic manifestations of illnesses that may present a psychological component as part of their etiology, the so-called psychosomatic disorders, from the direct physical manifestations of psychological conflict that emerge in the psychoanalytic situation under conditions of the activation of these conflicts. These latter physical manifestations of psychological conflicts, which may be properly called somatization in the narrower context of transformation of psychological conflict into somatic expression, include 1) the physical manifestations of anxiety and depression; 2) the symbolic expression of psychic conflict in the form of physical symptoms—that is, the broad spectrum of conversion reactions; and 3) the generalized hyperalertness and concern over physical illness in the syndrome of hypochondriasis. I am referring to hypochondriasis as a stable psychiatric syndrome, in contrast to the occasional hypochondriacal manifestations that are part of what are clearly manifestations of anxiety.

These physical manifestations of anxiety and depression, conversion symptoms, and hypochondriacal concern need to be interpreted in the context of the affectively dominant material that is the interpretive focus in the sessions. They need to be interpreted as part of the defensive and impulsive manifestations of the internalized object relations activated in the transference and are of particular importance in combination with the focus on acting out as combined efforts to avoid the emotional awareness of psychological conflict in the session. Physical symptoms as manifestation of anxiety and depression are most easily identified as part of the patient's total emotional reaction. Conversion symptoms tend to become prominent in the activation of the corresponding conflicts in the transference and, of course, have more complex relations to the unconscious conflict dominant at any particular time.

Chronic hypochondriasis constitutes a relatively rare but extremely difficult and prognostically reserved form of severe personality disorder, usually within the spectrum of borderline personality organization. Hypochondriacal symptoms typically represent the projection of paranoid defenses against aggression onto the interior of the body. These "internal enemies" protect the patient against imaginary external ones. An unstable equilibrium is achieved by fear of illness and magical procedures to control it. Medical professionals who attempt to assure the patient become allies of the internal enemies. The analytic interpretation of hypochondriacal symptoms typically transforms hypochondriacal pathology into severe paranoid transferences, at times to the level of psychotic regression in the transference. In fact, if an interpretive approach to hypochondriasis is attempted, the analyst or therapist needs to be aware of the extent to which the patient will be able to tolerate an analytic approach without a psychotic regression, which quite frequently may require a shift in the treatment approach to a supportive psychotherapeutic modality.

The Psychoanalytic Field

The "psychoanalytic field" is a relatively new addition to the repertoire of technical psychoanalytic concepts. It stems from the original contribution of Baranger and Baranger (1969) about "bastions," unconsciously conflictual areas that by unconscious mutual collusion of patient and analyst are excluded from analytic exploration in the sessions. This contribution signaled the importance of exploring the intersubjective processes in the treatment situation occurring in parallel and split off from other transference elements, an interest that also was fostered by Winnicott (1971), who pointed to the symbolic importance of the "frame" of the psychoanalytic situation. He stressed the importance of the stability of the analytic setting and its symbolic function in reproducing, particularly in severely regressed patients, the earliest "space" involved in the intersubjective relation between mother and infant. Ogden (1986, 1989), in turn, generalized the concept of the intersubjective space as an "analytic third" and described the intersubjective field, constructed by projective contributions of patient and analyst, asymmetrically insofar as projective identifications stemming from the patient by far predominate over those introduced to the field by the analyst. Ogden suggested a technical approach to this intersubjective field by utilizing the analyst's reverie, his or her fantasies involving the emotional experiences of this field, to gain access to the co-constructed "third subject" of analysis. The analysis of the intersubjective field was further expanded in relational psychoanalysis by the analyst's focusing on the importance of the contribution of the analyst's personality and countertransference to transference developments, so that a two-way street of transference/countertransference dominates the intersubjective space to be explored.

Neo-Bionian analysts, particularly Ferro (2009) and Civitarese (2014), have further developed the concept and analytic utilization of the psychoanalytic field, assigning major importance to the intersubjective creation of a constantly varying field of emotional experience that the analyst should attempt to capture by his or her alertness to the ongoing development in the analyst of "awake life dreaming" reflecting the transference/countertransference situation. The analyst's reverie or daydreaming becomes an important source of information determining the interpretive process. As mentioned before, the complementary consideration of the patient's free association as also representing a form of awake life dreaming to be understood as reflecting deeper unconscious thoughts contributes to an atmosphere of mutually induced narratives by patient and analyst that signals the potential for direct, mutual unconscious communication. The analyst's evocative, nonsaturated interpretive comments would foster this process. It seems fair to say that this theoretical and technical approach may be a significant departure from standard psychoanalytic approach to interpretation and transference analysis, separating from what I have called the psychoanalytic mainstream, including contemporary Kleinian analysis. In any case, as we have seen, both the relational approach and the neo-Bionians have underlined the importance of this analytic approach to the intersubjective field.

It remains an open question to what extent the analyst may or should rely on his or her reverie regarding the intersubjective field in which the analyst's relation with the patient is operating. Under certain conditions in which free association seems to be leading nowhere, or when it is not clear what the dominant transference relationship is, and there is a sense of disorientation dominating the analyst's countertransference, attention to the nature of reverie evolving as a "distracted" aspect of the analyst's reaction to the total situation may provide important information. At the same time, an excessive focus on his or her own reverie on the part of the analyst may distort his or her perception of what is affectively dominant and actively bring both the personality and the theoretical leanings of the analyst into the foreground.

In short, from a technical viewpoint, considering the activation of the intersubjective field as a temporary influence on the analyst's countertransference as a source of new information may represent an addition to the diagnosis of the presently dominant, workable transference/ countertransference bind. At worst, it may lead to the neglect of direct analysis of transference developments and of the activation of character patterns in the transference that reflect important problems in the patient's interpersonal life outside the sessions.

In TFP of severe personality disorders, chronic distortion of the therapeutic situation by rigid characterological patterns of the patient that constitute a veritable barrier to the establishment of a meaningful active interpersonal contact may bring about a situation of unreality and strangeness in the therapeutic relation that dominates the clinical situation. This situation may rapidly seduce the analyst into a defensive adaptation to that severe, chronic, ego-syntonic distortion of the relationship established by the patient. Here, the attention to the nature of the intersubjective field may be of particular interest, conveying an explanation in terms of object relations reflected in this situation that facilitates the analytic exploration of this severe, pervasive characterological defense. Sometimes the simple reminder to the analyst to question how a "normal" relation with a patient would be in similarly early stages of a psychotherapeutic treatment may bring into sharp focus the specific nature of the distortion of the relationship to be explored through analysis of the intersubjective field.

Termination

The psychoanalytic technical approach to termination deals with two main issues: the first issue is the criteria for the termination of the psychoanalysis, involving resolution of the pathology that brought the patient to treatment, normalization of the patient's personality functioning in all major areas of his or her life, and the assumption of autonomous growth and development. It has been abundantly documented in the literature that such an ideal goal often may not be achieved, and there are varying degrees to which the patient may obtain a significant improvement of his or her personality structure and functioning (Firestein 1974).

The second issue regarding termination is the process of termination itself. It has particular characteristics that must be evaluated and interpretively approached. Termination activates processes of mourning, the respective conflictual aspects regarding mourning derived from the general dynamic of the evolution of paranoid-schizoid defenses into depressive mechanisms, and the tolerance and elaboration of depressive defenses and related sublimatory functioning. Here, Melanie Klein (1950) has provided essential technical criteria in her proposal that, under conditions of the combined and alternating emergence of paranoid and depressive defenses connected with the analytic process following setting a date for termination, it is important to first analyze in-depth paranoid mechanisms and only later the corresponding or related depressive mechanisms. Premature focus on depressive mechanisms may drive paranoid defenses reactivated in the transference underground, whereas full elaboration of paranoid mechanisms and related unconscious conflicts linked to them permits a full-fledged emergence of the processes of the depressive position.

Ideally, the patient's capacity for analytic work should be reflected in a self-analytic function after the end of the analysis. The general criteria of symptomatic improvement, characterological change, and satisfactory functioning in love and sex, work and profession, social life, and creativity should become evident in concrete aspects of individual functioning. The tolerance of normal mourning processes; aggressive, sexual, and dependent impulses; anxiety; and conflicts around those impulses should go hand in hand with realistic self-affirmation, predominance of sublimatory mechanisms, affect maturation, and, of course, fully satisfactory object relations in depth.

The technical approach to mourning processes first involves their diagnosis. Psychotic intolerance of mourning—with loss of reality testing and emerging psychotic symptomatology—represents the pathological extreme of a spectrum of mourning reaction that includes, at the most severe but nonpsychotic end of the spectrum, the narcissistic incapacity for mourning reflected in the self-protective devaluation of object relations that must be abandoned, including the analytic one. We see this in narcissistic patients who report having no affective reaction to the ending of the treatment. Patients with borderline pathology (but with no narcissistic pathology) and unresolved mourning processes typically present predominantly paranoid reactions with severe separation anxiety, reflecting the unconscious experience of separation and loss of the analyst by projection, as an attack. They evince paranoid fears regarding the attitude of the analyst toward them.

Under the condition of healthier neurotic personality organization, mourning regarding termination may be present but excessive, with a development of idealization, clinging, and a sense of loss of an ideally needed object combined with feelings of unworthiness. When the patient reaches the capacity for more normal mourning, a more realistic mournful remembering of all the positive experiences of the treatment may be activated under the presence of impending separation and constitute the material that needs to be worked through. Mourning reactions at the end of analysis have already been analyzed preventively in patient's separation reaction to weekends, vacations, or illness during the treatment. The patient's affective reaction to separations such as depression, anxiety, or rage needs to be explored during the treatment in terms of the specific object relations activated in them. A patient's tolerance of normal ambivalence in intimate relations, also experienced in the relation to the analyst, is a good indicator of his or her capacity for working through of the depressive mechanisms of the mourning reaction. The analyst's corresponding countertransference reactions also indicate the extent to which paranoid-schizoid mechanisms have been shifting into depressive ones.

By setting a date for the end of the analysis within a prudent time period, the reactions of the patients may be observed, and a full-fledged analytic approach to the corresponding mourning processes achieved, in preference to a questionable "tapering off," or gradual reduction of the sessions of the treatment. The patient's mourning process will not end with the end of the treatment, and he or she must be prepared that under optimal circumstances a process of 6–12 months may be needed for full completion of the mourning over a successfully terminated analysis.

In psychoanalytic psychotherapy, because of the severity of the reactions to traumatic losses and separation and the severity of the incapacity to tolerate ambivalent feelings toward intensely hated parental objects, who quite often objectively may have presented important sadistic features, pathological mourning is frequently present. Narcissistic rage or paranoid reactions are more intense and frequent than those found with patients presenting neurotic personality organization, and these reactions practically become part of the ordinary treatment situation from the very beginning of the treatment. Paradoxically, then, the working through of the mourning reaction related to termination may offer lesser problems with severely ill inpatients. Traditionally, it used to be thought that very ill patients have greater difficulty to end the treatment than healthier ones, but for the reasons just mentioned—the importance of exploring separation reactions during the treatment, and the treatment of narcissistic pathology—we have found that this is not the case. In clinical practice in which severely ill patients are treated with psychoanalytic psychotherapy by therapists who see them as part of their training experience and as part of rotations and then transfer them to other therapists, the analysis of mourning reactions becomes much more important as part of these periods of transition, and the frequent neglect of such reactions is a major cause that determines these patients to stop treatment.

It is of great interest that contractually time-limited, brief psychoanalytic psychotherapies may permit the specific analysis of mourning reactions to termination as part of the overall approach in such a brief psychotherapy. In fact, there is clinical evidence for the effectiveness of such an approach, which constitutes an important application of present-day knowledge of the technique of dealing with mourning processes applied to termination in such brief therapeutic endeavors.

Conclusion

A broad spectrum of psychoanalytic techniques may be used in the conduct of psychoanalytically informed psychotherapies. There is a clear differentiation of the modification of some of these technical instruments required in the case of psychoanalytic psychotherapy, and an overall conceptual integration of the technical approach in psychoanalytic as well as in supportive psychotherapy based on psychoanalytic principles is needed. The basic components of psychoanalytic technique of interpretation, transference analysis, technical neutrality, and countertransference utilization have an important role in all psychoanalytic modalities of treatment, but they imply a precise awareness of the required modifications, particularly as far as depth of interpretation, degree of technical neutrality, and restrictions of transference analysis are concerned. The potentially contradictory effects of the use of psychoanalytic and supportive techniques are an additional important aspect of these applications of psychoanalytic technique to a broad spectrum of psychoanalytic psychotherapies. A supportive psychotherapy based on psychoanalytic principles may be more effective than a chaotic combination of techniques on an ad hoc basis, which is more prone to significant overrun by countertransference developments and problems in the setting up of indispensable protections for the therapeutic frame.

It is hoped that a clear and comprehensive definition of the instruments that characterize standard psychoanalysis and the modifications employed in psychoanalytic psychotherapies will contribute significantly to the empirical evaluation of the efficacy of the entire field of psychoanalytically based treatments and the possibility of its practical application to a broad spectrum of psychopathology. This chapter is a tentative, modest effort to move in the direction of these objectives.

References

Akhtar S: Comprehensive Dictionary of Psychoanalysis. London, Karnac, 2009
Auchincloss EL, Samberg E: Psychoanalytic Terms and Concepts. New Haven, CT, Yale University Press, 2012
Baranger W, Baranger M: Problemas del Campo Psicoanalitico. Buenos Aires, Argentina, Kargieman, 1969
Busch F: The ego and its significance in analytic interventions. J Am Psychoanal Assoc 44(4):1073–1099, 1996 8987011
Chused JF: The evocative power of enactments. J Am Psychoanal Assoc 39(3): 615–639, 1991 1719055
Civitarese G: The Necessary Dream. London, Karnac, 2014
de Mijolla A: Dictionnaire International de la Psychanalyse. Paris, Colmann-Lévy, 2002
Etchegoyen RH: Los Fundamentos de la Técnica Psicoanalítica. Buenos Aires, Argentina, Amorrortu, 1986
Fairbairn WRD: Psychoanalytic Studies of the Personality. London, Routledge, 1952
Ferro A: Transformations in dreaming and characters in the psychoanalytic field. Int J Psychoanal 90(2):209–230, 2009 19382957
Firestein SK: Termination of psychoanalysis of adults: a review of the literature. J Am Psychoanal Assoc 22(4):873–894, 1974 4421280
Freud S: Beyond the pleasure principle (1920), in Standard Edition of the Complete Psychological Works of Sigmund Freud, Vol 18. Translated and edited by Strachey J. London, Hogarth Press, 1955, pp 1–64
Green A: On Private Madness. Madison, CT, International Universities Press, 1993
Hinshelwood RD: A Dictionary of Kleinian Thought. London, Free Association Books, 1991
Joseph B: Transference—the total situation. Int J Psychoanal 66:447–454, 1985
Joseph B: Psychic change: some perspectives. Int J Psychoanal 73(Pt 2):237–243, 1992 1512113
Kernberg OF: Convergences and divergences in contemporary psychoanalytic technique. Int J Psychoanal 74(Pt 4):659–673, 1993 8407123

Kernberg OF: Contemporary Controversies in Psychoanalytic Theory, Techniques, and Their Applications. New Haven, CT, Yale University, Press, 2004

Kernberg OF: New developments in transference focused psychotherapy. Int J Psychoanal 97(2):385–407, 2016 27112823

Klein M: On the criteria for the termination of psychoanalysis. Int J Psychoanal 31:78–80, 1950

Laplanche J, Pontalis J-B: The Language of Psychoanalysis. London, Karnac, 1988

Mertens W (ed): Handbuch Psychoanalytischer Grundbegriffe, 4th Edition. Stuttgart, Germany, Kohlhammer, 2014

Mitchell S, Aron L: Relational Psychoanalysis: The Emergence of a Tradition. Relational Perspectives Book Series, Vol 14. Hillsdale, NJ, Analytic Press, 1999

Ogden T: The Matrix of the Mind: Object Relations and the Psychoanalytic Dialogue. Northvale, NJ, Jason Aronson, 1986

Ogden T: The Primitive Edge of Experience. Northvale, NJ, Jason Aronson, 1989

Reich W: Character Analysis. New York, Farrar, Straus & Giroux, 1933

Rockland LH: Supportive Therapy for Borderline Patients: A Psychodynamic Approach. New York, Guilford, 1989

Sandler J, Dare C, Holder A: The Patient and the Analyst. New York, International Universities Press, 1973

Skelton RM, Burgoyne B, Grotstein J, et al (eds): The Edinburgh International Encyclopaedia of Psychoanalysis. Edinburgh, Scotland, Edinburgh University Press, 2006

Spillius EB, Milton J, Garvey P, et al: The New Dictionary of Kleinian Thought. New York, Routledge, 2011

Winnicott DW: Playing and Reality. New York, Basic Books, 1971

Yeomans FE, Clarkin JF, Kernberg OF: Transference-Focused Psychotherapy for Borderline Personality Disorders: A Clinical Guide. Washington, DC, American Psychiatric Publishing, 2015

CHAPTER 7

New Developments in Transference-Focused Psychotherapy

What follows is a capsule description of the basic aspects of transference-focused psychotherapy (TFP) and new developments of this therapeutic approach that are derived from both our research findings and the clinical experience gathered in the various centers where it is being studied. Please keep in mind that this treatment is indicated for patients whose severity of illness, urgency of related life situations, and lack of capacity to participate in the therapeutic frame required by standard psychoanalysis would induce most experienced clinicians to carry out a supportive treatment. TFP, derived from psychoanalytic theory and technique, expands the realm of psychoanalytic therapeutic approaches with severely disturbed patients.

While abundant clinical evidence of positive developments in fundamental personality change with TFP is now available and justifies focused research efforts to study empirically these effects in long-term fol-

---

This chapter was originally published as Kernberg OF: "New Developments in Transference Focused Psychotherapy." *International Journal of Psychoanalysis* 97(2):385–407, 2016. Copyright © 2016 Institute of Psychoanalysis. Adapted with permission.

low-up studies, this chapter is an effort to update aspects of the basic techniques of TFP as described in the third edition of our manual (Yeomans et al. 2015). These developments essentially represent an expansion of the exploration of transference by focusing on sharply dissociated expressions of severely self-destructive tendencies in the patient's external life. This focus is reflected in various technical approaches to be outlined in this chapter. These new developments stem from our clinical observations of patients treated in our various research projects as well as from the consistent study of the most difficult cases in weekly group meetings of the Personality Disorders Institute in New York and with our colleagues there.

TFP is a manualized, empirically validated psychoanalytic psychotherapy derived from a synthesis of contemporary object relations theory and modifications of psychoanalytic technique to treat patients whose severity of pathology contraindicates standard psychoanalysis (Clarkin et al. 2007; Doering et al. 2010; Kernberg et al. 2008; Yeomans et al. 2015). The specific objective of TFP is the modification of the personality structure of patients with severe personality disorders, particularly borderline personality disorder but also narcissistic, paranoid, schizoid, and schizotypal personality disorders. We have also had success in treating personality-disordered patients with significant antisocial traits and behavior but not antisocial personality disorder proper, patients with milder borderline features (the infantile or histrionic personalities), and patients with a specific hypochondriacal syndrome.

TFP focuses on reducing the symptoms typically seen in severe personality disorders, such as chronic suicidal behavior, antisocial behavior, substance abuse, and eating disorders (Zanarini et al. 2010a, 2010b). It also has the ambitious goal of modifying the personality structure of the patient sufficiently to meaningfully improve the functioning in the arenas of work, studies and profession, and intimate relations, such that the patient develops a fuller capacity to integrate emotional commitment, sexual freedom, and tenderness. Such integration leads to improvements in the capacity for genuine friendships as well as investment in creative and cultural pursuits (Yeomans et al. 2015).

The treatment is conceptualized as applying basic strategies, tactics, and techniques (Kernberg et al. 2008) as outlined in this chapter.

Strategies

Our assumption was that patients with severe personality disorders or borderline personality organization have a chronic, fixed internal split reflecting the lack of integration of the concept of self and of the concept of significant others (*identity diffusion*) and that the ultimate cause of that syndrome is the failure of psychological integration resulting from the predominance of *aggressive* internalized object relations over *idealized* ones. In an effort to protect the idealized segment of experience, the ego is fixated at a level of primitive dissociative or splitting mechanisms that are reinforced by a variety of other primitive defensive operations (predating the dominance of repression)—namely, projective identification, omnipotence and omnipotent control, devaluation, denial, and primitive idealization.

The main strategy in the treatment of patients with borderline personality organization consists in the facilitation of the (re)activation of split-off internalized object relations of contrasting persecutory and idealized natures that are then observed and interpreted in the transference. TFP is carried out in face-to-face sessions, with a minimum of two, and usually not more than three, sessions per week. The patient is instructed to carry out free association while the therapist restricts his or her role to careful listening and observation of the activation of regressive, split-off relations in the transference and to helping identify them and interpret their segregation in the light of these patients' enormous difficulty in reflecting on their own behavior and often on the maladaptive, turbulent interpersonal interactions in which they find themselves. The interpretation of these split-off object relations assumes that each reflects a dyadic unit comprising a self representation, an object representation, and a dominant affect linking them, and that the activation of these dyadic relationships determines the patient's perception of the therapist. Not infrequently, rapid role reversals of idealized and persecutory aspects appear in the transference, providing the clinician with a vital window into the patient's internal world of object relations. Thus, the patient may identify with a primitive self representation while projecting a corresponding object representation onto the therapist, whereas 10 minutes later, for example, the patient identifies with the object representation while projecting the self representation onto the therapist.

This oscillation of the roles of the dyad must ultimately be differentiated from the split between opposite dyads carrying opposite (idealizing and persecutory) affective charges—that is, a surface dyad may be defending against a deeper, more dissociated structure. The final step of interpretation consists in linking the dissociated positive and negative transferences, which leads to an integration of the mutually split-off idealized and persecutory segments of experience with the corresponding resolution of identity diffusion. The overall strategy is facilitated by the fact that unconscious conflicts are activated in the transference mostly through the patient's behavior rather than in the emergence of preconscious subjective experiences reflecting unconscious fantasy. The intolerance of overwhelming emotional experiences is expressed in the tendency to bypass such emotional experiences, predominantly by acting out in the case of most borderline patients and somatization in some patients with other personality disorders (Green 1993).

Tactics

The tactics are rules of engagement that permit the application of a modified psychoanalytic technique that corresponds to the nature of the transference developments. The essential tactics are 1) establishing with the patient a treatment contract, 2) choosing the priority theme to address in each session from the material the patient is presenting, 3) maintaining an appropriate balance between exploring the incompatible views of reality between the patient and therapist in preparation for interpretation and establishing common elements of shared reality, and 4) regulating the intensity of affective involvement.

In the establishment of an initial treatment contract, in addition to the usual arrangements for psychoanalytic treatment, any urgent difficulties in the patient's life that may threaten the patient's physical integrity or survival, other people's physical integrity or survival, or the very continuation of the treatment, are taken up and structured with the patient in such a way as to give the treatment the optimal chance of succeeding. The combination of limit setting and interpretation of the corresponding transference developments is an essential, highly effective, and, at times, lifesaving tactic of the treatment. Yeomans et al. (1992) have described in detail the techniques and vicissitudes of initial contract setting, and the manual of the technical aspects of TFP (Yeomans et al. 2015) describes in detail the priorities to address in carrying out the therapy.

With regard to choosing which theme to address at any given moment, the most important tactic is the general analytic rule that interpretation has to be carried out where the affect is most intense: affective dominance determines the focus of the interpretation. The most intense affect may be expressed in the patient's subjective experience, in the patient's nonverbal behavior, or, at times, in the countertransference. One's countertransference reaction in the face of what on the surface seems a completely frozen or affectless situation can be especially helpful to understand what is going on. The simultaneous attention to the patient's verbal communication, nonverbal behavior, and the countertransference permits identifying what the dominant affect is at the moment—

and the corresponding object relation activated in the treatment situation. Every affect is considered to be the manifestation of an underlying object relation.

Still another tactical approach relates to certain general priorities that need to be taken up immediately, whether they reflect affective dominance or not, although they usually do. These priorities include, in order of importance 1) suicidal or homicidal behavior, 2) threats to the continuation of the treatment, 3) severe acting out that threatens the patient's life, 4) dishonesty, 5) trivialization of the content of the hour, and 6) pervasive narcissistic resistances that must be resolved by consistent analysis of the transference implications of the pathological grandiose self (Kernberg 1984; Levy et al. 2006). When none of these priorities seem dominant, the general tactic of privileging affective dominance and transference analysis prevails.

Techniques

Whereas *strategies* refers to overall, long range goals and their implementation in transference analysis, and *tactics* to particular interventions in the session, *techniques* refers to the general, consistent application of technical instruments derived from psychoanalytic principles. The main technical instruments of TFP are those referred to by Gill (1954) as the essential techniques of psychoanalysis—namely, *interpretation, transference analysis, technical neutrality,* and *countertransference analysis.* We have made some modifications to these techniques, but they otherwise define our treatment (see also Chapter 6, "The Spectrum of Psychoanalytic Techniques").

Interpretation is applied systematically but with heavy emphasis on its preliminary phases of clarification and confrontation, and the interpretation of the "present unconscious" (Sandler and Sandler 1987). It is only in the later stages of TFP that the "past unconscious" is prioritized and interpreted, although the therapist will remain attuned to ways in which it relates to the present unconscious.

Transference analysis in TFP differs from standard psychoanalysis in that it is always closely linked with the analysis of the patient's problems in external reality to avoid the dissociation of the psychotherapy sessions from the patient's external life. Transference analysis also includes an implied concern for the long-range treatment goals that, typically, are not the focus in standard psychoanalysis unless they emerge in the transference. In TFP, an ongoing concern regarding dominant problems in the patient's life is reflected in the occasional introduction of reference to major conflicts that brought the patient into treatment or that have been discovered during the treatment, bringing such conflicts into the treatment situation even if they are not transference-dominant at that point.

Technical neutrality is the optimal position from which to make interventions, but at times it must be abandoned when an urgent requirement for limit setting takes priority, such as when a threat arises to the patient or to the continuation of the treatment. Such deviation from technical neutrality may be indispensable to protect the boundaries of the treatment situation and protect the patient from severe suicidal and other self-destructive behavior and requires a particular approach to restore technical neutrality once it has been abandoned. Once the treatment situation is stabilized, it is very important to address with the patient the transference implications of the therapist's abandoning neutrality and the analysis of the implications and meaning of the crisis. Technical neutrality, in short, fluctuates throughout the treatment but is constantly worked on and reinstated as a major process goal.

Countertransference utilization as a major therapeutic tool has already been referred to as an important source of information about affectively dominant issues in the hour. The internal tolerance of countertransference permits its analysis in terms of the nature of the self-representation or the object representation that is being projected onto the therapist at that point, facilitating full interpretation of the dyadic relationship in the transference, so that countertransference is used in the therapist's mind for transference clarification.

As Green (1993, 2012) has pointed out, the avoidance of traumatogenic associations drives borderline patients to jump from one subject to the next, thus expressing their "central phobic position," and this may seem bewildering to an analyst used to expecting the gradual development of a specific theme in free association, thus leading to clarity about the subject matter that is being explored. Here, waiting for such a gradual deepening of free association is useless because of this defensive use of free association, which is also related to the splitting operations that affect the very language of the patient.

The corresponding technical approach in TFP consists of an effort to interpret the implication of each of the fragments as they occur in the therapeutic hours, with the intention of establishing continuity by the very nature of the interpretive interventions that gradually establish a continuity of their own. This approach may be compared with the interpretive work with dreams, in which the analysis of apparently isolated fragments of the manifest dream content leads gradually to the latent content that establishes the continuity between the seemingly disparate elements of the manifest content.

Relationship of TFP With Other Psychoanalytic Modalities of Treatment

TFP applies a contemporary psychoanalytic object relations theory approach but, in its application of an interpretive technique, differentiates itself from other versions of this general theoretical view. The basic TFP theory of pathology derives from the Kleinian developmental concepts referring to the paranoid-schizoid and the depressive positions. *Borderline personality organization* refers to the fixation at a primitive intrapsychic structure characterized by the predominance of defensive operations centering on splitting mechanisms. Idealized and persecutory internalized dyadic units of self and object representations constitute the building blocks of the later, tripartite structure based on the dominance of the depressive position. TFP conceptualizes the activation of dyadic relations in the transference, in the sense of not only projection of a representation of self or of an object (significant other) onto the therapist, but always a simultaneous enactment of the reciprocate object or self representation on the part of the patient. It needs to be stressed that what is being projected or enacted by the patient is an affectively charged representation, and in the reciprocity of the now-enacted object relation the entire intensity of the dissociated or split-off, conflictual unconscious relationship is played out.

Countertransference is an important source of information for understanding the patient's internal world of object relations and is used to interpret the total transference situation. We do not disclose these reactions to the patient. The therapist's capacity to contain, metabolize, and interpret the intolerable split-off aspects in ways that enable the patient to tolerate and reintegrate them in less toxic form profoundly engages the therapists' subjectivity, but requires continual meticulous monitoring of what belongs to the patient, the therapist, and/or their interaction. Insofar as neither patient nor therapist is free of internal relations with unconscious significant others, unconscious triadic situations enter the picture, in parallel to the triangulation described by Kleinian authors (Britton 2004). At the same time, insofar as the activation of these dyadic and triadic relations is split off from other experiences of the patient in his or her external world, TFP pays consistent attention to what is going on in the patient's external reality, particularly, of course, the split-off expression of destructive and self-destructive urges dominant in severe personality disorders.

We believe that in treatment it is a "relationship" that is activated and projected, and not just an "alien" part of the self. This view differentiates

TFP from an essential aspect of the mentalization-based therapy approach (Bateman and Fonagy 2004). TFP interprets conscious and preconscious defensively split-off experiences of the patient, rather than assumed "repressed" or "pretend mode" formulations, which bypass a patient's subjectivity. Our emphasis on attention to the patient's conflicts in external reality has the predominant objective not of raising the patient's mentalization process regarding these external circumstances, but of exploring the transferential significance of the dissociation of potentially dangerous developments in the patient's life from the treatment situation. Our efforts are not oriented toward directly influencing the patient's behavior through better understanding his or her motivation and those of others in such external situations; rather, they are oriented toward acquiring an awareness of the transferential significance of keeping potentially self-destructive developments from potentially therapeutic understanding and help.

TFP adopts an ego psychological approach in exploring defensive operations in the transference from a "surface-to-depth" perspective, evaluating the activated object relationship in the transference in gradual deepening of the patient's subjective experience. However, the systematic dyadic and triadic focus on primitive object relations and defenses differentiates TFP from the ego psychological psychoanalytic psychotherapies that also tend to combine interpretive and supportive technical techniques. This same difference applies with respect to German depth psychology–based psychoanalytic psychotherapy (*Tiefenpsychologisch fundierte Psychotherapie*), which in many ways is similar to the American expressive-supportive psychotherapy developed in the 1960s and 1970s (Rudolf 2002) and to recently developed short-term treatment, dynamic interpersonal therapy (DIT; Lemma et al. 2011), which seeks to modify symptomatology, particularly in affective disorders, by identifying and working with the dominant maladaptive self-object affect units that underlie and sustain both symptoms and personality pathology. DIT incorporates several TFP tactics and techniques, including in the early stages the identification of and consistent attention to a dominant object relational dyad (called, in DIT, the *interpersonal affective focus*) constituted by a self representation, object representation, and linking affect. In the middle stages, DIT pays attention to role reversals as the individual identifies alternately with both self and object poles of the dyad and to the defensive functions of the object relations dyad, and at all stages DIT focuses on the myriad ways the interpersonal affective focus manifests itself in both extratransferential and transferential relationships (the latter being particularly salient when the patient has comorbid personality disorder). However, the brevity of DIT treatment (16 weeks) and the consistent focus on one dominant object relational dyad necessarily limit the full exploration and interpretation of the panoply of regressive and often contradictory split-off object relations as they emerge in the transference. Previous research has confirmed that such consistent focus on the transference in TFP leads to the integration of polarized affect states and split, contradictory representations of self and others into a more coherent stable identity reflected in significant symptomatic improvement and increased capacity for reflective functioning (Fonagy et al. 1998). In addition, improvement has been found in narrative coherence and psychosocial functioning in work and intimate relationships (Clarkin et al. 2007; Levy et al. 2006).

TFP's technical approach is closer to the London Kleinian focus on primitive defensive operations and object relations. Apart from the systematic dyadic approach to the transference, the consistent focus on dominant problems in the patients' external reality—beyond the "total transference" interpretation of the patient's material—most clearly differentiates TFP from the London approach.

New Developments

GENERAL THEORY AND TECHNIQUE

In our efforts to test the therapeutic potential of TFP, we have expanded the selection of patients to include very severely disturbed patients whose functioning in their environment was marginal. We also discovered that patients who initially presented a façade of rather stable functioning were actually masking an ever more threatening deterioration of their psychosocial adjustment. What was most striking was how often the patients managed to keep the severity of their condition and of their deteriorating social adaptation dissociated from the material that emerged in the therapeutic situation. In most cases, this appeared to be an unconscious maneuver, a dissociated or split-off part of their destructive and self-destructive potential, often as an expression of an unconscious identification with an internalized sadistic/masochistic object relationship. At times, the discovery of this occurred too late to prevent disastrous consequences for the patient and for the treatment. Resisting the temptation to shift the treatment approach from an analytic to a supportive modality (many of these patients already had a history of failed supportive approaches to their pathology), we examined the transference implications of these developments.

Applying Betty Joseph's development of the Kleinian concept of the transference as a total situation, the central need to explore the patient's unconscious attempts to influence the analyst in the transference/countertransference bind (Joseph 1985, 1989) and the expansion of the analyst's evenly suspended attention into Bion's approaching the session "without memory or desire" (Bion 1967, 2013), we developed an expansion of our technical approach. We concluded that the focus on the total transference situation might not incorporate particular dissociated aspects of the patient's interaction in his or her environment, the unconscious acting out of severely destructive and self-destructive tendencies well sheltered from his or her awareness and capacity of concern. There was an effective primitive denial of any concern on the patient's part that emerged dramatically on discovering and elaborating that dissociated material. But how to incorporate that exploration without affecting the need to let the unconscious elements of the transference/countertransference bind emerge undisturbed in the initiation of each session? Our response was to acquire very solid, detailed information about every aspect of the patient's present life situation at the time of the initial diagnostic evaluation and then maintain an ongoing, current review of his or her present life situation as a constant background to our thinking about the patient. That meant occasional inquiry about strange moments of the patient's experience or a sense of significant gaps in our awareness of the external situation. An ongoing concern for the patient's life, the therapist's fantasy about what the patient might be doing to improve his or her lot in contrast to remaining paralyzed in his or her suffering, might be part of that concern.

The therapist must attempt to be completely open to what may emerge in the session and only draw on awareness of external factors when it is powerfully activated in his or her countertransference because of the transferential developments in the hour. In other words, it will have to enter the experiential subject matter that, in the therapist's mind, becomes affectively dominant because of the confluence of the patient's verbal communication, nonverbal communication, and the countertransference. It is, in short, an amplification or expansion of the awareness of the total transference situation. André Green's sober description of failed analytic cases (Green 2010) corresponded to our own experience that typically, in such cases, a significant self-destructive area of acting out had remained unrecognized or untouched during years of analytic treatment.

The question may be raised: How could the therapist's knowledge of an external life situation or crisis not influence the therapist's "memory nor desire?" Obviously, there are situations in which, given the severity of the illness of the patients under consideration, this may be an unavoidable occurrence. However, a solid knowledge of the patient's life situation at the initiation of the treatment, the establishment of individualized conditions for the treatment, and the firm demands that these conditions be met for the treatment to begin should provide the therapist with a sufficiently strong frame for the protection of the patient and the treatment to permit the therapist to maintain his or her position of technical neutrality and to have the mental space for working through countertransference pressures and face the individual sessions "without memory or desire." We believe that this paradox must be tolerated and elaborated continuously. It needs to be kept in mind that the patient population we are considering here have severe personality disorders with chronic failure and dangerous breakdown in their social life, work, and intimacy and have potentially catastrophic self-destructive behavior. A two-sessions-per-week frequency of treatment, which we have found to be a generally satisfactory arrangement, at times adds pressure to the concern for these patients' social and physical survival.

We have found that an attitude of starting each session "without memory or desire," in the sense of the therapist's honest openness to the new and unexpected elements that may evolve, is made possible and facilitated by the therapist's ongoing mapping and working through his or her countertransference to the patient's external life outside the treatment sessions. This contributes to maintaining or restoring a position of technical neutrality and facilitates the therapist's openness to the patient's communications. This stance is a limitation to the ideal "blinding" oneself to whatever is not emerging in the session, but it protects the therapist from excessive countertransference pressures given his or her possibility to elaborate in between sessions the implications of patients' dangerous, self-destructive acting out. Bion's (2013) ideal position is not reached, but technical neutrality—in the sense of intervening outside the transference/countertransference bind, from a position as "excluded third party"—is strengthened.

In this connection, it also needs to be stressed that technical neutrality refers not to what material is selected, but to the analyst's attitude of objective inquiry—that is, his or her trying to clarify an issue without taking a stance of either approval or disapproval. This requires freedom to experience and elaborate countertransference reactions internally and to use them as elements for interpretive interventions when such a point of technical neutrality has been reached or restored.

This paradox is much less intensively activated in standard psychoanalysis, in which the combination of higher frequency of sessions and less severe chronic regression and threats to the patient's social and physical survival shifts the material significantly from acting out to communication of subjective experience.

In what follows, some practical technical innovations reflecting the expansion of our theoretical frame are outlined.

PRACTICAL TECHNICAL INNOVATIONS

Initial and Continuous Evaluation of the Patient's Conflicts in Terms of Current Functioning in Social and Personal Life Outside the Sessions

We have found that it is essential in the initial diagnostic evaluation of patients to assess consistently four major areas of their present functioning: a) studies, work, or profession; b) love and sexuality; c) family and social life; and d) personal creativity. In fact, the evaluation of these areas during the initial diagnostic interviews not only contributes significantly to diagnostic precision in the assessment of the personality but also pinpoints where the patient stands in terms of overall present functioning, what the gap is between where the patient is now and where the patient might be ideally if he or she did not suffer from the personality disorder.

This Promethean attitude toward the patient is an important balance to certain countertransference reactions to the severity of the dysfunctionality of the patient, such as a sense of despair or even pity in the mind of the diagnostician, implying a sense of hopelessness about the patient. It can be difficult to resist a sense of pity in the presence of the most severely disordered patients, many of whom may seem to have destroyed almost all opportunities in their life and present with an aura of helplessness and resignation about the terrible life situation in which they encounter themselves. But such a reaction may limit the therapist's therapeutic evaluation of the patient's principal problems: What should be the goal of treatment in terms of resolving them, and where could this patient be ideally if he or she were not subjected to this pathology? I am not referring here to a *furor sanandi,* an unrealistic aspiration for perfection imposed on patients in terms of some abstract general therapeutic goal. I am referring to a realistic assessment of what a specific patient might have achieved and might still achieve if freed from the burden of illness, which would sharpen the diagnostic definition, therapeutic goals, and prognostic assessment. It would not be necessary to stress this point if, in practice, many severely ill patients were not able to create around them an atmosphere of pessimism and resignation that in turn may limit the efforts involved in therapeutic interventions.

This same assessment, however, becomes an important aspect of the psychotherapeutic technique with these patients in terms of the rapid evaluation, practically at the beginning of most therapeutic hours, of where the patient stands in terms of his or her relation to important domains of external life—love, work, social life, and creativity. The patient requires an alertness to urgent problems that he or she is ignoring or neglecting, or where self-destructive forces are active in undermining or destroying the patient's possibilities. It is a consistent finding in the intensive psychotherapy of patients with severe personality disorders and pervasive self-destructive tendencies that ongoing temptations to self-destructive behavior in those four areas are an almost unavoidable complication of the treatment. This naturally becomes a major area of transference acting out. The therapist's alertness to self-destructive temptations or acting out permits him or her to bring this subject matter into the focus of the hour, particularly the transference implications. This may make a fundamental difference in situations in which such acting out becomes a definite tragedy of opportunities lost or destroyed, life goals curtailed, and self-destructiveness achieving its purpose before it is detected in the content of the therapeutic hours.

We have learned that this attention to external life adds a crucial aspect in determination of the "selected fact" (Bion 1967) in the sessions (i.e., what urgent or threatening issue may be evolving in the patient's life that is being withheld, disguised, or ignored by the patient, particularly, the transference). Therefore, the selection of what is affectively dominant in each hour and each segment of the hour on the basis of verbal communication, nonverbal behavior, and countertransference must be enriched by the consideration of what, if any, issues are urgently developing and threatening the patient's life or the treatment. One implication of this ongoing diagnostic assessment is the question of what could be done about this particularly urgent, threatening issue. What would the therapist consider doing under identical conditions that the patient seems, at this point, to ignore, suppress, mask, or deny? The problem is complex, because the action the patient would need to undertake to avoid an urgent danger in his or her life outside the sessions may seduce the therapist into countertransference acting out, attempting to direct the patient to carry out certain behaviors or avoid certain behaviors and adopting a "supportive" stance, which in turn might correspond to a transference/countertransference acting out—the projection of the responsibility of the patient from himself or herself onto the therapist.

In our experience, shifting to a supportive, re-educative mode may be eagerly incorporated into the patient's self-destructive, and at times markedly masochistic, transference and gratify the patient's dependency needs, but there remains no authentic concern for himself or herself and an abdication of personal responsibility. It is important, under such circumstances, first, to bring the urgent issue in the patient's life that has been kept out of the manifest content of the hours into focus. We must analyze the reasons for which the patient may have been unaware, unconcerned, ignoring, or "hiding" an issue that seems of utmost urgency and importance. It is important to help the patient become aware of his or her collusion with the unconscious need to destroy opportunities and to examine the extent to which such awareness stimulates a real concern on the patient's part over what is occurring in him or her. The absence of such concern would be the first issue to explore, because only after the development of an authentic concern of the patient for himself or herself may it become possible to then explore the patient's thoughts or feelings about what he or she would need to do to avert danger, correct self-destructive behavior, or prevent some potential disaster from occurring.

A typical example of such situations is represented by one of our patients with significant narcissistic personality features and marked derogatory attitudes toward coworkers. He had entered a highly competitive new field of work within which, he trusted, his intelligence would bring about rapid promotion. However, his derogatory attitude and dismissive reaction to early criticism of his performance led to his being dismissed from this highly desirable and competitive situation before he even suspected that he was at risk.

Another patient, a woman with a borderline personality disorder and marked histrionic features, presented with chronic intense anxiety that precluded her from attending parties and participating in social life or even dating. She was able, however, to work efficiently in an office where her boss, a rather maternal woman, attempted to help her develop her expertise. This patient experienced crying spells at work, for no clear reasons, requiring the direct intervention of the boss to reassure her. Over time, aware that only the boss was able to reassure her, her coworkers decided to call the boss directly during the patient's inexplicable crying spells. The boss then would cross the large office space where several people were working and observing the scene to console the patient at her desk. It proved to be quite embarrassing for the boss. This brought about a gradual distortion of a realistic working relationship that seemed gratifying to the patient but, from an objective viewpoint, clearly indicated an unsustainable situation that over the long run threatened her position, which the patient ignored completely. At first, the therapist also ignored how those "little scenes" during business hours threatened the future of the patient's work situation, the only area in her life in which she had been functioning relatively well. The therapist was able to intervene, only at the very last moment, to clarify the risk that the patient's unstable behavior potentially would eventually lead to the end of her employment.

Another patient presented with the symptom of chronic lateness to all engagements, thereby threatening her employment, which was essential to permit her to continue financing her treatment. Yet another patient with profound ambivalence toward his girlfriend, toward whom he behaved in a childlike, chronically attention-demanding way, ignored the developments in their relationship indicating that she was getting tired of him and probably would leave him, thus repeating the traumatic experiences he had suffered with several women before.

In each of these cases, the most impressive, common element characterizing their sessions was the tendency not to discuss—to ignore, in fact—their self-destructive behavior, thus shielding the therapist from a growing awareness of an impending major crisis potentially induced by the patient's behavior.

In this regard, a general principle may be very helpful: the therapist should maintain a high degree of alertness and "impatience" with a patient's self-induced threats to his or her well-being within each hour while remaining patient over the long term in analyzing self-destructive and other major characterological problems of the patient. Patience over the long term and "impatience" in each session are complementary tactical approaches.

Life Goals and Treatment Goals

Many years ago, Ernst Ticho (1972) pointed to the importance of differentiating realistic treatment goals from patients' life goals. A typical example of a life goal would be the female patient who comes to treatment because she wants to get married and has not been able to find a mate. A thorough assessment of the patient's personality organization reveals a severely masochistic or narcissistic personality pathology that has interfered with her establishing gratifying relations or her willingness to settle down in a stable relationship and have a family. Now, concerned with the biological limits of fertility, she wishes to have a child or to get married with that purpose. Naturally, men with similar pathology may enter treatment with that objective as well, particularly men with narcissistic personalities and severe, chronic failure in previous marriages or love relationships. As Ticho pointed out, it is very important to clarify that the treatment may help the patient resolve whatever conflicts exist in the establishment of stable and satisfactory love relationships, but it can offer no guarantee that the patient will find such a person in external reality. This may sound trivial, were it not so often a manifest expression of negative transference or disappointment in the therapist who has not provided the patient with an appropriate mate.

In this connection, it has proved very helpful to clarify at the beginning of the treatment what the patient expects to get out of treatment and what the therapist thinks the therapy can reasonably accomplish. Common goals and expectations, along with a clear delineation of responsibilities, should be part of the treatment contract. This may also be a very good moment for the therapist to explore reasonable life goals that, for some reason, the patient has not considered and may present the first opportunity to help the patient envision a better life situation that may be within the realm of possibility. Such a discussion may be of help when the patient, under conditions of severe negative transference developments, threatens to interrupt the treatment or loses complete perspective of what initially the treatment was all about. Realistic, agreed-on treatment goals become, in short, an important component of the treatment frame and may be helpful under conditions of severe regression in the transference.

Patients' Potential Versus Reality of Their Life Situation

We have found that patients with borderline personality organization frequently present a remarkable discrepancy between their past—their background, education, family support, and the social and cultural environment of their childhood and adolescence—and their present existence as adults in a shadowy, nondescript, empty lifestyle that is devoid of meaningful investment in friendship, love relationships, or work. Not only do they present with a remarkable lack of ambition and concern over this discrepancy between past and present, but they do so unconsciously, with an attitude implying that any effort by the therapist to question where they stand in life represents an unwelcome invasion of their space and present reality. Sometimes one finds the opposite—a rather ambitious fantasy that is incongruent with the nature of their daily life or work and behavior and that stands for what could have been, given their potential and opportunities.

At the initiation of treatment, it is important for the therapist to consider whether the patient is really on the road to achieve what, given his or her background, personality, and potential, might be reasonable for success and gratification in life. Sometimes it helps for the therapist, when informed about the patient's apparently hopeless life conditions, to wonder how the therapist would deal with such a challenge if not compromised by the kind of pathology presented by the patient. There exists the danger, of course, of the therapist's imposing his or her own social biases and life goals on the patient and distorting the therapeutic relationship in that regard, so this concern also involves a self-reflective process in the therapist that requires careful attention. Over time, patients tend to "brainwash" their therapist into internally settling down with the patient's life as he or she presents it, particularly because chronic self-restrictive and self-limiting behaviors do not usually emerge in an active, conflictual way in the context of the transference.

Defenses Against the Sense of Personal Responsibility

As mentioned previously, a patient's denial of his or her own responsibility in creating and maintaining highly self-destructive situations in major areas of his or her life may become a major focus of the sessions once urgent issues in those areas have been discovered and brought into the transference analysis. Confronting the patient with his or her irresponsible behavior from the viewpoint of realistic survival, rather than from a "superego," moralistic perspective—the therapist must be moral but not moralistic (Ticho 1972)—may lead, nonetheless, to the patient's experiencing it as a moralistic assault. This may evolve particularly in the case of patients with significant antisocial features and corresponding projection of their own, intolerable superego functions. This situation requires working through of the patient's paranoid transference reaction before he or she becomes able to recognize his or her own responsibility in self-sabotaging behavior. Patients who present a chronically shifting, passive, parasitic lifestyle or a level of work that does not correspond at all with their background, education, intelligence, and social support system should alert the therapist to such a chronic acting out of self-destructive behavior and motivate the therapist to bring this issue into the analysis of the transference (Kernberg 2007).

The reference to the therapist's "moral but not moralistic" stance may be interpreted as a stress on correcting patients' "bad behavior," an obvious infringement of interpretive interventions from a technically neutral standpoint. The therapist's sense that his or her ethical convictions are being called into question by a patient's behavior constitutes an important alarm signal in his or her countertransference: Is the patient's behavior indicating an act of unacknowledged, potentially dangerous aggression against others or self? Or is the therapist being tempted to impose his or her own value system over the patient's value system? Are there objective dangers for the patient or others involved in what, at face value, appear to be unethical acts or intentions? These issues need to be examined, and the therapist's morality implies a diagnostic function, not an imperative to action. Patients' "immoral" behavior may have practical implications that they are denying and represent a defensive denial of reality. Confronting patients with the denial of reality, including the consequences of their actions for self and others, may be an important first step to investigate the unconscious functions of that behavior and should not be part of an effort to impose changes to the patient's behavior. Obviously, if there is a simple clash of culturally determined differences between patient and therapist, the therapist's task is to explore the countertransference. However, if the patient engages in concretely dangerous behavior—for example, one of our HIV-positive patients engaged in unprotected sex with partners whom he did not inform of his HIV status—the indication is for limit setting as a condition for carrying out TFP, combined with immediate interpretation of the transference implications of this radical abandonment of technical neutrality. This is the first step in later explorations of the unconscious meanings of this behavior and the interpretive restoration of technical neutrality. In short, setting limits is seen not as an end in and of itself, but as necessary precursor, under extreme circumstances, to exploration of the meaning of this behavior. This also may significantly reduce the therapist's anxiety over dangerous acting out.

In long-lasting treatments, the therapist needs to be alert to the possibility of being seduced into an implicit acquiescence with a stable, yet highly unsatisfactory life situation as if it were perfectly normal. It is helpful for the therapist to maintain a concerned attitude regarding what a "normal" person would do, under the patient's life circumstances, to enrich his or her experience, effectiveness, and satisfaction with life. This question may be raised in the therapist's mind with patients presenting a chronic parasitic lifestyle or a severely self-restricting lifestyle reflecting a defensive narcissistic isolation from their psychosocial reality, or with some severely masochistic patients, and with patients presenting the unconscious need to defeat the efforts of those who try to help them.

One patient with severely masochistic personality features functioning on a borderline level was an efficient lawyer at a leading law firm. After the end of a love affair with a high executive of the firm, she experienced herself as being pushed aside from participation in major strategic decisions and got involved in discussions with her ex-lover that escalated to the point of threatening her future at the firm. In one session, she mentioned casually that in a recent argument with the ex-lover, she had triumphantly told him that the leader of a major competing law firm had offered her an important job: other people, she told the now hostile and potentially dangerous executive, did appreciate her capacities. As she went on complaining over the present mistreatment at her firm, I raised with her whether she had considered the possibility of accepting the offer. No, she said, she had not thought about it and only used it as an argument. I confronted her with the combination of her worsening situation and prospects in her present job, the fears she had expressed about being fired, and her remarkable dismissal of what seemed to be an important opportunity. Obviously, there were significant transference implications to the patient's unconsciously "tempting me" to "force her" to overcome her self-defeating behavior, but it seemed important to keep the external reality in mind in detecting her masochistic acting out.

This contingency highlights the relationship between technical neutrality, ordinary common sense, and the therapist's image of the patient as capable of functioning at a higher level than perhaps the patient can envision. Keeping all this in mind will counteract the effects of a patient's relentless, chronic pathology and offer some protection from the temptation to give up on a patient, as well as help patient and therapist come to terms with life goals that the patient realistically would not be able to achieve. In any case, the principle that "psychotherapy starts where common sense ends" should be helpful to reevaluate, at least from time to time, where the patient stands within his or her overall relation to reality. To confront a patient's serious neglect of "real-life concerns" should not be confused with traditional "supportive" interventions made on the patient's behalf; rather, it provides the opportunity for exploration of the meaning of such neglect and how this can be understood.

Contract Breaches and "Second Chances"

What follows is a description of our technical approach to contract setting, extensively explored by Yeomans (Yeomans et al. 1992). We frequently find that therapists have a difficult time, after giving patients a second chance following a contract breach, systematically analyzing the risk of a second contract breach, and the related risk of sabotaging and ending the treatment, as part of transference interpretations. A typical example is the case of a patient who understood that if she experiences strong suicidal urges she should either discuss them in the following session or, if not able to control such an urge, consult or apply to a psychiatric emergency center or a general hospital emergency room, but who then carried out a severe suicidal attempt without having complied with this contractual understanding. The therapist, following protocol, offered her a continuation of the treatment with the understanding that a second breach of this contract would definitely end it. Both therapist and patient were clearly aware that this provided the patient with an omnipotent control: the means to dramatically and easily end the treatment. The temptation to do so may be a powerful aspect, for example, of a dominant negative transference, a negative therapeutic reaction, the impulsive acting out of aggression against third parties unconsciously displaced onto the therapist, and so on.

It may be difficult for the therapist to hold consistently in mind the urgency of this issue, despite its coloring all other aspects of the treatment developments, and it may in fact represent a chronic, yet acute, severe risk of interruption of the treatment, which is a "highest priority" issue codetermining the "selected fact" in any session. The patient may not refer again to the contract breach and may present other issues as affectively dominant, distracting the therapist's attention from a potential breach. Yet, remaining vigilant to this risk may be extremely helpful to the patient and prevent a failed treatment. Concretely, this implies linking the potential threat to the continuation of the therapy when it appears that transference developments are consonant with this threat, interpreting the implicit acting out of destructive transference impulses by repetition of the specific contract breach. Particularly in the case of patients with chronically suicidal tendencies, this concern needs to be maintained through all sessions until it becomes clear in the patient's material that suicide has become a completely irrelevant issue and that it is no longer meaningful in the context of the patient's present functioning. In short, the shifting transference implications of the same threat of a second treatment-ending contract breach need to be included, whenever appropriate, in the interpretive interventions of the therapist. When a patient convincingly tells a therapist that he or she should stop talking about suicidal threats and ideation because they have not been on the patient's mind for months, and which the patient no longer can imagine would be able to control him or her, the therapist may stop bringing up the subject again and again in different transferential contexts! However, as a safety measure, the therapist needs to maintain in mind the constant presence of the risk of temptations to end the treatment when a "second chance" period evolves in the treatment.

By the same token, these same considerations apply when new limit setting or modification of the initial contract is called for in light of new developments—for example, in the case of a patient with a severe anorectic disorder, in which a contract is set regarding the consequences of the weight of the patient fluctuating beyond mutually established limits, or in patients with drug abuse or dependency, with whom limit setting regarding drug abuse has become part of the overall structure of the treatment during the course of it.

Perhaps the most difficult, and quite frequent, situation is that of a patient who presents with chronic threats of suicidal behavior, who accepts the conditions of the treatment, which is either to discuss suicidal behavior in the sessions or to go to an emergency room, but who nonetheless continues to frighten friends and relatives with statements or actions implying that he or she has decided to commit suicide. This may be causing sufficient alarm to generate pressure on the therapist from outsiders as well as his or her own concern as to whether such limit setting around these threatening statements ought to be structured as a condition for continued treatment.

When faced with a patient's chronic suicidality or self-harm, we have found it most helpful to have a joint session with the patient and concerned family members (or friends). Such chronic self-destructiveness may necessitate a frank discussion with relatives about the unavoidable but serious risk, given that it is not a reflection of a depressive illness but, rather, deeply rooted in personality traits and characterological predisposition, and can be neither prevented nor predicted. Therefore, it constitutes a constant risk that must be accepted as one of the conditions required by this treatment. Alternatively, the family, in the face of this chronic unpredictable risk of suicide, may have to consider long-term hospitalization or residential treatment, but this provides only the illusion of safety.

The disadvantages of such a disruption of the patient's life, which interferes with the patient's carrying out his or her ordinary responsibilities instead of facilitating the normalization of functioning in all areas with the help of the therapist, would represent a major complication of long-term hospitalization. Therefore, despite the chronic risk of suicidal behavior, continuing in TFP (two times per week) may be preferable to long-term hospitalization. This kind of psychotherapeutic treatment can be carried out only if patient and relatives accept the risk that despite all efforts, the patient may end up committing suicide or suffer from self-destructive behavior.

Contracting around issues of severe lethality, wherein the patient accepts the conditions necessary to carry out the treatment and all parties accept the inevitable inherent risks, provides a degree of security to the therapist and an adequate frame to the treatment. This may permit the treatment to be carried out even if the patient continues behavior that may be upsetting or frightening to third parties. In the United States, given the litigious nature of the American culture, it would be absolutely essential to set down a written record of the full communication of these risks and the acceptance of these risks by the family. Sometimes, even a letter of understanding with family and patient may be indispensable. Behind these arrangements, then, lies the need to assure the security of the therapist in carrying out the treatment. The security of the therapist—physical, emotional, social, and legal—and the protection of his or her property and personal life are essential preconditions for the possibility of treating patients with severe personality disorders. The therapist must feel safe to conduct the treatment and free of the omnipotent control of the patient's destructive impulses, or the treatment may not be viable. If this is not possible, it may be preferable to discontinue the treatment and refer the patient elsewhere. One other important advantage of full discussion of the risks and corresponding contract arrangements is the effectiveness of this approach in reducing the secondary gain of the symptoms that prevents the symptoms from becoming a powerful mechanism of omnipotent control and transference acting out.

Technical Neutrality and Antisocial Behavior

We continue to confirm our experience that severity of secondary gain of illness and of antisocial behavior are the overriding indicators of negative prognosis. One might add to these two features the poor prognosis in cases of overwhelming, chronic wishes to die accompanied by chronic, severe, self-lacerating, suicidal, or parasuicidal behavior.

Patients with antisocial tendencies evince psychopathic transferences in the form of chronic deceptiveness in the transference (Kernberg 2007). Under optimal circumstances, the systematic analysis of dishonesty in the relation with the therapist transforms these transferences into paranoid ones: the open exploration of the paranoid reasons behind the patient's dishonesty. But there are cases in which a radical split evolves between antisocial behavior—now fully acknowledged and still ego-syntonic—and another segment of the patient's psychic experience in which feelings of guilt and anxiety over this antisocial behavior emerge. For example, a patient was stealing instruments and material from his workplace but professing guilt and shame over this behavior at other times. Similarly, the alternation between ego-syntonic, enjoyable sadistic abuse toward a sexual partner and feelings of guilt and shame over the abuse is not infrequent.

Here the authenticity and strength of concern that evolve during the exploration of the transference implications of this split crystallize cases in which the capacity for tolerance of superego functions and for a residual investment in the relationship with the therapist allows resolution through interpretation. To the contrary, other patients evince an unresolvable secondary gain from that split and behave as if expressed feelings of regret or concern over their antisocial behavior have redeemed them from further guilt or need to explore or change their behavior. This is a manifestation of the syndrome of perversity: the recruitment of love at the service of aggression (see Chapter 13).

One patient repeatedly presented his girlfriend with questions regarding her behavior and her understanding of the behavior of her family and friends. What at first seemed friendly inquiries regularly turned into sadistic attacks and merciless devaluation, leaving his girlfriend in tears. In the sessions, the patient acknowledged the enjoyment of his aggressive, provocative behavior and reflected on the possibility that it might relate to his past intense hatred of his mother. This understanding, however, did not influence his present behavior. It turned out that he was convinced that his past frustrations with his mother justified his present behavior toward his girlfriend. Although he presented himself as feeling guilty about his behavior, he expected the therapist to acknowledge that his suffering under periodic guilt feelings presented enough of an expiatory action to erase any need for future concern. For the therapist, the syndrome of perversity generates pressures on his or her position of technical neutrality: how can he or she maintain a moral stance without becoming moralistic? Some cases permit limit setting and subsequent analysis of the need for departure from technical neutrality. Other cases need to be terminated because the limits the therapist considers essential to the therapeutic relationship cannot be maintained. At bottom, it becomes a question of whether the patient, in not wanting to lose the therapist, is able to acknowledge his or her despair over an existence of total loneliness and abandonment, caused by his or her own aggression.

Sex and Money: Two Taboo Subjects

Two common problems we have frequently encountered in the training of therapists, even very senior therapists, are 1) a reluctance to fully explore the patient's sexual experiences, fantasies, and activities; and 2) a reluctance to discuss in detail the patient's management of his or her financial situation. The therapist's misguided avoidance of these important areas of the patient's overall functioning may develop into a transference/countertransference enactment that has the potential to limit the progress of, or even possibly threaten, the continuation of the treatment. It is extremely important to get a comprehensive picture of the patient's sexual and love life as part of the initial evaluation. The patient's capacity or incapacity to fall in love and to establish satisfactory love relations, to experience fully a sexual intimacy, to integrate or to keep strictly separate tenderness and emotional relations from sexual gratification; the nature of the patient's masturbatory fantasies; and the relation between the masturbatory fantasies, sexual activities, and predominant nature of sexual dreams—all provide important information about the patient's psychological organization. The patient's expression of sexual behavior and sexual fantasy in the transference is, generally, more easily thought about and conceptualized but, again, sometimes difficult to fully explore, particularly under conditions of highly sexually seductive behavior on the part of the patient. Perhaps, particularly with severely narcissistic patients for whom sexual seduction may become a way of asserting their superiority or control over the therapist under the guise of sexual interest, this may lead to an inhibition in the therapist's full exploration of the patient's sexual conflicts.

Similarly, we have found great reluctance on the part of therapists to discuss in detail the patient's financial circumstances, particularly with patients who have great difficulty in dealing with their financial needs and commitments and who present significant irresponsibility, secondary gain, or even antisocial behavior in the management of their finances. When financial problems affect the treatment situation itself—for example, a patient's rationalizing his or her wishes to interrupt the treatment due to financial difficulties—the therapist's countertransference reactions, derived from his or her own anxieties over finances, may inhibit full exploration of the transference situation and from clarifying objective reality and its potential distortion in the light of transference developments (Berger and Newman 2012). It is essential to assure realistic conditions for carrying out the treatment from the very start and to be alert to masochistic behavior being acted out by unrealistic commitments on the part of the patient, and the potential for narcissistic and antisocial features to be manifested in the patient's exploitive tendencies.

Conclusion

The primary new development in the technique of transference-focused psychotherapy consists of an expansion of the concept of the *total transference situation* to include exploration in the transference of dissociated and apparently "unaware" expressions of severely self-destructive tendencies in the patient's *external life*. The subtlety and slowly accumulating gravity of this acting out may be detected by an ongoing in-depth exploration of the patient's functioning outside the treatment situation. The therapist's alertness, concern, and common-sense approach to analysis of apparently confused or confusing "innocent" or "trivial" episodes or developments may provide essential cues that illuminate a dangerous reality. The clarity and firm stability of the treatment frame facilitate the therapist's maintenance of technical neutrality while he or she remains consistently concerned for the patient and aids in approaching each session "without memory or desire." Systematic transference analysis, under such circumstances, is more effective than the countertransference temptations to supportive shortcuts of problematic, threatening acting out.

The development of new ways to approach severely regressive narcissistic transferences constitutes an additional important area of new technical TFP developments. These are explored in Part III of this book.

References

Bateman A, Fonagy P: Psychotherapy for Borderline Personality Disorder: Mentalization-Based Treatment. New York, Oxford University Press, 2004

Berger B, Newman S (eds): Money Talks: In Therapy, Society, and Life. London, Routledge, 2012

Bion WR: Second Thoughts: Selected Papers on Psychoanalysis. New York, Basic Books, 1967

Bion WR: Los Angeles Seminars and Supervision. Edited by Aguayo J, Malin B. London, Karnac, 2013

Britton R: Subjectivity, objectivity, and triangular space. Psychoanal Q 73(1):47–61, 2004 14750465

Clarkin JF, Levy KN, Lenzenweger MF, et al: Evaluating three treatments for borderline personality disorder: a multiwave study. Am J Psychiatry 164(6):922–928, 2007 17541052 17541052

Doering S, Hörz S, Rentrop M, et al: Transference-focused psychotherapy v treatment by community psychotherapists for borderline personality disorder: randomised controlled trial. Br J Psychiatry 196(5):389–395, 2010 20435966

Fonagy P, Steele M, Steele H, et al: Reflective-function manual: version 5.0 for application to the adult attachment interview. July 1998. Available at: http://www.mentalizacion.com.ar/images/notas/Reflective%20Functioning%20Manual.pdf. Accessed June 30, 2017.

Gill MM: Psychoanalysis and exploratory psychotherapy. J Am Psychoanal Assoc 2(4):771–797, 1954 13211443

Green A: Le Travail du Négatif. Paris, Les Éditions de Minuit, 1993

Green A: Illusions et Désillusions du Travail Psychoanalytique. Paris, Odile Jacob, 2010

Green A: La Clinique Psychanalytique Contemporaine. Paris, Les Éditions d'Ithaque, 2012

Joseph B: Transference—the total situation. Int J Psychoanal 66:447–454, 1985

Joseph B: Psychic Equilibrium and Psychic Change. London, Routledge, 1989

Kernberg OF: Severe Personality Disorders: Psychotherapeutic Strategies. New Haven, CT, Yale University Press, 1984

Kernberg OF: The almost untreatable narcissistic patient. J Am Psychoanal Assoc 55(2):503–539, 2007 17601104

Kernberg OF, Yeomans FE, Clarkin JF, et al: Transference focused psychotherapy: overview and update. Int J Psychoanal 89(3):601–620, 2008 18558958

Lemma, A, Target M, Fonagy P: Brief Dynamic Interpersonal Therapy: A Clinician's Guide. New York, Oxford University Press, 2011

Levy KN, Meehan KB, Kelly KM, et al: Change in attachment patterns and reflective function in a randomized control trial of transference-focused psychotherapy for borderline personality disorder. J Consult Clin Psychol 74(6):1027–1040, 2006 17154733

Rudolf G: Konfliktaufdeckende und strukturfördernde Zielsetzungen in der tiefenpsychologisch fundierten Psychotherapie [Gaining insight and structural capability as goals of psychodynamic psychotherapy]. Psychosom Med Psychother 48(2):163–173, 2002 11992326

Sandler J, Sandler AM: The past unconscious, the present unconscious and the vicissitudes of guilt. Int J Psychoanal 68(Pt 3):331–341, 1987 3667083

Ticho EA: Termination of psychoanalysis: treatment goals, life goals. Psychoanal Q 41(3):315–333, 1972 5047036

Yeomans FE, Selzer MA, Clarkin JF: Treating the Borderline Patient: A Contract-Based Approach. New York, Basic Books, 1992

Yeomans FE, Clarkin JF, Kernberg OF: Transference-Focused Psychotherapy for Borderline Personality Disorders: A Clinical Guide. Washington, DC, American Psychiatric Publishing, 2015

Zanarini MC, Frankenburg FR, Reich DB, Fitzmaurice G: The 10-year course of psychosocial functioning among patients with borderline personality disorder and Axis II comparison subjects. Acta Psychiatr Scand 122(2):103–109, 2010a 20199493

Zanarini MC, Frankenburg FR, Reich DB, Fitzmaurice G: Time to attainment of recovery from borderline personality and stability of recovery: a 10-year prospective follow-up study. Am J Psychiatry 167(6):663–667, 2010b 20199493

CHAPTER 8

A New Formulation of Supportive Psychodynamic Psychotherapy

What follows is an effort to make use of the new knowledge and experiences that we have acquired at the Personality Disorders Institute of Weill Cornell Medical College regarding the application of transference-focused psychotherapy (TFP) to the treatment of severe personality disorders. Two major concerns have moved us to reexamine the concept and techniques of supportive psychotherapy based on psychodynamic principles.

First, would it be possible to develop an updated method of supportive psychodynamic treatment for cases that have traditionally been treated in a supportive modality? These include cases of such minor degree of severity that brief psychodynamic psychotherapies are sufficient to treat effectively. At the other end of the spectrum are more severe cases that have not responded to, are contraindicated for, or otherwise do not present sufficient conditions for carrying out TFP or other intensive psychodynamic psychotherapeutic treatments. These latter cases include a significant number of severe personality disorders that have not responded to a wide spectrum of psychodynamic and cognitive-behavioral treatments carried out with appropriate expertise over a sufficiently extended period of time (Rockland 1989).

Our second concern is a very practical one: the societal and financial pressures for reducing the frequency of treatment to one session per week, which presents an impediment for carrying out TFP, which requires a minimum of two individual sessions per week. In fact, therapists whom we have trained to carry out TFP with patients with severe personality disorders have attempted, under the pressure of socially determined constraints, to maintain this treatment on a once-per-week basis ("TFP light"). Whereas some patients seem to have responded to once-per-week TFP, many other patients ended up in long-term treatments without adequate therapeutic response. This calls for further empirical research to determine patient–therapist characteristics that might predict successful once-per-week TFP. In practice, under the circumstances referred to above, supportive psychotherapeutic techniques became necessary to deal with transference developments that could not be explored from a technically neutral viewpoint. Given the urgency of multiple problems reflecting these patients' poor social functioning and requiring rapid interventions under the conditions of a once-per-week treatment situation, interfering transference resistances could not be interpretively resolved.

Our encounter with these obstacles has motivated us to reexamine the possibility of developing a supportive psychotherapeutic approach that could be carried out on a once-per-week basis, making use of our experiences in treating severe personality disorders with TFP while maintaining an internal coherence of the treatment that would provide an adequate frame for the therapist's interventions within a clear theory of technique.

Traditional Definition and Changes in Psychodynamically Based Supportive Psychotherapy

The model of traditional supportive psychotherapy based on psychoanalytic theory and psychodynamic techniques centers on the effort to help the patient achieve a better equilibrium between defenses and impulses, strengthening ego functions by reinforcing adaptively useful defensive operations and making use of positive transference developments in fostering the patient's identification with the therapist's healthier ego functions (Gill 1954). This conceptualization, developed in the 1950s and

1960s in the United States, expanded further in later decades under the influence of the findings of the Menninger Foundation's Psychotherapy Research Project (Kernberg et al. 1972). It eventually led to the manualized supportive psychotherapy for borderline conditions carried out under the leadership of Lawrence Rockland and Ann Applebaum at our Personality Disorders Institute, and was explored in a randomized controlled treatment that showed both positive effects and limitations of that approach (Kernberg et al. 2008; Rockland 1989).

The following influences from our ongoing development of TFP seemed important in terms of a contemporary review of supportive psychotherapy. First, we noted the contributions from contemporary psychoanalytic object relations theory. It became evident that primitive defensive operations based on splitting mechanisms, including projective identification, denial, omnipotent control, devaluation, primitive idealizations, and severe splitting of self and object representations, had significantly weakening effects on ego functioning. The concept of "reinforcing adaptive defenses" became less relevant than the need to reduce the dominance of these primitive defensive operations. The awareness of these defenses replaced the older concept of the assumed "frailty" of the patient's ego. The apparent frailty of the patient's self experience and self-concept was a consequence of these primitive defensive operations, in the same way as the patient's distortions of his or her experiences in the relations with significant others. A supportive psychotherapeutic approach would have to focus on these negative effects of the patient's habitual defensive operations.

Second, the use of modified psychoanalytic techniques in TFP opened the possibility of using some aspects of these technical modifications in combination with other, supportive techniques as part of an essentially supportive approach that would reflect our experience with the severe life problems and crises of severe personality disorders.

Third, we had become acutely aware how crucial was an ongoing monitoring of the patient's functioning in the major areas of daily living—that is, in work and profession, in love and sex, in social life and creativity. We had to assess the urgency of the patient's life problems at any time, along with the corresponding need for shifts in the priority of the therapeutic interventions.

Last, our experience with constant attention to transference developments permitted us to diagnose more appropriately the activation of manifest (in contrast to latent) negative transferences that, in a supportive approach, necessarily would have to be dealt with to maintain a minimal therapeutic alliance in carrying out the tasks as agreed on in the patient–therapist relationship.

A Newly Defined Strategy of Treatment

The strategy of supportive psychotherapy we developed involves an effort to improve the patient's overall functioning without attempting to resolve identity diffusion (Kernberg 1999). We focused on helping patients to become aware of the many ways in which their dysfunctional responses to emotional tensions and triggers perpetuate their difficulties, and how alternative ways of dealing with these tensions may improve their functioning and well-being. The main objectives of this supportive treatment refer to the patient's better functioning in the major areas of work and profession, love and sex, social life, and creativity, but with a clear recognition that improvements in love and sex may have the greatest limitations without the benefit of a more traditional psychoanalytic approach. Supportive psychotherapy may not be able to resolve the profound limitations in these patients' capacity to love and to integrate tenderness and sexual desire. This limitation notwithstanding, modifications of behavior that can be achieved in the areas of work and profession, social life, and creativity should provide a broad spectrum for areas of improvement.

Practically, therefore, the strategy of treatment would depend on highly individualized goals derived from a full assessment of the patient's present difficulties and the evaluation of his or her potential for resolving them to a lesser or greater extent. This relates to an immediate tactical aspect of the treatment at its very start, namely, the patient's potential in the therapist's fantasy. In other words, what does the therapist construct in his or her fantasy about the possibilities that this particular patient has to improving his or her limitations? What would the patient be able to do if he or she were not tied down by his characterological and symptomatic restrictions? A related countertransference issue involves the question: What would the therapist do if he or she were in the patient's body, exactly in his or her present position, but with the therapist's capacity to assess the situation and the knowledge of what he or she could do to improve it? These questions illustrate the importance of the initial countertransference reaction in terms of sympathy and antipathy, hope and skepticism, interest, or pity and despair that the patient may evoke for the therapist before more subtle aspects of transference developments take over—in short, a realistic establishment of treatment goals in the mind of the therapist, which then can be discussed and negotiated with the patient. These agreed-on priorities are a modification of TFP in that the therapeutic goals from the outset are more modest than the aim of resolving identity diffusion and structural change.

Major Treatment Techniques in the Application of Supportive Psychodynamic Psychotherapy

A MODIFIED INTERPRETIVE APPROACH

Preliminary techniques of interpretation—that is, clarification and confrontation—are freely used to help the patient become fully aware of the meaning of his or her communications and interactions in the sessions, signaling both appropriate and inappropriate and clear versus problematic or confused aspects of the patient's narrative in an effort to clarify both the immediate reality of the therapeutic interaction and the reality of the interactions that the patient establishes in his or her environment. An important reminder to the therapist doing this work is, if you don't understand something, ask until you do. At this point, supportive psychodynamic psychotherapy (SPP) is modified from TFP in that the therapist would stop short of interpreting the unconscious meanings of the interactions and their relation to the patient's unconscious past. Interpretation at this level would be limited to one aspect of the transference, as follows.

TRANSFERENCE ANALYSIS

In contrast to standard TFP, transference analysis is *not* carried out systematically, and positive transference is used to sustain and reinforce the patient's capacity to respond positively to the supportive techniques that will be dominant in the therapist's repertoire. Used only in the case of manifest negative transference, full clarification and confrontation of it would be followed by an effort to explore its origin, inasmuch as the patient is able to do at a preconscious level, in order to reduce it. The therapist also would clarify the reality of the treatment situation, reducing the patient's misconceptions of their relationship and acknowledging his or her potential contribution to the patient's misconceptions. The therapist also must be alert to the degree to which the negative development in the transference might correspond to parallel negative interactions in the patient's external environment, to highlight them, and to attempt to reduce them in parallel to the reduction of the manifest negative transference in the treatment situation.

For example, one patient who presented significant difficulty in maintaining his erection during intercourse with his girlfriend assumed that I, in trying to obtain detailed information of the circumstances under which the patient would lose his erection, was being ironic and evinced an attitude of superiority, implicitly making fun internally of the patient's difficulty in his sexual life. The patient felt that I was questioning his manliness. As this became quite evident to me, I confronted him with the fact that this was a fantasy on his part and that as far as I could tell, there was no questioning in my mind of his masculinity, only an effort to find out what might be inhibiting him. This led to him talking about his parents' extremely critical attitude about his masturbatory behavior. I did not explore any further the evident transference implication of his fear of my critique but further explored in what way this fearfulness might have something to do with what happened to him in the relationship with his girlfriend. The patient then told me that when he would lose his erection she would smile, and he felt that she was looking down on him, not considering him fully as a man. He saw in her the same attitude he attributed to me of devaluing him because of his sexual difficulty. At that point, I told him that it seemed to me the most reasonable way to think of this was that she herself might feel insecure because she might feel that she was not able to attract him sufficiently for him to maintain his potency and that she might interpret his difficulty as if it reflected her insufficiency as a woman. The patient confirmed this, saying that occasionally when he had difficulty in achieving an erection and she had that same smile, it was true, now that I mentioned it, there was something helpless regarding that smile in her expression. Thus, the combination of exploration, "reduction" and "export" of the manifest negative transference complemented the utilization of a predominantly positive transference in carrying out this supportive technique.

ABANDONMENT OF TECHNICAL NEUTRALITY

Insofar as the therapist uses cognitive information and affective support, he or she is no longer in a position of technical neutrality and may at times clearly indicate to the patient what might have been a more appropriate behavior on the patient's part, or what indeed, in the therapist's view, was an inappropriate reaction of the environment, to which the patient reacted frightfully. One problem with this approach is the risk of infantilizing the patient by providing the patient with an excess of advice giving or guidance, thus bypassing the patient's responsibility for his or her own behavior; additionally, there is a risk that the abandonment of technical neutrality may foster countertransference acting out.

COUNTERTRANSFERENCE UTILIZATION

The therapist's ongoing internal explorations of countertransference reactions to the patient and to the specific transferences enacted in the treatment situation are crucial elements of the treatment, guiding the therapist in his or her reaction to the positive and negative transference developments and providing him or her with ongoing information about affective dominance in the therapeutic hours. This is an important component of the priority setting of interventions. In essence, countertransference exploration in SPP does not differ from its use in TFP (Yeomans et al. 2015).

CONFRONTATION OF PRIMITIVE DEFENSIVE OPERATIONS

The predominance of splitting-based defensive operations in severe personality disorders emerges clearly in the treatment developments of patients with borderline personality organization. Pervasive acting out, dissociated affect storms, severe paranoid transference developments, and somatization, all related to primitive defensive operations, also threaten the social survival of these patients and, not infrequently, the very continuity of the treatment.

Here, a reality-oriented, predictive discussion with the patient of the risk that his or her present reactions or planned behavior entails may directly address the potential consequences of behavior based on severely distorted assessment of internal and external reality. For example, a patient's provocative challenging behavior under the effects of projective identification may be reduced by pointing out the self-fulfilling risk of such behavior, the need for him or her to be alert to others' motivations that may not be related to the patient, alerting the patient to his or her demonstrated proneness to attribute negative intentions to the reaction of others.

One patient mentioned her frequent reactions with crying spells to critical observations of her supervisor at work. I became concerned with the effects of this behavior on the evaluation of her work performance. My pointing to her denial of the potential negative consequences of her emotional outburst at work (i.e., the threat of being fired as such regressive behaviors accumulate) helped her to exert more control over these outbursts, without my attempting to explore the patient's deeper unconscious wishes to provoke the supervisor and to be mistreated in turn. Another narcissistic patient's repeated tendencies to idealize women who then "disappointed" him after a few weeks could be "slowed down" by exploring the price he was paying for his desperate search for the "perfect" woman.

A supportive psychotherapeutic approach cannot bring about a fundamental change in a patient's capacity to love, but it can reduce the destructive effects of the denial of this emotional limitation. The general aspect of the technique of confronting primitive defensive operations may be defined as a "common sense" approach to the patient's characterological behavior pattern while respecting the unconscious roots of these defensive operations and their chronic and repetitive features. It is an effort to strengthen the adaptive behavioral potential of the patient by increasing his or her awareness of the destructive effects of the repetitive problematic behavior.

So far, we have discussed the application of the derivatives of basic psychoanalytic techniques within a supportive psychotherapeutic treatment. In the next subsection, we describe the specific supportive techniques that complement this treatment.

SUPPORTIVE TECHNIQUES

Supportive techniques include cognitive information and support, affective support, facilitating emotional abreaction, and direct or indirect interventions in the patient's social reality by means of orientation and advice to the patient or to auxiliary caregivers. When indicated, third persons involved in providing the patient support outside the sessions may be activated and their work reinforced. The therapist should feel free to interact directly with others in the patient's life if that seems indicated in terms of the overall strategy of the treatment, the general condition being that the patient either participates or is completely informed of the therapist's intervention with such third parties.

Supportive techniques involve ongoing detailed monitoring of the patient's life tasks, the completion of the recommended tasks set up in the treatment situation, and his or her participation in expected collaborative ways with the therapist's effort. All these supportive techniques relate directly to the initial contract setting, the conditions for limit setting, and identifying specific tasks that the patient is expected to carry out as part of the treatment arrangements.

Treatment Tactics

ASSESSMENT

An essential aspect of our supportive psychotherapeutic approach is a careful, detailed evaluation of the patient's present personality, mapping out all the symptoms, difficulties, and problems that the patient may have in any areas of living. We also try to obtain information about his or her physical condition, medical history, and ailments, and assess the responsibility that the patient takes toward his or her physical health. The method of structural interviewing that we have developed as part of TFP applies perfectly to the initial study of patients who will enter a supportive psychotherapeutic treatment.

ESTABLISHING PRIORITIES OF OVERALL INTERVENTIONS, PROGNOSIS, AND LIMITATIONS OF THE TREATMENT

It is essential to make a realistic assessment of what the patient's possibilities are and what his or her limitations are, and to have a full discussion with the patient regarding what in the therapist's view the patient can expect from the treatment. The patient's responsibilities in participating with the work of the treatment and under what conditions the treatment may achieve the desired changes should be clarified and agreed on. Later, under conditions of severe acting out, particularly with problems regarding the continuity of the treatment and risks of premature disruption, these initial discussions and clarifications may become useful in reminding the patient—again and again, if necessary—what the reasons for the treatment are and under what conditions the treatment may succeed.

On the basis of all the information initially obtained, the therapist may establish general priorities for his or her interventions, and these overall treatment tasks determine important criteria for interventions that are combined in each session with the priorities derived from the momentary affectively dominant subjects. In contrast to TFP, the highest consideration in SPP for the therapist's interventions is no longer only what is affectively dominant but a combination of such affective dominance and general treatment priorities.

CONTRACT SETTING AND TREATMENT FREQUENCY

The general conditions of treatment, its frequency, and ways of dealing with missed sessions should be discussed at the outset. Supportive psychotherapy may be carried out on a once-per-week basis but also at a higher—or lower—frequency. The consistent adherence to a predetermined minimal frequency becomes even more important than in TFP with its higher frequency.

FREE ASSOCIATION

The patient should receive instructions for carrying out modified free association. In practice, we tell the patient that in each session he or she should feel free to bring in whatever is worrying him or her most at that point, how his or her present difficulties are evolving, and, if there are no important issues on his mind, to talk freely about whatever emerges in the patient's mind in the session itself. In other words, the patient is instructed not to come with a fixed agenda while still being invited to talk freely about whatever worries he or she wants to bring up. The general intention is to help the patient come as close as possible to carrying out free association, knowing that it will be limited by pressures from the patient's immediate reality issues as well as by the therapist's selective interventions in terms of the therapist's own criteria.

SELECTED FACT

As mentioned previously, the therapist's criteria for intervention include the combination of the priorities for the treatment set at its initiation and the presently affective dominance, which are derived from the patient's verbal communication, nonverbal communication, and the countertransference that emerges in the session itself. From a practical viewpoint, the following are frequently competing priorities in the interventions of supportive psychotherapy:

a. Urgent issues in the patient's work or profession, determining his or her "social survival"
b. Problems in the patient's physical care, including the patient's not dealing appropriately with illness and his or her difficulty with preventing medical complications—in other words, "physical survival"
c. Problems in the patient's intimate relations, or "relationship survival," an area particularly difficult because of the limitations in supportive psychotherapy in affecting the patient's subjective, emotional reactions to partners and sexual objects in general[1]
d. Control of aggression against the self or others, or "control of self-destructiveness," which becomes particularly relevant in patients with severe, chronic self-mutilation[2]

---

[1]It is particularly in the case of patients with narcissistic personalities, with severe limitations in their capacity to love and to engage in stable intimate relations that integrate eroticism and tenderness, that the limitation of supportive psychotherapy becomes evident. This is a practical issue that may require the therapist to spell out in his or her own mind what can be expected in the treatment of this patient, and that, in turn, may involve serious, ongoing clarifications of existential decisions the patient may have to make on his or her own.
[2]This often involves certain narcissistic personalities, in which self-mutilation may reflect the gravity of illness and negative prognostic outlook of the case.

e. Control of antisocial behavior, or "legal survival" (may become an urgent task of the treatment)[3]

TRANSFERENCE MONITORING AND MANAGEMENT

As mentioned earlier, it is important to be alert to and to ventilate manifest negative transference to restore or maintain a workable positive transference relationship; this may take an extended time in some patients with very severe personality disorders who have already failed to respond in previous psychodynamic and cognitive-behavioral treatment models. Sometimes, open defiance and challenge dominate the sessions, and the patient may triumphantly confront the therapist with his or her assumed incapacity to help the patient. The reality-oriented reduction of manifest negative transference may include the therapist's pointing out repetitive aspects of the patient's behavior that replicate his or her conscious behavior toward others in the past. It is a clarification and deflection of the transference that is perfectly commensurate with a supportive approach. Under these circumstances, the main task is to discuss the situation in realistic terms, fully and patiently. It is important that the therapist be open, direct, tactful, and honest in his or her communications and not attempt to artificially foster a "therapeutic alliance."

Sometimes the task is to explore systematically with patience and respect for the patient all the reasons for the patient's convictions that he or she cannot be helped and that lead the patient to oppose actively all the interventions of the therapist. At times, it is helpful to make it very clear to the patient that, in effect, if the patient, for whatever reason, persists in rejecting everything that comes from the therapist, the treatment will not help. Acceptance of the fact that the treatment may not help the patient without manifestations of negative countertransference reactions or a sense of failure on the part of the therapist may help. To the contrary, the therapist's internal, tranquil acceptance that the treatment may not work, while still being interested in the possibility of studying whether something might still make it work despite everything, would reflect the therapist's appropriate way to deal with a rejecting onslaught.

It may become necessary for the therapist to also convey his or her questioning attitude regarding whether this treatment will be helpful to

---

[3]At times, this issue raises problems for the therapist in terms of his or her own risks and responsibilities in a particular case and may signal the need to obtain legal advice about the limits of the therapeutic situation.

the referral source, the patient's family, and/or any third party that would appear to exert pressure on the therapist to help the patient despite the patient's consistent rejection of help.

In other words, the therapist needs to be in emotional control of the situation, rather than under the combined pressures of therapeutic expectations from the social environment and an active opposition of the patient, who has the fantasy that he or she is defeating the therapist by resisting the treatment. The therapist may use selective communication of aspects of his or her countertransference reaction as part of the therapeutic intervention, if that would serve to reduce the emotional distortions the patient is inducing in the interaction, as part of the therapist's effort to reduce the intensity of the negative transference and to facilitate an improvement in the immediate therapeutic interaction.

This would seem a perfectly appropriate way of using one's countertransference under extremely negative conditions in an initial evaluation, but it raises the risk of the patient's exploiting this way of obtaining information about the therapist by escalating his or her own negative reactions. Accusations of the therapist's hostility, indifference, callousness, and so on may serve this purpose; therefore, the therapist must limit carefully such countertransference communications where they serve the obvious purpose of the patient's exercise of omnipotent control. While countertransference communication generally would not be indicated in supportive psychotherapy, selected communication of countertransference reactions either to deal with severe manifest negative transference or as part of a focused re-educative approach on the part of the therapist may be indicated, as long as the therapist is aware of the risks of the patient's exploiting this communication in the transference.

Under ordinary circumstances, in which, at least on the surface, there seems to be no urgent problem that requires immediate intervention regarding any aspect of the patient's external reality and positive transference manifestations seem affectively dominant in the session, the ventilation of the conscious aspects of the transference may be indicated. This includes the therapist's acknowledging the patient's good feelings toward him or her while realistically reducing excessive idealizations that increase the patient's feelings of inferiority and incompetence, and thus contributing to mitigation of the severe splitting processes that are typical of patients with severe personality disorder. There are other times in which, despite presence of transference manifestations in the hour, the urgency of a conflict in external reality may deter the therapist from bringing up the transference at that point unless it can be linked at a conscious level with the urgent issue enacted in the external environment.

THE THERAPIST'S RELATIONSHIP WITH THE EXTERNAL ENVIRONMENT

The degree to which the therapist requires information about the patient from the external environment in SPP is variable. There are patients who have no antisocial features and are honest and direct in reporting what is going on in their environment, and the therapist has a realistic feeling that he or she has a good sense of the ongoing developments in the patient's life. In other cases, particularly with patients who present severe antisocial features, who are dishonest, withhold information, or frankly lie, it may be indispensable to maintain an ongoing contact with family members or other important people in the patient's life. The therapist must make the decision as to what extent he or she needs to have periodic contacts with third parties to obtain information about the patient's life outside of sessions. This is a crucial aspect of the treatment of certain patients and must be made an indispensable condition for the treatment to take place. The treatment may stand or fall on the patient's authorization to the therapist for maintaining such a contact. As mentioned earlier, if such contacts are available and used freely, it is important to keep the patient fully informed and not to do anything for which the patient has not given full consent.

This issue is particularly relevant with adolescents with personality disorders, in which an open communication with parents, school, and other authorities must be shared with the patient. Assuming outpatient treatment is the appropriate level of care, it is important for the therapist to keep in mind that the adolescent patient's aggressive behavior toward others or self should, in theory, be or come under the patient's control, whereas the patient's subjective feelings of love and hatred cannot be manipulated behaviorally. The patient must be free to feel whatever he or she feels, but the patient is also responsible for his or her behavior, and this continues to be true throughout the entire treatment.

A prominent problem encountered in SSP is the presence of secondary gain of illness, a prognostically negative feature that is often, but not always, coupled with severity of antisocial behavior, another prominent problem seen in the context of severe personality disorders. Either of these features bodes ill for successful treatment, the more so if they are found to be co-occurring. It is important for the therapist to attempt to control and eliminate secondary gain as far as is possible. Secondary gain is involved most frequently in exploitation of the patient's family and/or state and social service agencies. The therapist may be of help to the family in reducing exploitation by the patient by being very direct in expressing his or her views and recommendations in this regard, again, with full awareness on the patient's part of what the therapist is doing. In the case of patients who obtain chronic subsidies from state or other social service agencies, it may be more difficult for the therapist to intervene, and patients may successfully exploit such systems under the erroneous assumption that severe personality disorders limit or contraindicate the possibility of work or studies.

It is important for the therapist to keep in mind that there is no reason why a patient should be declared unable to carry out ordinary work or studies because of a personality disorder. This is a general principle that may run against conventional understandings in certain subcultures and may provide a social reality militating against the possibility of treatment. There are cases in which the patient's passivity, supported by a long-standing external supportive declaration of his or her incapacity to work, maintains him or her in an inactive condition that serves as an obstacle to overall improvement. At a certain point, this societal or familial undermining of the patient's potential will limit what can be expected from the treatment and even may end the treatment.

One alternative to ending the treatment under such negative circumstances is the consideration of the patients as "lifers." If treatment continues, expectations must be sharply reduced. The treatment now requires a shift toward accepting the patient's limitations, with the therapist complementing social support by providing the patient with advice, prescribing medication if indicated, and fostering the patient's ability to make the best of what his or her life situation and personality permit. This treatment may be carried out at a reduced frequency—for example, once or twice per month—geared to deal with immediate life problems for which the patient may require and be able to benefit from some help, but without any further attempts to change the overall nature of the equilibrium between acting out of unconscious conflicts and the predominant defensive operations that maintain the status quo. It is desirable, if such a state of affairs is reached, to make very clear that the patient is being maintained in a chronic supportive counseling status that is not to be confused with the very active treatment ordinarily implied in SPP.

THE PATIENT'S RESPONSIBILITIES

A central aspect of SPP is the establishment of specific goals that focus on improving the patient's functioning in the major areas of his or her life: work and profession, love and sex, social life, and creativity. Realistic goals derive from the patient's potential, from his or her external reality, and, very importantly, from the therapist's expectations and confidence in what this patient might achieve if he or she were not limited by his or her characterological illness. These overall objectives may translate into complex tasks that must be fulfilled for their achievement, such as the patient returning to work, obtaining additional education or training, or completing or returning to school. In the interpersonal realm, treatment goals might involve, for example, the patient learning to function independently, learning ways in which serious conflicts in the relationship with a partner can be managed and crises avoided. The therapist's own life experience and his or her technical expertise and full, detailed assessment of the patient's present personality are crucial determinants in setting up concrete treatment goals and tasks for which the patient has to take responsibility. Supportive psychotherapy, therefore, is always a joint effort, a joint task, and not something that the therapist is doing while the patient is the passive recipient of it.

For example, one adolescent patient with an infantile personality disorder, less than average intelligence, chronic school failure, sexual promiscuity, and drug abuse assumed that her limited intellectual capacities would never get her through college. She was interested in becoming a nurse but thought she would never be able to achieve that. After discussing with her the nature of her intellectual difficulties and the fact that this meant that her efforts would have to be much greater than those of people for whom intellectual tasks came much easier, I insisted that she might be able, if she worked hard, to achieve a college education. She did enter college with the financial support of her parents, and during the treatment managed to do the very hard work that permitted her to successfully complete a college education. The confidence of the therapist that, given the right motivation, she would be able to do the very hard work necessary to keep up with college demands despite her intellectual limitations seemed a crucial feature in this case.

At the same time, it became clear that the sexual promiscuity of this patient involved an infantile effort to obtain a boyfriend, a dependent wish to fight off loneliness. We addressed, without exploring the profound masochistic features of her personality, how she would have to proceed about finding a boyfriend who might be interested in her beyond simply having sex on a few occasions. This became possible by "forcing her" to carry out hard studies while stimulating her openness and freedom in relating to men, which helped her to develop better criteria about who would be more acceptable and thus improved both of these areas of major difficulties. In the process, I also obtained her compliance with the strict requirement that she stop the use of all drugs ("You won't be able to make it in college while high on drugs"). A subtle but clear erotic transference was not explored, except in the indirect approach of reducing her guilt feelings related to her sexual life. This patient became used to the fact that, at least once a month, I would discuss with her in great detail her grades, difficulties in studying, and the number of hours she had spent doing the work. It became clear to her that therapy became another subject in which she had to perform in order not to fail. Her reward was the sense that the therapist shared with her the triumph around every grade and class that she successfully mastered.

In short, setting up of realistic tasks and ongoing monitoring of these tasks, together with attention to what is affectively dominant in the sessions, determines the priority of interventions in the therapeutic hours and summarizes the tactical approaches for this kind of treatment.

Overview of General Indications, Contraindications, and Frequency

As mentioned previously, SPP would be indicated for the lightest and the most severe cases of personality disorders, particularly for the very severe patients, in which various contraindications may be present regarding carrying out TFP such as practical impossibilities of treatment beyond one session per week or a history of no response to a broad spectrum of both psychodynamic psychotherapies and cognitive-behavioral therapies. At our hospital, we quite frequently see patients who have been treated with the usual type of generally supportive-expressive psychodynamic psychotherapy, TFP, mentalization-based therapy, dialectical behavior therapy, or cognitive-behavioral therapy. Usually, the severity of patients' aggression, severe antisocial features, uncontrollable secondary gain, and destructive factors in the family or the social environment contribute to these negative developments, and supportive psychotherapy along the lines mentioned here might become the treatment of choice or considered as a treatment of last resort.

The objectives of SPP are highly variable, from efforts to bring about radical improvement, to chronic support that is individually tailored, to the possibility of an alternative, final shift into maintenance counseling for "lifers." The antisocial personality proper represents, in our experience, a contraindication for any kind of psychotherapeutic treatment, but there are cases in which it is not clear whether this diagnosis can be confirmed at the beginning of the treatment. SPP may represent a diagnostic trial under such uncertain circumstances to explore the possibility of whether the patient still can be helped. Some patients with uncontrollable secondary gain may be started in treatment with the understanding and agreement that elimination of that secondary gain is a treatment goal. The patient's capacity to work collaboratively toward that goal will provide an answer as to whether he or she still might be helped with SPP. Finally, there are patients who, without presenting an antisocial personality proper, suffer from antisocial behavior that interferes to such an extent with honest communication in the therapeutic hours that a psychotherapeutic approach becomes practically impossible.

As mentioned before, SPP may be carried out on a once-per-week basis. The basic rationale for this position is that, insofar as the transference is not expected to be fully deployed and systematically interpreted, supportive measures may be employed quickly to deal with major crises and urgent life problems. We try to help the patient to manage his or her ongoing conflicts while monitoring his or her capacity to do that by ongoing review of the accomplishment of the jointly agreed-on tasks or the failure to achieve them. Supportive psychotherapy based on these principles may be carried out at a higher frequency. The question then arises as to whether this might not be an indication, after all, to attempt to change personality more radically using TFP proper.

Comparison of Supportive Psychodynamic Psychotherapy and Transference-Focused Psychotherapy

It may be helpful to summarize commonalities and differences between these two related treatments. Both TFP and SPP are based on an equally extended, in-depth diagnostic evaluation, with a crucial mapping out of all the patient's life problems in the different areas of the patient's functioning. Both treatments attempt to establish priorities of interactions that need to be explored and potential limitations given the nature of the pathology, the patient's personality, and the treatment situation. Both treatments have as major prognostic limitations the negative effects of secondary gain and antisocial features, particularly patients' dishonesty, that may limit the capacity for the therapist to contain the total therapeutic situation.

Major differences between these treatments include the following: In SPP, the need for information about the relations with the external environment becomes maximal, much greater than in TFP. Within the treatment sessions, SPP has a more complex set of priority of interventions in each session. In TFP, affective dominance is the main criterion for priority setting, except under certain well-defined emergencies. In contrast, in SPP, the therapist needs to be aware of affective dominance as well as how the patient is carrying out the major treatment tasks, and what the present emergencies in his or her real life are (i.e., the "survival" issues). The interference in the sessions by the enactment and acting out of manifest negative transference needs to be reduced and/or deflected. SPP may require faster decision making and crisis intervention, and any disruption, such as a cancellation of sessions for whatever reason, creates a longer and more risky gap in the treatment.

SPP requires the therapist continuously to evaluate what has been learned and what has changed from session to session and to recognize when the therapy is at risk because basic conditions for carrying it out have been affected. SPP is very much geared to improve the patient's functioning but is not invested in basic personality change. Intense consultations involving external reality and monitoring of the patient's tasks and difficulties tend to eliminate technical neutrality, an essential aspect of supportive psychotherapeutic treatment that creates the danger of countertransference acting out and patients' infantilization. Patient and therapist will have to assess and live up to "common sense" to a maximum in SPP, and the therapist must be aware of the risk that his or her own value system may pose in the areas of ethics, sex, religion, and so on. The direct environmental intervention by the therapist also differentiates SPP from TFP.

Finally, there are basic similarities between SPP and TFP, namely, the ongoing monitoring of the transference, and even the selective management of potential role reversals in the transference in SPP, so long as the general rule of lack of transference interpretation is followed. Both these treatments are characterized by intense and sophisticated monitoring of countertransference and by the awareness of the dominance of splitting mechanisms in the case material. In SPP, the therapist partially accepts splitting mechanisms in the sense of the patient's identification of the therapist with a positive segment of internalized object relations while still encouraging the patient's reducing excessive idealization on the one hand and accepting the reality of manifest aggression in the transference on the other. This reduction of inappropriate idealization and limited tolerance of manifest aggression in the transference reduce the dominant primitive defenses based on splitting mechanisms.

References

Gill MM: Psychoanalysis and exploratory psychotherapy. J Am Psychoanal Assoc 2(4):771–797, 1954 13211443

Kernberg OF: Psychoanalysis, psychoanalytic psychotherapy and supportive psychotherapy: contemporary controversies. Int J Psychoanal 80(Pt 6):1075–1091, 1999 10669960

Kernberg OF, Burnstein E, Coyne L, et al: Psychotherapy and psychoanalysis: final report of the Menninger Foundation's Psychotherapy Research Project. Bull Menninger Clin 36:1–275, 1972

Kernberg OF, Yeomans FE, Clarkin JF, et al: Transference focused psychotherapy: overview and update. Int J Psychoanal 89(3):601–620, 2008 18558958

Rockland LH: Supportive Therapy for Borderline Patients: A Psychodynamic Approach. New York, Guilford, 1989

Yeomans FE, Clarkin JF, Kernberg OF: Transference-Focused Psychotherapy for Borderline Personality Disorders: A Clinical Guide. Washington, DC, American Psychiatric Publishing, 2015

PART III

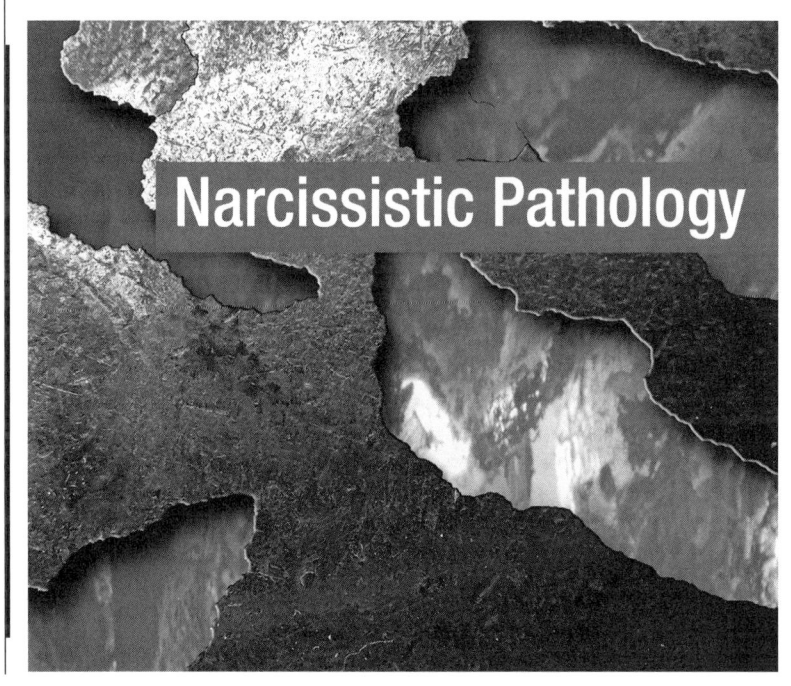

Narcissistic Pathology

CHAPTER 9

An Overview of the Treatment of Severe Narcissistic Pathology

This chapter is an overview of the pathology of severe narcissistic personality disorders, the common features of their transference developments in psychoanalysis and transference-focused psychotherapy (TFP), as well as differences in their clinical presentations and the corresponding implications for the technical approaches. It represents an expansion of both the theoretical framework and the clinical field explored in earlier contributions (Kernberg 2004, 2007) and reflects the technical developments of my approach to these patients, particularly in the interpretation of specific constellations of transference developments and the detailed interpretive integration of external reality into transference analysis. In this chapter, I present the various narcissistic syndromes that I will describe in order of increasing severity, beginning with narcissistic transferences at a high, stable level of functioning; next considering narcissistic transferences at a fluctuating, borderline level;

This chapter was originally published as Kernberg OF: "An Overview of the Treatment of Severe Narcissistic Pathology." *International Journal of Psychoanalysis* 95(5):865–888, 2014. Copyright © 2014 Institute of Psychoanalysis. Adapted with permission.

then considering extreme nondepressive suicidality and self-destructiveness; and finally turning to the antisocial dimension.

The integrated clinical-theoretical frame that I have constructed over several decades draws on the work of a number of authors who have described different constellations of severe narcissistic pathology and their clinical manifestations. As I outline the development of my own conceptual model, I will place my own thinking in relation to these authors' contributions and show how I have linked aspects of their work together with my own to form an integrated theoretical framework. I will also place this integrative model in relation to work of other authors who have contributed significantly to the delineation of clinical constellations of severe narcissistic pathology.

This work represents the experience of the Personality Disorders Institute of Weill Cornell Medical College in recent years and is an effort to integrate conceptually clinical syndromes, transference developments, and therapeutic approaches from a common theoretical perspective. It is based on the Personality Disorders Institute's experiences in carrying out both standard psychoanalysis and TFP with a broad spectrum of narcissistic patients, and exploring their commonalities and differences (Clarkin et al. 2006).

Our basic assumptions have evolved in the context of our experiences in treating a range of narcissistic pathology as follows: the so-called thin-skinned patients described by Rosenfeld (1987), patients with the syndrome of malignant narcissism described in earlier work (Kernberg 2007), chronically suicidal and self-mutilating patients with narcissistic pathology (Kernberg 2004), and patients with the "dead mother" syndrome described by André Green (1993b).

Before spelling out basic commonalities and specific differences of various constellations, I wish to summarize briefly a theoretical frame arrived at in the context of this work and applied to the understanding of the relationships of these syndromes. This frame should be considered a tentative hypothesis to be explored further regarding its validity, and the outline that follows should be considered as a tentative working document.

Our theoretical model is linked to a general hypothesis regarding the relationship of narcissism and aggression, and we believe that our clinical examples provide support for this hypothesis. Our views of basic Freudian drive theory are similar to the later formulations of André Green (Green 2007; Kernberg 2009). Green suggested that the gradual disappearance of references to narcissism after Freud's formulation of the dual drive theory reflected his awareness that the destructive nature of self-directed aggression, what Green has called the "narcissism of death," coincides with the death drive. In other words, the dual drive theory of libido and death implies that both libido and aggression are invested in the self (thus constituting elements of narcissism) and also invested in object relations (thus determining the profound struggle between love and hatred that lies at the bottom of object relations) as well as in the constitution of the self. Under normal circumstances, the shift from the schizoid/paranoid into the depressive position guarantees the dominance of libidinal investment in the self as well as in the relations with significant others. Under conditions of predominance of aggression, this may be reflected in a fixation at a level of primitive defensive operations and the corresponding identity diffusion typical of borderline personality organization. Alternatively, aggression may be condensed within the structure of a defensive, pathological grandiose self, constituting the basis of the most severe constellations of pathological narcissism.

Pathological narcissism is always characterized by the crystallization of a pathological grandiose self, but libidinal dominance in such a pathological structure gives origin to the better-functioning narcissistic personalities with effective defenses against the direct manifestation of aggression in their world of object relations. In contrast, the most severe cases of narcissistic personalities present a dominant infiltration of the pathological grandiose self with aggression. This may be reflected in the syndrome of malignant narcissism, in which aggression is still mostly directed against internalized object relations reflected in conflicts with the external world. In the most severe cases, aggression is directed not only against all internal relations with significant others but against the very self. Here we find the radical de-objectalization of the "dead mother" syndrome (discussed later in this chapter) and the severely self-mutilating narcissistic personalities.

Common Transference Features Reflecting the Pathological Grandiose Self

Although the clinical characteristics of narcissistic patients may vary widely depending on the degree of severity of the pathology and the regressive features of these patients, there are certain common transference developments that remain constant. They include the activation of a dominant transference relationship between a grandiose, entitled, superior self and a depreciated object that reflects the patient's pathological grandiose self, and a complementary, devalued, inferior, paralyzed counterpart that is usually projected onto the therapist but sometimes enacted by the patient himself or herself. This devalued object corresponds to the patient's own devalued, dissociated, projected, or regressed infantile self. In contrast to the typical activation of dissociated internalized relations between aspects of the patient's infantile self and his or her internalized dissociated object representations (i.e., self representation–object representation dyads), here the dyads were constituted by the relation between the pathological grandiose self and devalued self representations.

This constellation of grandiose and devalued self, however, may appear in different forms, depending on various associated characterological features. These features determine the types of narcissistic personality disorders described in the literature as the "thick-skinned" and "thin-skinned" narcissists, the "syndrome of arrogance," chronic nondepressive suicidality and parasuicidality, and narcissistic pathology with antisocial features.

In addition, patients in the narcissistic spectrum cannot depend on the therapist or analyst. His or her interventions are discarded, ignored, or distrustfully examined for anything "new" that the patient thinks he or she has not heard before. The patient does not feel understood or helped by the therapist's manifestation of interest and concern, and is unable to explore with curiosity what the analyst's comments may evoke in his or her mind. The patient talks either to himself or herself in the presence of the therapist or to the therapist to influence him or her in the direction the patient desires. As mentioned in earlier work (Kernberg 1984), this affects the countertransference reaction of the therapist in that it conveys the impression that the therapist really is alone in the room.

These two features (i.e., the activation of this particular self–self relationship in the transference and the patient's incapacity to depend on the therapist) differentiate narcissistic patients at all levels of severity of illness from the usual type of primitive, dissociated object relations activated in the psychoanalytic approach to patients with borderline personality organization. These narcissistic transferences, when dominant, require lengthy and consistent working through. What follows are particular forms these transferences take in different patient constellations and technical approaches to them that we have found helpful. In describing these constellations in a sequence of degrees of clinical severity, the emergence of predominant infiltration of the grandiose self with aggression in the severe realm of this pathology and the gradually predominant direction of this aggression against the self in the most severe cases will become apparent.

NARCISSISTIC TRANSFERENCES AT A HIGH, STABLE LEVEL OF FUNCTIONING

Standard psychoanalysis is generally indicated for narcissistic patients functioning at a relatively high level if some symptomatic difficulties motivate them to enter treatment.

Typical Transference Development

The dominant experience of the analyst with this type of narcissistic patient, initially, is as if there was no transference. In fact, the transference is between the pathological grandiose self that denies all dependency and an unimportant outsider, who might be useful as a source of admiration but is also potentially dangerous. The analyst, in the patient's mind, might replicate the patient's grandiosity, devaluing the patient in the process, or, under the effect of the patient's implicit devaluation of him or her, crumble and give the patient a sense of wasted time, emptiness, and disappointment in the treatment. It is as if the patient were defending himself or herself against the double danger of either being depreciated by somebody who acts superior to the patient, or wasting his or her time and money with a worthless therapist. Efforts to control the analyst—who should be as good as the patient but not better, because this would evoke envy or, worse, devaluation—characterize this transference. This dominant transference may remain stubbornly unchangeable over an extended time.

Narcissistic patients may perceive the treatment as "cognitive learning." They may be curious about interpretations as knowledge that they must learn and incorporate in order to not have any further need of the analyst and that typically, once absorbed, tends to be unconsciously devalued, with no felt need for further exploration by the patient. One patient carefully repeated my interpretations to him, "checking" their correctness or questionable nature. The same patient repeatedly experienced questions emerging in his or her mind about whether this particular session or a segment of a session was "good" or "useless." These patients are forced to carry out omnipotent control of the analyst to keep him or her within an acceptable range of value for them, and behind this control and distancing are powerful defenses against profound envy and resentment of having to depend on what the analyst presumably has to give and the patient needs.

This dominant relationship between the pathological grandiose self and an outsider to be controlled so that he or she does not become a replica of the devalued part of the self-concept may oscillate into its opposite (i.e., periods of feelings of inferiority, failure, and humiliation on the part of the patient, and fantasies of the analyst's grandiosity and contemptuous superiority now may dominate the picture). Upon systematic analysis of this transference, the relationship between the pathological grandiose self and the devalued self is gradually dismantled into its components, which are idealized representations of self and others that are enacted and/or projected by the patient.

As the pathological grandiose structure is dismantled, we see subtle shifts toward transferences that seem more object related, while they have a more primitive and predominantly paranoid character as the patient projects grandiose and threatening aspects of significant others of his or her past onto the analyst. One patient, a mental health professional whom I was treating in a relatively small town where the entire mental health community was familiar with one another, was spreading derogatory comments about me to a few colleagues. A few weeks later, he heard these same comments repeated by others, became frightened, and confessed them in a session. On exploration of this behavior, it turned out that he had been acting out an identification with his mother, whose chronic feelings of inferiority had motivated her to spread derogatory gossip regarding friends within her social circle. The patient then became afraid that I might be discussing his case with other colleagues.

The task now becomes to explore the gradual development of periods of rupture of the pathological grandiose self into these component internalized part-object relations and the correspondent unconscious conflicts involved. The treatment, over time, becomes more like that of ordinary borderline patients, in terms of split-off activation of idealized and persecutory relationships. Gradually, the underlying conflicts beneath the defensive structure of the pathological grandiose self may emerge, typically as intense primitive aggression linked to feelings of envy, a condensation of pregenital and oedipal conflicts, and the activation of traumatic early experiences against which the pathological grandiose self had become a major defensive structure.

Thick-Skinned Narcissists

There are other cases, however, where even careful, consistent interpretation of the defensive function of the grandiose self does not lead to a gradual shift into its internalized ideal self and ideal object components. Instead, severe splitting between periods of unremitting grandiosity and brief, dissociated, devastating experiences of self-devaluation, depression, and suicidal tendency requires very long term interpretive dismantling of a sadistically infiltrated grandiose self. The "thick-skinned" narcissistic personalities described by Rosenfeld (1987) belong to this group of patients.

These are patients who generally function quite well in their social and work life, but who are so bereft of an internal world of object relationships that they seem to be completely closed to the possibility of fantasy and daydreaming. They live in the concrete reality of their interactions with the analyst, which do not lead to any development of fantasy, desire, fear, or deeper conflict. The patients themselves may state freely that they see no reason why they should develop any particular emotional reaction to a relationship that, after all, follows the principles of a commercial contract in which "one person gets paid to take care of the problems of the other." A patient assured me that although I seemed like a nice person, if I died suddenly, he would have no particular feeling about it.

The patient's efforts to carry out free association may be severely distorted by his or her unwavering need to keep the analytic situation under control. Free associations are so well structured and orderly in sequence that they reveal an intentional effort to direct the analyst's attention in a certain direction, preconsciously planned by the patient. Or the patient's "checking" on the meaning of what he or she is saying while communicating it to the analyst may provide the patient's discourse with an empty, intellectualized quality.

I have found it helpful to analyze the defensive function of this way of associating by focusing on the patient's reactions to the analyst's interpretive interventions. The patient may simply ignore what the analyst says, resuming his or her monologue after a respectful brief silence, or examine carefully all the implications of the analyst's comments, speculate on their meaning, express agreement or disagreement, or dismantle the analyst's statement altogether—anything, really, to avoid being impacted by the analyst in a way that is not totally under the patient's control in an attempt to avoid a humiliating indication of his or her dependency on, and therefore inferiority to, the analyst. The interpretation of this constellation may allow the patient to become aware of his or her need to control the analytic relationship implied in the style of carrying out free association.

An additional helpful technical approach to these patients may be to analyze in great detail their difficulties outside the transference situation, the details of their difficulties in work, in intimate sexual relations, in their social life, and with their families. It is usually not difficult for patients, by sharply focusing on the areas of daily conflicts in their lives, to gradually open up their understanding of aspects of their interactions that are motivated by emotional pressures and deeper fears or desires, which can then be linked to similar manifestations that in subtle ways emerge in the transference. The "microscopic" analysis of extratransferential relations allows for gradual exploration of the transference itself. For example, behind the indifference toward their partners, one may detect the emergence of envy of the other person's capacity for love and friendship and the freedom to have an interesting daily world of experiences from which the patient is excluded.

The indifferent patient I referred to above bitterly resented his wife talking animatedly for hours with her friends by phone, comparing it with his own restrictions and limitations in such interesting interchange with acquaintances. Similarly, behind the admiration and sexual excitement involved in their transitory infatuations, one may discover and highlight for the patient resentment of an exciting, teasing, and withholding other, and its repetition of past similar experiences with significant objects of childhood and infancy. The development of negative therapeutic reactions in the sessions, reflecting unconscious wishes to devalue the treatment following moments of envious recognition of the therapist's capacity to help and be interested in them, offers another entrance into this transference development. Above all, these patients constantly need to compare themselves with others. The fluctuations between triumphant superiority and anxious fear of being devalued are dominant issues in the extratransferential relations to be explored, providing a bridge to the later exploration of similar issues in the transference.

NARCISSISTIC TRANSFERENCES AT A FLUCTUATING, BORDERLINE LEVEL

In our research projects studying the treatment of borderline personality disorders with TFP, we found a significant number of borderline patients with predominant narcissistic transference developments, and became more able to identify patients with narcissistic personality disorders functioning at an overt borderline level as well as patients whose symptoms centered on inordinate arrogance and aggressiveness and patients with the syndrome of malignant narcissism (Clarkin et al. 2006; Kernberg 2004, 2007).

Patients with severe clinical syndromes may present indications for psychoanalysis or psychoanalytic psychotherapy, but when they appear as descriptively "borderline"—that is, with a general chaos of behavior patterns and breakdown in social life, work, love, and sex—they may optimally be treated with TFP (Clarkin et al. 2006). This is particularly true when they present prognostically negative features such as the infiltration of the pathological grandiose self with severe, ego-syntonic aggression toward others or self, chronic suicidal behavior, and, particularly, antisocial behavior.

The contribution of aggression directed against others or self, severe paranoid traits, and antisocial behavior constitutes the syndrome of malignant narcissism (see Chapter 11, "The Differential Diagnosis of Antisocial Behavior"). Although malignant narcissism is at the boundary of treatability, TFP may be indicated if a clear framework and structure for the conduct of the treatment can be established and maintained.

Within this most severe group of narcissistic patients we find other typical developments in the transference that correspond to the thin-skinned narcissistic personalities (Rosenfeld 1987), the syndrome of arrogance (Bion 1967), or an almost psychotic level of social functioning by patients who have zero tolerance for any triangulation (Britton 2004). Some of these patients present a severe, chronic self-destructiveness with a significant risk of suicide (Kernberg 2007). Indications for specific treatments and complications in the treatment, prognosis, and technique are affected by the variables of the degree of superego integration, antisocial behavior, paranoid tendencies, the ego-syntonic nature of aggression, and chronic manifest self-destructive suicidal and parasuicidal behavior.

Thin-Skinned Narcissists

Thin-skinned narcissists are more severely regressed and often fail in analytic treatments but respond well to TFP. They present both severe infiltration of the pathological grandiose self with aggression and a structural weakness of the pathological grandiose self, so that shifts from states of arrogance, superiority, and contemptuous feelings about the analyst to severe feelings of inferiority, humiliation, depression, self-accusation, and suicidal tendencies may occur frequently and rapidly. Such shifts, sometimes, are motivated by minor sources of triumph or defeat, and their hypersensitivity to any experienced criticism, real or fantasized. Their clinical presentation evinces severe characterological depression or chronic dysthymic reactions, suicidal tendencies, and marked identity diffusion—despite the pathological grandiose self, reflected in absence of goals, uncertainty, and confusion about their life direction and relations. Ego-syntonic sadistic features are both expressed and projected onto the therapist, who is frequently perceived as a seductive, scheming, and dishonest persecutor. These are patients with rapid changes in transference developments, extreme frustration for not being able to totally control the therapist in terms of his or her thinking or behavior, and angry outbursts of total devaluation of the therapist and wishes to interrupt the treatment. Their contemptuous attitude may take the form of accusing the therapist of not understanding anything, projecting onto the therapist the confusion in their own relationships with significant others, and heightened paranoid tendencies in the transference.

Often these are patients who have been severely traumatized by physical or sexual abuse or gross neglect in their infancy or early childhood. Their unconscious tendency to reactivate these traumatizations in the transference both conveys important information about the past and poses difficulties because of their high potential for acting out. These are the patients for whom John Steiner (1993) recommended to interpret "in the projection," clarifying their experiences and views of the analyst rather than interpreting what is being projected into the analyst. This corresponds to an extremely effective technical approach of TFP whereby the therapist points out, at every opportunity, the kind of relationship that the patient's experience is activating in the transference, with attention to how the same relationship tends to get activated, again and again, with role reversals. In the role reversal, the patient experiences himself or herself in the role of the internal object representation, a role that he or she had previously projected onto the therapist while remaining identified with an aspect of his or her self. Now, however, the self-aspect is projected into the object, the patient can experience what he or she had previously projected into the object, and the full nature of what had been projected may become available to the patient's subjective experience.

For example, a patient thought that the therapist showed a sarcastic and depreciatory behavior toward him. Enraged, he became extremely critical and derogatory toward the therapist, treating the therapist as totally worthless, dishonest, and not understanding. Again, 10 minutes later, the patient had a sense that he was being treated in exactly the same way by the therapist. By highlighting the patient's grandiose, devaluing experience with a perceived worthless or despicable therapist, without attempting to directly explain this as a projection, but showing that it was a reversal of the patient's experience of having been attacked by the therapist in similar superior and derogatory ways that preceded it, the role reversals could be interpreted and the interpretation of projective identification thus completed. Feelings of having been attacked motivated the counterattack by the patient, and the counterattack motivated fears that the therapist, in turn, would take revenge in the same way, so that vicious cycles were generated by which the same relationship got enacted, again and again, with such role reversals.

The patient's contemptuous, derogatory attitude toward the therapist could gradually be interpreted as a protection against the activation of an opposite role relationship. It also became easier to interpret brief periods of idealized relations with the therapist as a combination of actual recognition of something good going on in the relation and an effort, on the patient's part, to protect himself against the bad and frightening experiences at those other moments of alternating, mutual devaluation. In our experience, a consistent interpretation of the split transferences, with particular consideration of the involvement of an easily fragmented pathological grandiose self, has been very helpful with thin-skinned narcissistic patients. At the same time, whenever what occurs in the transference seems to be a practical repetition of past experiences that the patient has been conscious of at different moments, this lends itself to a complete interpretation of the genetic aspects of the patient's conflicts that have become an emotional reality rather than a defensive intellectualization of the patient's remembered or reconstituted past.

Rosenfeld (1987) suggested that thin-skinned narcissistic patients who had experienced severe traumatizations in their past might be retraumatized by the analyst's interpretations of their aggressive conflicts in the transference. In our experience, the clarification of the dominant transference "in the projection," without full interpretation of the projective identification at that point, permits completion of the interpretation once the reciprocal activation of self and object representation in the transference has taken place. This TFP-derived technique permits the therapist to carry out a systematic interpretive approach to extremely negative transferences without the patient's experiencing this interpretation as an attack. Here, I agree with Steiner (2008), who questions Rosenfeld's excessive caution in interpreting negative transference developments in these patients.

The Syndrome of Arrogance

Bion (1967) has described the *syndrome of arrogance* in severely regressed patients, consisting of 1) an openly aggressive and extremely arrogant behavior toward the therapist; 2) incapacity for any cognitive reflection, so that the patient appears to be "pseudo stupid"; and 3) an inordinate curiosity about the therapist rather than one's self. Bion describes the projection of these characteristics into the analyst and proposes as an essential dynamic of this situation: the activation of the frustrated baby's rage at an impatient mother who would talk to him or her without really understanding the baby and "stupidly" expects the baby to respond as verbally as she addresses the baby. It implies the projective identification of a destructive, sadistic object interfering with the communicative aspects of projective identification. The analyst's containing this projection of an extremely destructive internal object geared to eliminate all verbal communication would be the key to managing this situation. In our experience, it reflects the chronic enactment in the sessions of primitive hatred and envy, but with the characteristic that the aggression is acted out without the patient's having any self-reflective awareness of it. The arrogant behavior expresses his or her combative aggressive needs: the need to not demonstrate any capacity for cognitive communication with the therapist, the desperate effort not to have to acquire any awareness of the significance of his own behavior, and the need to control the therapist to avoid the projected and feared aggression to return in the form of counterattacks from the therapist.

I have found that the best way to manage this syndrome, which presents in some of the most severe types of narcissistic regression, is a combination of interpretation and maintaining firm boundaries of the treatment situation. The therapist needs to set very clear limits regarding how far the patient may express his or her aggression verbally, without attacking the therapist, or the office, physically or invading the therapist's space outside the sessions, so that the attacks are limited to an extent that can be contained in the therapeutic sessions. At the same time, the therapist's focus needs to be on the patient's intolerance to recognize the sadistic pleasure that he or she obtains from the aggressive behavior. The defense against the fear of recognition of the pleasure in his sadistic behavior, when it is overcome, permits the patient to accept that pleasure without fear of retaliation or guilt. By the same token, this acceptance tends to reduce the intensity of the aggression, opening the possibility of studying the origins of that reaction in the transference.

One of our patients cut the plants in her therapist's office and abused him verbally in public spaces, but eventually she was able to acknowledge and explore her pleasure in these attacks as an unconscious identification with a sadistic aunt who had dominated her childhood and had been extremely physically abusive. The decomposition of the pathological grandiose self into its component internalized object relations—in this case, the activation of the sadistic aunt identification—signals the resolution of the structure of the pathological grandiose self during transference interpretation.

There are patients who function at a much higher level, with much better control of their behavior inside and outside the sessions, but in whom the attitudes of contempt, devaluation, and depreciatory competition with the therapist go with periods of self-contempt, despair, and suicidality under the effects of this self-contempt. These patients usually have strong paranoid tendencies and tend to justify their contemptuous behavior through intellectual debates with the therapist that are expressed in combatively arrogant attitudes. This same contempt creates severe conflicts at work, in the social sphere, and in intimate relations. With these higher-functioning patients, the contemptuous behavior and arrogance is less intense and overwhelming than in the regressed arrogant patients; nonetheless, it is very clear to the analyst that he or she is being treated contemptuously and clear to the patient that he or she is doing that, so that, in the short run, this is open to transference exploration. However, the extended duration of unrelenting contempt may undermine the analyst's positive disposition toward the patient, which is one of the unconscious objectives of this transference development: both revenge against hated parental images and, at bottom, a desperate effort to still maintain a good relationship with the analyst and not be abandoned, despite this behavior.

One such patient came to us after a series of previous analysts, all of whom she ridiculed to other persons outside the treatment. Upon settling to work with a member of our group, she was highly contemptuous of him as well and bad-mouthed him for quite some time before this behavior became evident and could be explored in the transference. Another patient secretively bought a complete set of CDs to train therapists in cognitive-behavioral psychotherapy, cheerfully arguing with the therapist over weeks about the limitations of his analytically oriented approach. The working through of these issues in the transference and the consistent interpretation of all the implications and features of the patient's arrogance and contempt may resolve the problem, but at a significant cost of the analyst's working through the corresponding countertransference reactions. Over time, these patients manage to significantly challenge the analyst's self-regard and confidence in his or her work.

In fact, the tolerance of the countertransference may become quite a central issue in such cases. When patients involve third parties (e.g., complaining to relatives and to other therapists, requesting consultations to protest about the way they are being treated), it is particularly difficult to maintain a technically neutral stance. It may become necessary in some cases to establish limits to the patient's behavior, geared to permit the indispensable sense of security—physical, emotional, professional, legal—the therapist needs to maintain his or her position of concerned objectivity. The therapist's capacity to evaluate what enactments and projective identifications are activated in the transference/countertransference developments needs to be protected.

At all levels of narcissistic pathology, the mechanism of omnipotent control represents an important unconscious effort on the patient's part to prevent change to occur—to "freeze" the therapeutic situation—as a crucial attempt to protect the patient's identification with his or her pathological grandiose self. At "higher" levels of narcissistic pathology, this may take the form of idiosyncratic convictions such as political ideologies or highly personal thought systems, even in persons with otherwise excellent reality testing. At the borderline level of narcissistic pathology examined here, these personal thought systems may take on a quasi-delusional quality and may serve to protect the patient's conviction of his or her intellectual superiority. One patient was convinced that any love for a woman signified an inferiorizing weakness; another patient was convinced that he was the greatest artist in his field and that all experiences to the contrary were engineered by fellow artists who envied him. These beliefs had the effect of preventing the therapy from having any impact on the patient and protecting the grandiosity. The development of "incompatible realities" in the transference, and the technique used under this condition that has been described in earlier work (Kernberg 2004, 2007), may become an important aspect of transference analysis of these cases.

Intolerance of Triangulation

An extreme form of omnipotent control may evolve as part of the intolerance of triangulation (Britton 2004) in very regressed narcissistic patients. *Intolerance of triangulation* refers to a particularly severe distortion of internalized object relations, a regression within which the patient cannot tolerate any thoughts that are different from his or her own. The role of the therapist is to confirm the view of the patient and to assure the patient of the reality and stability of that shared experience. Any contribution from the therapist that is at variance with the patient's thinking is destabilizing to the patient's grandiose self and carries malignant implications. At bottom, it is the search for a perfect symbiotic relationship within a dyad that does not tolerate the disruption by a third, excluded object and represents the fragile omnipotence of a pathological grandiose self that attempts to maintain absolute control over experienced reality. Here, archaic oedipal conflicts (i.e., the intolerance of the relation between the parental couple from which the infant feels excluded) surface in the transference as the envious resentment of the therapist's relation to an internal object of his or her own (his or her independent thinking, theory, or reflection about what is going on in the relation with the patient), making different perspectives intolerable to the patient.

Efforts by the therapist to bring in views different from that of the patient are experienced either as a total abandonment and rejection or as a sadistic intrusion, an aggressive effort to control the patient's mind. This situation, originally described by Britton (2004), may even be observed in patients functioning at a relatively high level within the spectrum of narcissistic pathology, in which it is revealed in very subtle ways of rejection of the therapist's independent thinking by highly sophisticated maneuvers that reassert the patient's initial views and force the therapist into a temporary emotional retreat. But this condition emerges as well with extremely regressed narcissistic patients functioning on an overt borderline level, in which the patient's experience of reality has such an extremely distorted quality that it is close to psychotic.

In this latter case, the patient may be totally convinced of the realistic nature of an emotional experience, within which the patient's behavior may have been extremely inappropriate and practically psychotic in the context of its social surround. Here, any effort of the therapist to probe reality testing may be experienced as an attack, bringing about a rageful effort by the patient to shake off the intrusion.

One patient maintained an almost delusional conviction that a man, who was obviously exploiting her and showed his indifference at every turn, was in love with her. In turn, she treated the therapist who was trying to confront her with her illusions as if *he* had a totally unrealistic view of reality. This woman functioned remarkably well in other areas of her life. Another patient with severely overt borderline functioning created such a disruption at a family funeral that family members escorted him away from the grave. In the subsequent sessions, he raged against his family's callous indifference to his intense suffering and would become incensed by any effort by the therapist to tactfully question whether, under the circumstances, the expression of his mourning had acquired characteristics that were, in fact, quite problematic and socially inappropriate.

A technical approach that has been helpful with these conditions is enormous patience and consistency in pointing out to the patient the fact that any view that is different from his or her own creates an intense pain, as if the patient's thinking or very capacity to deal with reality were questioned, so that the patient has to protect himself or herself against such a dangerous assault. To the patient, it seems to be a case of the therapist trying to drive the patient mad. The analyst needs to spell out gradually the nature of the danger that is creating panic in the patient: the fear of a total disqualification of his or her capacity to think, of total abandonment and loneliness, and of the patient's own intense enraged reaction to this dangerous situation, along with his or her fantasies of the sadistic intention of an imaginary outsider—who seems to be committed to destroying the safety of the patient's earlier experience—and the therapist's collusion with such an enemy. By its absence, in these cases the situation described points to the importance of the existence of a "three-person psychology," which constitutes the basis of a therapeutic relationship, and the resolution of this severe regression marks an important improvement for these patients.

The concept of the *three-person psychology* refers to the consideration of the therapeutic relationship as determined by, at a minimum, the transference, the countertransference, and the analyst/therapist's position as an "excluded third party"—that is, that part of the analyst's personality able to explore the transference/countertransference relationship without being immersed in it (Kernberg 2012). It is a reflection of an internal split in the analyst's ego in relating to the patient that gets "obliterated" again and again in countertransference enactments and in the developments of projective counter-identifications (Grinberg 1979). At a deeper, symbolic level, the three-person psychology refers to the oedipal structuralization of the analytic relationship and the potential for intolerance of the oedipal situation in regressive, symbiotic transferences. At this symbolic level, the patient becomes the excluded third party, the infant excluded from the relationship of the parental couple. This is the case of the patients described by Britton (2004).

EXTREME NONDEPRESSIVE SUICIDALITY AND SELF-DESTRUCTIVENESS

Severe Narcissistic Suicidality

It usually is not difficult to differentiate the chronic suicidal and parasuicidal behavior of patients with severe personality disorders without dominant narcissistic features from that of narcissistic personalities functioning on an overt borderline level. Nondepressive suicidal behavior of patients with borderline personality disorders usually is impulsive, an equivalent or symptom of an acute affect storm, related to a frustrating, enraging, or traumatizing experience, or an effort to influence or control a close family relative or love/hate object. Conversely, chronic suicidal or parasuicidal behavior of patients with narcissistic personality disorders evolves slowly and in a determined way over a period of weeks or months and is prepared and carried out in what impresses an observer as a cool and deliberate plot, quite often in the context of surface behavior that is seemingly friendly and relaxed. Patients with this extreme degree of severity of narcissistic pathology differ from the constellation in whom suicidal behavior is part of severely disturbed, aggressive, and shifting moods with strong depressive features. Here, in contrast, suicidal and parasuicidal behavior—even severe self-mutilation—punctuate a generally stable, seemingly normal behavior.

From a psychodynamic and transferential perspective, this behavior reflects a deep and consistent aggressive devaluation of the external world, a radical devaluation of significant others and the self, a "negative narcissism," in Green's (1993b) terms, with a patient's profound sense of superiority derived from overcoming all feelings of fear of pain and death, all feelings of needs involving others, and a sense of omnipotence by controlling one's own death as a final, absolute power and freedom. This general transference disposition takes many different forms. The therapist's capacity, within his or her countertransference reaction, to empathize with this terrible psychological reality of the patient, with that part of the patient identified with a self-murderous grandiose self, may become a crucial aspect of transference interpretation. The therapist is a natural enemy of that internal object, and a major question arises as to whether the therapist has any ally in the patient's mind: Is there some way to contact the patient's oppressed, tenuous wish to survive? Highlighting this potential internal conflict in the patient's mind as it becomes activated in the transference, a true struggle between the death drive and the wish to live, is a major therapeutic task in these cases.

For example, one of our patients chronically ingested rat poison to try to kill herself. Despite careful searches, carried out during her hospitalization at our service, it was not possible to find the source for obtaining the poisonous substance. The patient denied her continuous ingestion of the poison, while the serum prothrombin gradually increased over days. She had a history of severe internal hemorrhages that required extensive diagnostic and therapeutic interventions, and, in the middle of all this, she maintained an apparently calm and almost cheerful attitude that belied the extreme gravity of her condition.

Another patient carried out severe self-mutilations, cutting tendons, which led to the loss of fingers, and attempted to set herself on fire, creating a near catastrophe that threatened the life of numerous people living in her apartment building. Sometimes her self-destructive attempts were serious parasuicidal behaviors, such as profound self-cutting that occurred in the middle of what seemed perfectly relaxed and adaptive behavior by the patient. Still another patient went out with her sister to go shopping, spent what appeared to be a very pleasant afternoon with her, and, after getting back home, retired to her bedroom. Her sister approached her to share with her some of the objects they had bought and found her sister with multiple cuts on both arms, bleeding heavily, and requiring major interventions at an emergency service.

There are patients who deny their suicidal intentions and preparations and convey a sense of triumph in their capacity to shock the unsuspecting therapist with their behavior. Other patients may talk freely about their suicidality, while implying that it is beyond their control and that for the time being they are not in touch with that part of themselves that wishes them to be dead. The implicit attack on family and on the therapist in such behaviors often remains unconscious, but at times is accompanied by a sense of sadistic satisfaction and triumph. At the same time, patients may unconsciously bring about situations in which their suicidal behavior would seem to reflect some neglect or insufficient alertness on the part of the therapist, and families may become enraged at what they perceive as the therapist's failure to contain or prevent the patient's behavior. Some patients triumphantly point out that their behavior is not only not under their own control but not under the therapist's either and thus reflects the therapist's impotence and incompetence. We have all seen cases in which family members unwittingly collude with the patient to blame the therapist and then move on to find another. The patient, in the role of a "serial killer" of therapists, thus experiences an unconscious sense of triumph at having "killed off" another therapist.

The combination of severe self-destructive tendencies and antisocial tendencies may be expressed in provocative and litigious behavior, blaming the therapist for not having been attentive to the risk of a severe suicidal attempt by the patient, indirectly exerting an omnipotent control over the therapist by means of induction of paranoid fears and guilt feelings. Here, the aggressively infiltrated pathological grandiose self provides the patient with an illusionary power, not only over the therapist, but over life and death over pain and suffering, and opens an escape into a "liberating" death from a world that cannot be controlled.

In a randomized controlled trial comparing TFP, dialectical behavior therapy (DBT), and supportive psychotherapy based on psychoanalytic principles (SP), we found that TFP was as effective as DBT in reducing suicidal and parasuicidal behavior, in contrast to SP, which was less effective. Only TFP increased mentalization (Kernberg et al. 2008).

I believe that it is important that the therapist accept honestly, in his or relationship with the patient and the patient's family, and in the elaboration of his or her countertransference, the possibility that the patient may commit suicide and that the treatment may not be able to prevent it. The therapist may have to acknowledge openly, in diagnostic sessions with the patient and the family, that outpatient psychotherapeutic treatment carries a serious and unavoidable risk of suicide, given the patient's severe condition, and yet may be still preferable to the long-term, indefinite duration of hospitalization. The fact that here suicide is neither predictable by the presence of severe depression nor preventable because of its deep characterological basis may have to be made explicit verbally and, at times, in documentation that protects the therapist legally. At the same time, the patient's knowledge that he or she will not be able to blackmail the therapist with suicidal threats may reduce the secondary gain of this symptom and limit the patient's sense of omnipotence. The therapist needs to be assured of his or her own physical, psychological, and legal safety to be able to be dedicated to helping these extremely difficult patients.

In all these cases, one must interpret openly and calmly that the patient, while willing to undergo a psychotherapeutic treatment that he or she hopes to bring about improvement of his or her condition, is nonetheless under the sway of powerful and destructive internal forces. An acknowledgment of objective concern (the excluded third) for the patient's self-destructiveness conveys the possibility of discussing destructive impulses openly to assure the patient that one respects the severity of his or her condition and the power of this part of him or her. The need to protectively dissociate the destructive part of himself or herself from the apparently "cheerful" participation at other moments in the treatment can be clarified and resolved, and the patient's open acknowledgment of his or her dominant self-destructive motivation becomes the main issue to be explored in the sessions.

An important related technical requirement is the exploration of the patient's apparent absence of concern over this terrible control that the part of him or her wishing to die has over whatever part wishes to remain alive and the reasons for the devaluation and implicit hatred of that part that wishes to be alive. Here, the gradual discovery of the dangers of remaining alive, the terrible suffering related to the implied loss of control and superiority that is implied in identification with death, having to experience oneself alone and abandoned, having to face envy toward people not condemned to such self-induced destruction—all may emerge in the context of more specific aspects of the patient's infantile and childhood history. Sometimes, the patient unconsciously hopes for an omnipotent good object that will rescue him or her from that desperate state and projects his or her own omnipotence to an illusional godlike rescuer. This fantasy, in turn, needs to be explored for its potentially self-destructive implications.

The "Dead Mother" Syndrome

A related group of patients, who on the surface seem much less severely ill but at a deeper level evince a relentless determination to destroy all relationships, the efforts of the therapist, and even their own sense of being alive, is reflected in the syndrome of the "dead mother" described by André Green (1993a, 1993b). Under these conditions, there is a rejection of any significant relationship out of identification with an internalized imago of a dead mother, frequently derived from the early experiences with a severely depressed, unavailable mother. The patient unconsciously attempts to maintain the relationship with this absent, nonresponsive mother, unconsciously enacting the fantasy that in his or her own emotional death and loss of self, he or she will be reunited with an idealized mother and protected from any further suffering. To give up one's own existence as an autonomous self, one's own need to depend on anybody else, to devalue completely all representations of significant others would, in the fantasy of these patients, provide definite restfulness, security, and equanimity. These are patients who may, on the surface, attentively listen to the therapist's interpretations and then react, saying, "All this is very interesting, but doesn't touch me at all." Their attitude of "So what?" in response to interpretations is persistent and unmovable. By the unconscious dismantling of all relationships, what Green (1993b) calls "de-objectalization," they obtain the same effect as patients whose repeated severe attempts at self-destruction reflects their dominant motivation in life.

De-objectalization refers to an extreme manifestation of the death drive, whereby an attack is leveled against the very structures of the mind that sustain introjective processes and permit the establishment of representation of self and object within an internal space. As an ultimate defense against intolerable dominance of aggression over libidinal investments, the patient's very capability to experience an internal world is attacked: the sense of time is frozen, the aggressive and libidinal investments of object and self are dismantled, and a total void occupies the mind (Green 1993b, 2010). This self-destructiveness, in Green's view, goes far beyond masochism. In our experience, these patients are remarkably free of conscious awareness of both aggressive and libidinal impulses. Often effective in their work and superficial social relationships, they are basically loners and convey a sense of total isolation and lack of interest to live. They are not depressed, and the initial depressive countertransference reaction they evoke in the analyst shifts, over time, into a sense of exhaustion and emptiness. If it becomes possible during lengthy treatment to unmask their unconscious efforts to deaden the relation with the analyst as a defense against severe frustrations in their need for love and dependency, and to explore the aggressive resentment of the analyst's alleged indifference, self-centeredness, and unconcerned enjoyment of his or her own life, there may be hope. Under the most favorable circumstances, intense primitive hatred and envy may become reactivated and a "revival" of internalized object relations possible.

Severe Sadomasochistic Transferences

Another group of patients, who are somewhat less severe in the manifestations of their self-destructiveness, unconsciously attempt to transform all relationships into hostile interactions, or severely sadomasochistic involvements. It is as if the only way in which they can trust that someone cares about them is to provoke an attack from that person. Within the frame of a psychotherapeutic treatment, this need to provoke attachment through hostility may lead to disastrous stalemates and breakdowns. These patients, at least, still attempt to maintain some sort of relationship with the therapist, in contrast to patients with the "dead mother" syndrome (discussed below), in which the destruction of all relationships seems to be the overriding goal. Here, the therapist's interpretive clarification of this consistent attempt to provoke the therapist to attack the patient may open the possibility of modifying this pattern. These cases, in fact, represent the most severe form of negative therapeutic reaction.

Regarding these most severe cases described, we have found that technical requirements include, first, the establishment of realistic conditions under which the treatment can be carried out. The structure of the treatment, as determined through contract setting, must create conditions in which the therapist is protected physically, psychologically, socially, and legally. The involvement of the family in the process of setting up the conditions for the treatment is essential. During the treatment itself, it may be necessary to maintain ongoing family contacts to maintain and reinforce the treatment frame and realistic expectations. In a litigious culture such as the United States, it is particularly important that the therapist be solidly protected from any risk of being involved in threatening lawsuits related to a patient's attempted or completed suicide. If the safety of the therapist cannot be established and maintained, the treatment is not possible.

Amid all these struggles, the patient's attempt to destroy the therapist, spoil his or her reputation, expose his or her impotence, and blacken his or her image to his or her family members needs to be explored as an expression of that part of the patient that, at bottom, is attempting to destroy himself or herself. The exposure of a sadistic, murderous internal object and the patient's fascination with, submission to, and identification with that object, and the savage suppression of his infantile self and aspirations for love, are frightening aspects of the transference. They also may emerge as very disturbing aspects of countertransference developments. This, again, requires a combination of objective security of the therapist and "space" for working through one's countertransference reactions. The therapist's survival despite a patient's consistent unconscious efforts to transform him or her into a sadistic and devalued object and the tolerance of the feelings of frustration, delusion, envy, triumph, and loneliness dominant in the intersubjective field, are the heavy price for carrying out these treatments, as well as the material on the basis of which understanding may be gained, and both success and failure evolve.

THE ANTISOCIAL DIMENSION

Although narcissistic pathology with antisocial features reflects a higher level of engagement with the external world than the most severe group of narcissistic constellations examined previously, the practical absence of protective superego functions facilitates uncontrollable acting out of aggression that may easily destroy the therapeutic relationship and represents a negative prognostic feature for any therapeutic intervention. A high degree of secondary gain and/or the presence of severe antisocial features represent negative prognostic indicators in the treatment of the narcissistic pathology we are exploring (Kernberg 2007). We have found that it is essential for the therapist to carry out an adequate diagnosis at the beginning of the treatment, to differentiate antisocial personality proper from narcissistic personalities with significant antisocial behavior and from the syndrome of malignant narcissism. The latter conditions may be psychotherapeutically treated, in contrast with antisocial personality proper (see the criteria outlined by Hare [Hare et al. 1991], Stone [1993], and Kernberg [2004]).

Once the decision has been made that, although the prognosis may be guarded, TFP would still be indicated, it is important to set up a treatment arrangement by which not only family are involved, but the therapist has the assurance of adequate outside information that may protect the patient, the therapist, and the treatment from severely destructive behavior that is kept split off from the sessions and reflects a long-standing unresolved dishonesty of the patient. Antisocial behavior with deceptive communications by the patient in the treatment hours may still be treatable if the patient does not present an antisocial personality disorder in a strict sense. The systematic analysis of dishonest behavior becomes a central precondition for structural change in these patients. Often a team structure may be necessary to assess the patient, as well as to protect him or her from severe acting out of antisocial behavior, and the therapist must be prepared to analyze all symptoms of deceptiveness as the highest priority of his or her interventions. The fact that patients cannot be trusted to convey honest information about what is occurring in their lives, what they think and feel, must be accepted as a given reality whose conscious and unconscious motivation needs to be explored in the sessions. Obviously, deceptiveness and dishonesty protect the patient from imagined dangers that would occur if, in his or her mind, he or she were not to deploy such dishonest behavior.

This means that severely paranoid features are constantly present as conscious and unconscious motivation protecting antisocial behavior in the transference, and the transformation of "psychopathic transferences" into "paranoid transferences" is a major tactical aim in these treatments. Often the atmosphere during sessions, at least initially, is apparently friendly and distant, only to become extremely paranoid and hostile when this transformation is achieved. The patient seems to be worse, acting out may intensify, the treatment may appear more at risk, and yet a more realistic relationship may be taking place. The combination of antisocial defenses and the pathological grandiose self makes this transition from a psychopathic into a predominantly paranoid transference much more difficult and laborious.

During this process, patients may attempt to seduce the therapist into colluding with some of their deceptive behavior under the guise of a more honest collaboration with the therapist. It is important, of course, to resist this temptation, and it is under such circumstances when the therapist's responsibility to the patient, to his or her own moral values, and to society may enter into conflict. In all cases, any collusion with antisocial behavior carries a heavy price and, eventually, the risk of treatment failure. It may be preferable to interrupt a treatment when therapeutic conditions are no longer compatible with the therapist's commitment to an honest and moral relationship. Once again, the therapist's safety represents the first condition that determines whether a treatment is viable, and psychoanalytic psychotherapy is no place for inordinate heroics.

Some patients' antisocial behavior is expressed under dissociated conditions. For example, one patient would physically abuse his wife in the middle of rage attacks, a behavior rationalized as part of a patriarchal ideology that required her to accept orders from him without raising questions. This behavior, infused with sadistic pleasure, gradually became ego-dystonic outside such crises, but the behavior persisted despite professed guilt feelings at other times. It was as if the expression of guilt and concern, instead of influencing that behavior pattern, contributed to stabilize it by serving to replace any reparative action based on these guilt feelings. In another example, a research scientist falsified the data derived from his experiments and then replicated these experiments to annul the impact of the false results previously communicated. Sometimes the antisocial behavior is rationalized as part of the entitlement professed by the pathological grandiose self: one patient refused to pay taxes, disobeyed parking laws, and ignored his incoming mail to the extent of seriously damaging consequences for him.

The transference implications of these behavior patterns vary widely: from generalized projection of superego precursors to enactment of identification with specific dishonest or poisonous representations of infantile objects, to provocative testing of the therapist's commitment to the patient. The countertransference developments in such cases, in turn, challenge the analyst's commitment to the patient and sometimes tend to induce a paralyzing denial of the gravity of the situation. The analyst's sense that the unremitting nature of the antisocial behavior of his or her patient threatens to make the analyst an accomplice of a sort may contribute to a realistic consideration as to whether the treatment is still viable.

As mentioned previously regarding several cases, the systematic working through of the transference related to the pathological grandiose self gradually unmasks the component self and object representations of that pathological self-structure. A female patient presented a syndrome of malignant narcissism, with chronically deceptive social behavior, exploitive relationships, paranoid reactions, exhibitionistic behavior, and sexual promiscuity. She had a history of childhood sexual abuse by close relatives, an intensely ambivalent and symbiotic relation with her mother, and a seductive but distant father. In analysis, the transference shifted gradually from a grandiose, aloof demandingness and devaluation of the analyst to an intense negative therapeutic reaction whenever she felt helped by him. In her four-sessions-per-week analysis, these episodes of feeling worse as a result of her treatment, lasting for weeks, seemed at first to reflect unconscious envy over the analyst's capacity to help her. Gradually, however, they reflected increasing paranoid fears over the analyst's presumed seductive intentions involved in helping her, representing the projected identification with the sexual abusers of her childhood. It also reflected the projection of the patient's own seductive and promiscuous behavior. Later on, severe aggressive conflicts over the dependency on an unavailable, teasing, and withholding mother emerged. Her irresponsible handling of money increased, and she fell behind in her payments for the treatment, linked to the developments of resentful depressions over any frustrations in the therapeutic setting, enacting the relationship between a hungry infant and a withholding mother, with corresponding role reversals in the transference. Now the withholding, sadistic mother representation reflected another of the patterns of the pathological grandiose self, initially expressed in her teasing and withholding behavior toward men with whom she would get involved. At this stage of her treatment, for the first time, guilty feelings and depressive reactions evolved as a consequence of her becoming aware of the deceptive behavior in the transference of lying and withholding important information to maintain an illusory superiority over the analyst. All these transference developments could be explored gradually in her chaotic relations with men, leading to more stable and deepening love relations. She was able, eventually, to obtain a very profound change in her characterological structure, with normalization of her capacity to achieve a gratifying, stable love relationship and an effective improvement in her professional function and social life.

While the chronic dishonesty in this patient's social interactions and irresponsibility regarding financial matters were subtle and relatively minor and did not constitute a major objective danger to others or to herself, this is not always the case. Many narcissistic patients with severe antisocial behavior or passive exploitive or aggressive behavior may, indeed, threaten other persons, society at large, and/or themselves. Whenever the patient's behavior seems to pose a threat to his or her physical, psychological, or legal survival, clear limits may be required as a condition for the treatment. In some cases, it may be necessary to have access to corroborating information from external sources, with the patient's permission, of course. For example, patients who are chronically deceptive and who carry out violent behaviors against sexual partners or other members of their family that they avoid communicating to the therapist, or patients involved in stealing, drug dealing, or other severe conflicts with the law that reflect serious risks to themselves or others but that they are withholding from the therapist, may require such interventions. Such arrangements may be limited to early periods of the treatment. The technical approach in TFP for such severe cases includes the combination of setting appropriate limits, availability of external sources of information, open communication with the patient regarding all involvement with third parties, and ongoing interpretation of the transference implications of the therapist's temporary abandonment of a position of technical neutrality, should circumstances warrant the therapist's having to take a more active intervention.

In cases of severe secondary complications such as alcoholism, drug addiction, or severe eating disorders, we have found that psychoanalysis or TFP is not effective without first getting these obstacles to treatment under control. There are alternative ways to achieve this, depending on the nature of the complication, the degree of pathology of the patient, and the actual danger that such a complication presents.

As a general rule, alcohol or drug abuse, but not dependency, may be tolerated as a complication that can be dealt with in ordinary therapeutic settings. In contrast, definite dependency requires either that treatment by detoxification and rehabilitation before a psychoanalytic psychotherapy or psychoanalysis be started or that the therapy be timed to coincide with the start of a rehabilitation program that allows open communication between the treatment team and the therapist. Ancillary arrangements such as regular attendance at 12-step programs or ongoing work with an eating disorder specialist are part of the general strategy of setting up a therapeutic contract and free up the therapist to focus on the patient's object relational world. Again, if the major problem is deceptiveness, but without chronic behavior outside the sessions threatening the patient and/or his or her psychosocial environment, ordinary treatment arrangements and the therapist's preparedness to deal with the dominance of psychopathic transferences in the early stages of the treatment usually are sufficient.

Conclusion

I have attempted to provide an overview of different constellations of narcissistic personality disorders as they present clinically along a spectrum, from the relatively best functioning and organized forms of pathological narcissism to the most regressive and potentially most threatening to the patient's psychosocial and physical survival, that may yet be helped within our present clinical understanding and therapeutic approaches.

I would place the general approach to the treatment of narcissistic pathology represented in this chapter as very close to Kleinian theory and, particularly, to the contributions of Herbert Rosenfeld (1987), John Steiner (1993), Ronald Britton (2004), and Wilfred Bion (1967) to the study of narcissistic personality, and the clinical and theoretical contributions that André Green (1993a, 1993b) has provided throughout the years developing the concept of narcissism of death, the psychology of the negative, and de-objectalization as a manifestation of severe narcissistic pathology. My own contributions to the technical approach of narcissistic personalities, particularly the most severe cases, in which functioning is at a borderline level, represent a significant aspect of this therapeutic approach, as well as the technical implications of the development of TFP as a general treatment approach to severe personality disorders (Kernberg 1984, 2004, 2007). Within this general technical approach, I believe that the treatment of patients with severe narcissistic pathology, as well as patients presenting borderline personality organization in general, should be approached with an interpretive psychoanalytic stance from the very beginning of treatment. The early analysis of the alternation of primitive unconscious dyadic relations in the transference in the most severe cases facilitates their psychoanalytic treatment. This particular technical approach facilitates mentalization and constitutes an important aspect of the technical approach at severe levels of transference regression (Kernberg 2012). In short, I have presented an approach that reflects the application of psychoanalytic theory of pathology and technique to a broad spectrum of patients and expands the realm of classical psychoanalysis with its extension of a specific type of psychoanalytic psychotherapy.

References

Bion WR: On arrogance, in Second Thoughts: Selected Papers on Psychoanalysis. New York, Basic Books, 1967, pp 86–92

Britton R: Subjectivity, objectivity, and triangular space. Psychoanal Q 73(1):47–61, 2004 14750465

Clarkin JF, Yeomans FE, Kernberg OF: Psychotherapy for Borderline Personality: Focusing on Object Relations. Washington, DC, American Psychiatric Publishing, 2006

Green A: On Private Madness. Madison, CT, International Universities Press, 1993a

Green A: Le Travail du Négatif. Paris, Les Éditions de Minuit, 1993b

Green A: Pourquoi les Pulsions de Destruction ou de Mort? Paris, Éditions du Panama, 2007

Green A: Illusions et Désillusions du Travail Psychoanalytique. Paris, Odile Jacob, 2010

Grinberg L: Countertransference and projective counteridentification. Contemp Psychoanal 15:226–247, 1979

Hare RD, Hart SD, Harpur TJ: Psychopathy and the DSM-IV criteria for antisocial personality disorder. J Abnorm Psychol 100(3):391–398, 1991 1918618

Kernberg OF: Technical aspects in the psychoanalytic treatment of narcissistic personalities, in Severe Personality Disorders: Psychotherapeutic Strategies. New Haven, CT, Yale University Press, 1984, pp 197–209

Kernberg OF: Aggressivity, Narcissism, and Self-Destructiveness in the Psychotherapeutic Relationship. New Haven, CT, Yale University Press, 2004

Kernberg OF: The almost untreatable narcissistic patient. J Am Psychoanal Assoc 55(2):503–539, 2007 17601104

Kernberg O: The concept of the death drive: a clinical perspective. Int J Psychoanal 90(5):1009–1023, 2009 19821849

Kernberg OF: Mentalization, mindfulness, insight, empathy, and interpretation, in The Inseparable Nature of Love and Aggression: Clinical and Theoretical Perspectives. Washington, DC, American Psychiatric Publishing, 2012, pp 57–79

Kernberg OF, Yeomans FE, Clarkin JF, et al: Transference focused psychotherapy: overview and update. Int J Psychoanal 89(3):601–620, 2008 18558958

Rosenfeld H: Impasse and Interpretation: Therapeutic and Anti-Therapeutic Factors in the Psychoanalytic Treatment of Psychotic, Borderline, and Neurotic Patients. London, Tavistock, 1987

Steiner J: Psychic Retreats: Pathological Organizations in Psychotic, Neurotic, and Borderline Patients. London, Routledge, 1993

Steiner J: A personal view of Rosenfeld's contribution to clinical psychoanalysis, in Rosenfeld in Retrospect: Essays on His Clinical Influence. London, Routledge, 2008, pp 58–84

Stone MH: Abnormalities of Personality. New York, WW Norton, 1993

CHAPTER 10

Narcissistic Defenses in the Distortion of Free Association and Their Underlying Anxieties

In this chapter, I examine distortions in the characteristics of free associations of patients with narcissistic personality disorders. I propose that the dominant narcissistic transference developments typical of the early and middle phases of the analytic treatment of these patients are reflected in these distortions of free association and proposes technical interventions geared to deal with them.

A frequent finding in narcissistic personalities treated with standard psychoanalysis or transference-focused psychotherapy (TFP) is their persistent difficulty in carrying out free association. They may show a particular type of association that reflects an ongoing critical evaluation of what comes to mind, rather than any curiosity about what is un-

---

This chapter was originally published as Kernberg OF: "Narcissistic Defenses in the Distortion of Free Association and Their Underlying Anxieties." *The Psychoanalytic Quarterly* 84(3):625–642, 2015. Copyright © 2015 Wiley-Blackwell. Adapted with permission.

known or not understood, or about the unexpected and surprisingly new ideas that may emerge. The prevalence of intellectual speculation over what does come to mind gives their associations an obsessive-compulsive quality. Although they may appear much freer than obsessive patients to engage in intense affective reactions, the matter-of-fact, nonreflective assertion of their feelings also indicates a great difficulty in exploring the unknown in their mind.

When the analyst draws these patients' attention to peculiar ideas, behavioral reactions, or questions that arise during their apparent efforts to do free association, their reactions take the form of intellectual speculation, theoretical musings, or reflections about the analyst's intentions. They present, in short, with what may be called an ongoing self-supervision of what emerges in their mind or in reaction to the analyst's interpretive interventions.

This is the nature of the problem with free association that I wish to explore. It affects, particularly, the "thick-skinned" narcissistic patients (see Chapter 9, "An Overview of the Treatment of Severe Narcissistic Personality"), including those who represent the relatively less severe degree of pathology within the wide spectrum of narcissistic personality disorders (Kernberg 2014).

In earlier work (Kernberg 2007), I have stressed the dominant defensive operations geared to protect the narcissistic patient from any authentic dependency on the analyst as the most important expression of the activation of the patient's pathological grandiose self. In a recent publication (Kernberg 2014), I have related my overall approach to those of other authors. Authentic dependency on the analyst would mean recognition of the importance of his or her capacity to provide the patient with psychological understanding and help. That, by the same token, would evoke intolerable envy and resentment, and feelings of inferiority and humiliation. As a result, it is as if the patient, while carrying out free association, seems to be talking to himself or herself in the presence of the analyst, or to the analyst in order to influence him or her. As a result, the analyst's countertransference is as if he or she were alone in the room, with a painful lack of contact or meaningful interaction with the patient that, typically, may cause a sense of boredom and a chronic temptation to distraction. Although this development is present in all types of narcissistic personality, it is most clearly observable over an extended period in cases of the thick-skinned narcissistic personality (Rosenfeld 1987).

This defensive avoidance of true dependency is matched frequently by a complementary defense of omnipotent control, which is a conscious effort on the patient's part to influence and control the analyst's behavior to avoid both the emergence of feelings of inferiority (stemming from the newness or recognized importance of what the analyst is saying) and a complete devaluation of the analyst (as a consequence of the activation of the patient's contemptuous grandiosity.) If the analyst is completely devalued, there remains no possibility of receiving any help or any useful consequence of the treatment; if the analyst expresses anything potentially useful, however, this is intolerable and the resentment may be unavoidable.

The two mutually complementary operations—denial of dependency and omnipotent control—may evolve in several ways, expressed in the influence on the process of free association rather than in any specific fantasy or other material emerging concretely in the content of the sessions. It is on the effects of these defensive operations on free association that I wish to focus in this chapter.

The instructions given to the patient in explaining the fundamental rule of free association include the invitation to try to say whatever comes to mind, in whatever form that occurs (e.g., thoughts, fantasies, observations, relationships, fears, dreams, memories) without attempting to order all these contents in any way. The patient is instructed to try to verbalize what goes through his or her mind regardless of whether that seems easy or difficult, something to be proud or ashamed of, something important or trivial, and so on. The patient is often told that this may seem difficult at first but may gradually be learned, and that the analyst will be attempting to help the patient in this regard. Narcissistic patients quite frequently present what comes to mind in an organized way, similar to what would be typical for obsessive patients, but may "learn" to disperse such organized communications with some words, thoughts, feelings, or questions that convey a spontaneity that feels more uncontrolled but is then followed by an orderly communication of what the patient was trying to present in the first place.

Typical "organizing" comments may include a clarification of what the patient is trying to communicate by enumerating it, or by commenting "I will clarify this later." The result is a clearly ordered sequence of subjects repeatedly activated, with a focus on different angles from which the patient considers this material as part of his or her self-analysis. The total sequence results in an "imitation spontaneity" that makes it difficult for the analyst to perceive what, if anything, is emotionally relevant—other than the patient's control of the process.

Some patients express concern over whether what comes to their mind will be helpful and question repeatedly if the analyst understands it. They may wonder, throughout the session, whether it is going to be a "good" or "bad" session, or initiate the session with such a comment.

Free association is accompanied by a continuous evaluation regarding the extent to which what is coming to their mind right now will foster the analytic process.

The patient's reaction to the analyst's interpretive comments may show some typical repetitive qualities. The patient seems to consider very thoughtfully what the analyst has said and may repeat it to assure himself or herself that he or she has understood it correctly and therefore is able to "work" with it. The patient may frequently express agreement or disagreement with what the analyst has said, or ask for further clarification. What seems to be missing is a spontaneous expression of the emotional response to what the analyst has said. The patient conveys an impression of being an attentive and interested participant in a dialogue, rather than open to an effort to experience anything new in himself or herself. It usually takes some time for the analyst to become aware of this subtle way of the patient's protecting himself or herself against any unexpected emotional impact of what the analyst is saying. Narcissistic patients have enormous difficulty understanding that the analyst's interpretations are hypotheses that only will be proven right or wrong from whatever they stimulate in the patient's awareness of his or her emotional reactions to them. Rather, the patient will treat them as theories or oracles.

Sometimes the analyst may have the experience of an important breakthrough or change, something unexpectedly understood by the patient that sheds new light on a particular problem. This new emotional understanding, however, disappears without leaving a trace in the days and weeks that follow. This development may be considered a form of negative therapeutic reaction or an unconscious devaluation, or may even reflect a silent, conscious dismissal of what the patient has received from the analyst. What is impressive, however, is the patient's reaction when the analyst returns to this event because it fits the material of a later session, and when the analyst wonders whether the patient remembers what occurred in that past session. Often a patient may respond "Yes, of course," and repeat almost verbatim the interaction, saying that he or she remembers it very well and that, in fact, it involves an issue that in different ways has been discussed a thousand times, with the implication that he or she has heard it, remembers it, and therefore has nothing else to say about it. This sequence of events clearly illustrates the intellectual "learning" of interpretations that do not really touch the patient. The patient incorporates the new knowledge and devalues it in the process.

Beneath this pattern lies the defensive constellation of omnipotent control and the need to avoid any authentic emotional dependency on the analyst, with the patient's ongoing monitoring of his or her free association and the analyst's comments to develop, on his or her own, an analytic understanding of what evolves in the sessions. What may be most helpful at this point is to focus the patient's attention on the risks involved in just listening to what the analyst is saying, with an open question as to whether that will bring about any reaction in the patient. Will the analyst's intervention foster his or her own superiority, putting the patient down, or will it confirm the patient's feared demolition of the analyst? One may point out to the patient his or her frequent concern as to whether the analyst's comment is "good" or "bad," "correct" or "not," whether it implies that the analyst is accepting or rejecting the patient. In other instances, it may help to focus on the patient's paranoid attitude regarding the analyst that emerges as a consequence of pointing to the patient's lack of spontaneity in his or her response to the analyst's comments.

The development of "filler" subjects in the patient's discourse also may alert the analyst to an underlying difficulty in free association. The patient comes back, again and again, to the same subject matter—for example, a detailed reference to the technical aspects of his profession, or some particular work project he or she needs to carry out at home, and similar repetitive contents—without any reference to any human interaction. This is in sharp contrast to the repetitive narrative about the dominant conflicts in the patient's life, which, even if repetitive on the surface, usually imply live transferential implications. Thus, repetitive discussion about, for example, the various concrete tasks involved in gardening may serve as a protective avoidance of uncontrolled emergence of new material. One patient returned, again and again, to technical details regarding his scientific research in an area totally unknown to the analyst. Eventually it became clear that his apparently obsessive concern served the function of asserting his superiority over the analyst.

A frequent—and, for the analyst, quite disturbing—development may be the patient's appropriation of the analyst's language or theory when reporting emotional reactions or conflicts, so that analytic explanations may be included in the patient's discourse without reflecting any authentic emotional learning. Obviously, the analyst should attempt to talk in concrete, ordinary language rather than introducing technical terminology reflecting his or her own theories. However, even if interpretive comments are presented in very simple language, the analyst's underlying theoretical orientation may be perceived clearly by the patient and be reflected in the content of his or her associations. In peer supervision, this development in the patient's discourse may lead to amusing identification by the group of the analyst's theoretical preferences.

The ongoing effort to monitor, absorb, and store the analyst's comments in a continuous learning process also reflects the narcissistic patient's need to be admired, rather than any authentically loving or dependent relationship. Where does the patient stand regarding the analyst's interest in him or her? Does the analyst appreciate and feel impressed by the patient's communications? Is the analyst bored, distanced, indifferent, or angry, resentful, or dismissive and contentious? The patient may be projecting aspects of his or her own pathological grandiose self onto the analyst, including the need for admiring confirmation from the patient, as well as devastating hostility or humiliating contempt. At the same time, the patient cannot build up an awareness of those aspects of the analyst's personality that ordinarily would come through in any long-standing therapeutic relationship, in terms of the analyst's concern, empathy, and interest and his or her emotional sensitivity to the patient's needs. All this may be unavailable to the narcissistic patient. Under the dominance of the pathological grandiose self, the patient is reduced to evaluating how the analyst's behavior affects him or her, rather than being capable of an authentic interest in the analyst as a person, an interest that would grow and develop in consonance with a developing dependent relationship, and the development of appreciation and gratitude for what he or she receives from the analyst. By the same token, the patient cannot believe in the analyst's authentic interest and concern for him or her.

This same difficulty to empathize with the personality of the analyst shows, of course, in the relation between the patient and all other people in his or her life. It leads to the stereotyped description of the most important persons in his or her life and the persistence of these stereotypes throughout lengthy periods of the analysis. Typically, these patients present a fixed, rigid view of their family and of their own past, with an impressive lack of curiosity or reflection on the wishes, experiences, and motivation of significant others. This conveys to the analyst the painful experience of emptiness that these patients must contend with in all their interactions, and against which fantasies of grandiosity and superiority and self-sufficiency provide an illusory protection. The stereotyped panorama of the patient's life combines with the rigid cognitive control in the patient's free associations to convey an arid emotional experience that can only be penetrated by the analysis of its replication in the transference. The analysis of the patient's fear of listening without his or her controlling safeguards opens up the analysis of his or her difficulty to listen to others as well, and the consequent ignoring or misunderstanding of communications, an emotional ignorance caused by the underlying paranoid stance to protect the patient against threats to the pathological grandiose self.

Under these conditions, the patient brings narratives about brilliant, exuberant, exciting, overwhelming experiences that may have a dramatic or exhilarating quality. These reports, in which the patient experiences himself or herself as the center of attention, have a grandiose quality and serve to reassure the patient and impress the analyst, but they have a strangely empty quality. The patient may enthusiastically communicate an experience that, however, leaves no trace of permanence in terms of some emotional relationship and, in the analyst's countertransference, leaves him or her cold or uninvolved despite all efforts to empathize with the patient. Narcissistic patients, however, may find an escape from emptiness in such experiences of exuberance, as they do in unusual sexual involvements, drug-induced emotional states, or dangerous sports.

The lifeless quality of communication conveyed by the repetitive descriptions of interactions that show very little or no change throughout time is reinforced by the patient's reaction to the very comments of the analyst indicating that what is being referred to now seems to be a replica of what has been discussed before, but with no reference to the contribution made by the analyst in previous discussions of the same material. It is as though these, or similar matters, have never been previously discussed. A confrontation with this fact may trigger the patient's sense of being attacked or, to the contrary, professed agreement with the analyst, with the implication that the patient is communicating precisely the understanding that was reached in the previous discussion. The naturalness with which the patient may assert the latter may dovetail with another aspect of the communication that reflects the omnipotent control of the interaction. Some narcissistic patients are prone to the repetitive use of semiautomatic statements such as "as you know," "that we have discussed before," or "that we have seen before," implying a harmonious bit of work with the analyst in terms of the confirmation of the patient's view or interpretation of an experience. In essence, the unchanging repetition of an experience that had been explored earlier in some depth expresses the patient's stress on maintaining his independence from the analyst's interference.

With some frequency, after an extended narrative of what the patient wishes to communicate to the analyst and often expressing an unconscious effort to influence the analyst in some specific way, the patient may remain silent and then make a statement such as "I've said all I've had to say. Now it's your turn." Such a statement perhaps reflects, better than anything else, the subtle transformation of free association into a shared, alternating communication of the respective thinking of patient and analyst, or the patient's implicit reminder to the analyst that it is now his or her task to make sense of what the patient has been saying and to add something new to it. Questions directed to the analyst regarding his or her agreement or disagreement with what the patient is saying may disrupt the patient's free association from time to time, with the implication of assuring himself or herself that there is no disagreement or implicit critique, or any negative reaction of the analyst that may have threatening implications for the patient. Or, the patient wonders, is there in the analyst's contribution something new, not already known to the patient, which could be a source of humiliation?

Obviously, these efforts to maintain control to defend against dependency or any real influence from the analyst affect long-term countertransference developments with narcissistic patients who show a strong combination of these defenses. The analyst's very commitment to the patient may suffer by the patient's unconsciously undermining everything that comes from the analyst and the chronic absence of an authentic connection with the patient.

The intensity of negative countertransference under those circumstances may take many forms. One analyst, with very good understanding of her patient although still somewhat limited clinical experience, found herself frequently contrasting, with a revengeful enjoyment, her own satisfactory love life with the emptiness of the patient's sexual exploits. It was as if she obtained a particular satisfaction with this comparison, and the analyst clearly recognized this as an expression of her hostile, resentful feelings in the countertransference.

The artificial, manipulated quality of the patient's communications tends to evoke a sense of meaningless triviality and monotony, and may induce boredom in the analyst that requires an ongoing attention to the subtle, transitory shifts in the interaction that may become noticeable in response to the analyst's interventions. As mentioned previously, the patient's experience of the analyst's comments may be that of an assertion of the analyst's superiority and dominance over the patient or of an expression of hostile indifference. At other moments, the patient may experience the analyst as ignorant, incompetent, or helpless, with a sense of superior security that then turns into worry that the patient is wasting his or her own time, given the uselessness of this treatment.

Pointing to this rapid, and at first relatively subtle but gradually more obvious, oscillation between the patient's sense of triumphant superiority and humiliating inferiority in his or her relation to the analyst may help the patient to become aware of projecting the activation of his or her pathological grandiose self and identifying himself or herself with devalued aspects of the self when confirmation of his or her omnipotence fails. This is an important step in the exploration of the narcissistic transference. It opens the patient's awareness to his or her deeper sense of total ignorance regarding the realistic attitude he or she encounters on the part of the analyst and of the patient's deep conviction that the best that can be expected is an analyst who is basically indifferent, thus confirming the patient's aloneness in the world.

At this middle stage of the treatment, the patient's heightened interest in the analyst's relationship to him or her may clarify the correspondent identifications with the pathogenic experiences from the past, the gradual attributing to the analyst of features that replicate aspects of parental figures that reflected the sources of the conflicts with, and the power of, the parental couple. By the same token, the patient now enacts his or her identification with such parental imagos while projecting his or her corresponding self experience onto the analyst. In the countertransference, moments of relatively quiet interest in pursuing the development of the patient's experience in the hour may be followed by a sense of sudden openness to an authentic emotional experience, a live intensification of an internal relationship with the patient, that may then be almost brutally dismantled by a subsequent expression of disdainful disqualification of everything that has been evolving in this relationship. Against the background of consistent efforts to deepen transference analysis over a long period, months of hopefulness and occasional experiences of emotional closeness may shift again into disappointing disengagement by the patient, and the analyst is faced with a new wave of empty trivialities filling the sessions. Here, the dynamics of disappointment, disillusionment, and despair in the countertransference described by Lucy LaFarge (2015) may enter the picture.

The patient's incapacity to experience himself or herself in any relationship where he or she is being loved may become an important issue at this point: the patient may feel that any positive interest and commitment to him or her on the part of the analyst is the product of the patient's seductive efforts and the analyst's weakness and naïveté, and therefore justifies the patient's contemptuous devaluation. The unconscious efforts to provoke the analyst into a consequent counter-disqualification of the patient may help the patient to reconfirm the lack of trust in the analyst and the worthless quality of that apparent emotional investment in him or her by the analyst. The clarification of this issue may highlight the patient's unconscious envy of the analyst's capacity to love, and that resonates with the patient's unconscious envy and resentment of those in his or her early life who might have become a source of ordinary and trustworthy love and commitment.

Narcissistic patients' typical incapacity to commit themselves emotionally to a loving partner is reflected in these complex dynamics in the transference, and highlighting them in working through these issues would seem essential for changing this fundamental aspect of their pathology. The analyst's tolerance of the patient's expression of arrogance and consistent devaluation precisely at points at which the analyst has given evidence of his or her deep wish to understand and help and his or her emotional commitment to the patient may be crucial to avoid falling into the trap of a reactive devaluation of the patient in response to his or her contempt. In short, the patient's rejection of moments of the analyst's intense investment in him or her and the reinforcement of the patient's distancing himself or herself emotionally in a grandiose way from the analyst may be a crucial precondition for the discovery of those hidden moments of recognition of the analyst's authentic interest, which, however, the patient cannot tolerate. Boredom in the countertransference may represent a defensive smokescreen against the resentment following an active effort on the patient's part to destroy the analyst's recognized interest and commitment to him or her.

I have found it helpful, at times, to share with the patient my thoughts about what is going on in the patient at this point in his or her relationship with me, or what I think might have been going on in relation with someone else as an expression of the displacement of the envious devaluation in the transference. I might communicate these thoughts to the patient even though I am quite certain they will be depreciated or incorporated intellectually in a destructive way. In doing this, I am treating the patient "as if" he or she were a "normal" person who would be able to be interested in listening to me and imagining what goes into my saying what I said. And yet, I would be open to expect the forthcoming devaluation of what I have to contribute. I might be right or wrong in what I am saying, but that would only emerge in the patient's reaction: if what I am saying were to be taken seriously, this would reflect at least the patient's momentary awareness of a concerned expression of my interest in him or her.

The patient may surprise me by reacting to what I am saying without immediately "analyzing" it or qualifying it for its value or uselessness, and may experience an emotional reaction that he or she now communicates to me. That would indicate a "normal" attitude that we expect from free association and would indicate that I was wrong in my pessimistic assessment of the patient. More frequently, the patient indeed will react in the disqualifying manner described. I would then interpret this as the patient's way of avoiding *reflecting* on what I have just been saying, but rather assessing my comments in terms of whether I have said anything new, therefore confirming my superiority or uselessness.

As an indication of the working through of a prevalent narcissistic transference, the patient's increased capacity to depend on the analyst will emerge. Patients now may evince reactions to separation over weekends or other extended absences. These reactions may have a predominantly paranoid quality but may also coincide with the beginning of awareness of the aggressive, devaluing behavior as an issue to be examined. They give hope of some potential for feelings of concern for the analyst. There may be times when a patient provocatively insists that nothing has changed, stating that he or she is worse than ever, and flaunts the repetition of old symptoms as an indication of the incompetence of the analyst while also beginning to be aware that such repetitive provocativeness also has the function of testing the extent to which the analyst is still available to him or her and has not given up. Fear that he or she has exhausted the therapist may be another expression of concern and tolerance of a dependent relationship.

Naturally, parallel behavior in relation to others in the patient's life may provide further evidence of some change in his or her capacity to love and to be authentically interested in what happens inside other people, and change in his or her concern over other people's reaction to the patient. The patient's developing fantasy life regarding the experiences of the analyst may reflect a deepening of the activation of specific object relations in the transference, in contrast to the long-standing, fixed nature of the relationship between the grandiose self and the devalued aspect of the self. The analysis of dreams will reflect a broader and deeper space of associations that creates a new dimension of dialectic tension between manifest and latent dream content not available in early analytic stages, in which the patient's associations to elements of the dream were simply new versions of intellectualized interpretations of his or her experiences.

The achievement of the depressive position—the patient's capacity to realize that the intense hatred and resentment of his or her objects have been preventing the patient from perceiving any valuable and loving engagements that he or she had received in life, and what the patient might have received from those who loved him or her if the patient had not been so resentfully envious of their capacity to love him or her—may become a very painful experience. Mourning over the rejection and squandering of potentially good relationships, over the mistreatment of those who love him or her, and the realization of time lost indicate the tolerance of the depressive position. As the patient can increasingly tolerate the exploration of his own mind and feelings, he or she now becomes aware of and interested in the feelings and intentions of others. The experience of guilt over the aggression toward those who love him more and more now motivates impulses to repair relationships and to salvage what is good, and a new capacity to experience gratitude for the good in life may emerge.

Success or failure in the treatment of narcissistic pathology can be most clearly assessed in these patients' capacity to love, to be committed to life-enriching interests and commitments that are not bound to their narcissistic self-assurance or grandiosity, and the capacity to identify with a value system that transcends their own existence. Regarding the degree to which patients are able to achieve such a development, we have been reviewing the case material of the Weill Cornell Medical College Personality Disorders Institute faculty. The range of outcomes makes it clear that there are differences in the nature of the analytic experience of these patients based on their personality and life situation that affect the treatment and that remain to be clarified. To say the least, it seems that the extended experience in the earliest year of life of at least one stable relationship with a parental object that provided a consistent source of love, care, and concern is a prognostically important positive indicator. A person having achieved, throughout life, some understanding and enjoyment of the emotional values of art, literature, or science; a value system not centered in personal triumph or based on a rationalized system of hatred; and the availability, at some time, of a love object that did not have to be devalued and rejected seem to be significant positive features. Sometimes the emergence of the wish to be taken care of, the experience of being taken care of by the analyst without the analyst's expressing his or her superiority or making any demands on the patient, may indicate the potential for dependency that, dissociated from severely destructive tendencies, might imply a positive potential in extremely lonely patients. At the end, the achievement of the capacity to love without experiencing this development as a potential source of weakness or inferiority, and without basic self-regard being affected by the painful possibility that this love will not be reciprocated, indicates the transformation of pathological narcissism into the achievement of a normal capacity for object relations in the context of normal narcissistic development.

Perhaps the most significant issue regarding free association of these patients is the analyst's recognition that the patient's capacity to free associate has been distorted by the narcissistic pathology to the extent that suggesting to the patient to associate to any apparently significant subject matter will not lead to deepening awareness of emotionally significant material. The nature of the transference must be clarified and worked through systematically before the deeper functions of free association may emerge in treatment. Such extreme cases of narcissism illustrate the importance of the analysis of the process of the analytic relationship rather than assumed repressed contents, without losing sight of the eventual emergence of those contents once a more normal object relation evolves in the transference.

In short, all the defenses against the exploration of the pathological grandiose self and, particularly, against the development of a dependent transference relationship protect the patient against the anxieties of underlying conflicts between the pathological grandiose self and the projected devalued aspects of the self in the transference relationship. In essence, this is the conflict between a grandiose, self-sufficient, arrogant, and devaluing representation of an omnipotent self relating to a projected, devalued, depreciated, inferior, aspect of self—each, in essence, reflecting condensations of more primitive internalized object relations under the dominance of early aggressive conflicts.

The defenses operating through distortion of free association are not the only ones that protect the patient from the activation of these conflicts in the transference. Split-off acting out of these conflicts in extratransferential relations and subtle expression of these conflicts in the fantasy material produced by the patient during the sessions, as well as dreams and somatization, may reflect deeper aspects of these problems that have not reached the patient's preconscious and conscious awareness.

The systematic analysis of all these defensive operations tends to activate intense negative affects, including nonspecific anxiety, paranoid fears, experiences of humiliation and shame, and, at the end, the emergence of the potential for authentic feelings of guilt and concern as the patient recognizes the nature of his or her involvement in these transferential developments.

The nature of the anxieties that emerge in the transference reveals the degree to which the activation of the pathological self and the defenses against a dependent relationship in the transference are being worked through and resolved. To begin with, what usually predominates in the early stages of psychoanalytic treatment of narcissistic patients are paranoid anxieties linked to the projection of the grandiose self onto the analyst, a sense that the analyst is a cold, rigid, harshly critical authority who loathes and despises the patient, or is sadistically provocative. These early experiences rapidly turn into fantasies that the analyst is trying to put the patient down or humiliate him or her, with the surface rationale of confronting the patient with his or her difficulties disguising the analyst's true intent of asserting superiority and enjoying the humiliation of the patient, whose inferiority confirms the mighty position of the analyst. Defenses against experiences of humiliation may dominate the analytic situation for a significant period, together with the patient's defensive efforts to ignore and devalue the analyst's interventions. On the surface, fears of being humiliated and the reactive reinforcement of the distortions in free association may predominate at that point.

As the treatment progresses, and the patient is able to tolerate the realization that part of his or her fantasies and behavior reflect a problematic exaggeration of his or her importance and superiority, feelings of shame may replace those of being humiliated and put down. The patient may begin to realize that his or her efforts to assert superiority represent attempts to protect himself or herself against the experience of envy of competitors or rivals, who represent threats to the patient's assumed greatness. The activation of intense conflicts around envy in the transference, usually at first displaced onto extratransferential objects—in the middle of enormous resistances to acknowledge envious feelings toward the analyst—may dominate the treatment situation. As the patient begins to realize how the unrealistic nature of his or her grandiose fantasies and aspirations negatively affects his or her daily life, causing chronic suffering and feelings of failure, shame may become painfully prevalent.

Shame as a normal, quite prevalent early experience is related to the small child's gradual realization that some spontaneous, naïve interests, habits, and behaviors—particularly, exhibitionistic and self-affirmative behaviors—may be rejected and powerfully suppressed by those whom he or she loves. This includes the early enjoyment of oral incorporation of "dirty" objects, and the enjoyment of anal play and fecal deployment, and, later on, of infantile masturbation as well as polymorphous sexual impulses. Critique and rejection of these behaviors lead to conflicts between the ideal representation of the self, loved by an ideal object, and a shamefully devalued, criticized self, cognizant of the discrepancies between this new, unexpected reality and the ideal representation of self (Lansky 1994; Wurmser 1981, 2004). In this regard, shame is an early affect activated in negatively valenced interactions with infantile objects, which then determines powerful efforts to live up to the critical, newly incorporated aspects of the ego ideal. Under ordinary circumstances, shame is gradually replaced by the development of guilt over unacceptable behavior. This includes the painful recognition that one has failed in one's own responsibility in maintaining the relationship with the ego ideal and with ideal objects, the recognition of unacceptable sexual and aggressive impulses that are part of normal ambivalence in relations with significant others. The development of guilt feelings reflects the integration between the prohibitive aspects of the superego and the ego ideal, a reflection of the integration of the superego and a key aspect of the integration of the self in the development of normal identity.

Shame normally acquires a particular, specialized function to protect the privacy and secrecy of infantile sexuality, of sexual desire and activity, the infantile reaction to, and replication of, the secretive life of the parental couple. This secretive internal sexual life increases the intensity of erotic impulses in the later achievement of an intimate sexual relation with a realistically available object, the erotically exciting "shamelessness" of the intimate sexual encounter (Kernberg 1995).

In the case of the narcissistic personality, however, shame acquires a particularly important function as an expression of discrepancy between ideal self and real self. Here, what evolves is a discrepancy between the pathological grandiose self and the gradual acceptance of emotional reality, the previously denied, projected, and unacceptable aspects of the self geared to protect the totally idealized nature of the pathological grandiose self. Thus, in early and middle stages of psychoanalysis or TFP with narcissistic personalities, shame may become prevalent, gradually replacing feelings of humiliation as an intermediate stage between the paranoid nature of early anxiety and the beginning of the capacity to tolerate guilt, concern, and depressive anxieties and defenses. Shame, in short, stands between paranoid fears and painful humiliation, on the one side, and development of recognition and guilt over one's own aggressive impulses, on the other.

Obviously, given progressive and regressive moments of analytic treatment, these sequences are not that clear in individual cases, and these affects may appear in combination or apparently reversed sequences. Their differentiation, however, is helpful in leading to a clearer picture of the nature of working through of the pathological grandiose self in the transference, and the gradual transformation of the grandiose self–devalued self relationship into the more specific object relations that characterize the general transference developments of borderline personality organization. At this point, the treatment begins to reveal the history of the patient's internalized object relations, the conflictual and traumatic nature of which originated the pressures in the direction of the establishment of a pathological grandiose self in the first place.

References

Kernberg OF: Love Relations: Normality and Pathology. New Haven, CT, Yale University Press, 1995

Kernberg OF: The almost untreatable narcissistic patient. J Am Psychoanal Assoc 55(2):503–539, 2007 17601104

Kernberg OF: An overview of the treatment of severe narcissistic pathology. Int J Psychoanal 95(5):865–888, 2014 24902768

LaFarge L: Disappointment, disillusionment, and despair in the analytic situation. Presentation at the Midwinter Meeting of the American Psychoanalytic Association, January 2015

Lansky MR: Shame: contemporary psychoanalytic perspectives. J Am Acad Psychoanal 22(3):433–441, discussion 443–448, 1994 7844020

Rosenfeld H: Impasse and Interpretation: Therapeutic and Anti-Therapeutic Factors in the Psychoanalytic Treatment of Psychotic, Borderline, and Neurotic Patients. London, Tavistock, 1987

Wurmser L: The Mask of Shame. Baltimore, MD, Johns Hopkins University Press, 1981

Wurmser L: Superego revisited. Psychoanal Inquiry 24:183–205, 2004

CHAPTER 11

The Differential Diagnosis of Antisocial Behavior

A Clinical Approach

The Spectrum of Antisocial Behavior

What follows is a clinical approach to the differential diagnosis of antisocial behavior as a significant symptom in a patient's psychopathology. *Antisocial behavior* may be defined as actively damaging or aggressive behavior directed against other individuals or society at large, typically expressed without guilt feelings and classifiable as either passive-parasitic type (e.g., lying, stealing, irresponsibility regarding money, exploitation of others) or aggressive type (e.g., destruction of objects, physical assault, armed robbery, sadistic sexual behavior, murder). While both types of antisocial behavior may be combined, most frequently patients are involved mainly in one or the other. The practical importance of making this differential diagnosis resides first in the assessment of the

---

This chapter was originally published as Kernberg OF: "Differenzialdiagnose antisozialen verhaltens unter klinischen gesichtspunkten," in *Handbuch der Antisozialen Persönlichkeitsstörungen*. Edited by Dulz B, Briken P, Kerberg OF, et al. Stuttgart, Germany, Schatthauer, 2017, pp 259–270. Copyright © 2017 Schatthauer. Adapted with permission.

dangerousness that the patient represents for his or her immediate psychosocial environment and for society at large, and second in the prognostic implications for treatment that sharply separate different types of pathology in which antisocial behavior is present or dominates. From the viewpoint of antisocial behavior as an aspect of severe personality disorders, it constitutes one of the two most important negative prognostic indicators for psychotherapy, the other one being the degree and type of secondary gain of illness.

In what follows, I describe succinctly the various psychopathological entities that have to be considered in the differential diagnosis of this syndrome, starting with the most severe and prognostically most negative diagnosis, and proceeding along a continuum of character structures in which antisocial behavior dominates, from the most severe to the least severe, the latter having a more positive prognosis. The practical implication of this list resides in the relative ease with which the corresponding differential diagnostic evaluation may be achieved in the context of detailed, extensive, complete mental status examinations.

PSEUDOPSYCHOPATHIC SCHIZOPHRENIA

The diagnostic category of *pseudopsychopathic schizophrenia*, which was used clinically in the 1950s, has fallen into disuse but deserves renewed attention because of the influence that psychopharmacological treatment of schizophrenia has had on the clinical manifestations of these patients (Bender 1959; Durst et al. 1997; Holmesland and Astrup 1984). This designation originally referred to schizophrenic patients who, in the course of psychotic episodes, carried out violent and often strange destructive behaviors, committing murder with bizarre features in the context of delusional and hallucinatory symptomatology. The extreme severity and bizarre nature of criminal behavior carried out under these circumstances drew attention to this, fortunately rare, type of patients.

What is remarkable is that with the advent of effective psychopharmacological treatment of schizophrenia, these patients might become free of their psychotic symptomatology but persist in antisocial behavior of an aggressive and sometimes a combined aggressive- and passive-parasitic type. Under such nonpsychotic conditions, they appear to have a presentation typical of antisocial personality disorder. These patients are usually treated within a forensic-judicial context in specialized hospital services for the criminally ill. Clinical experience has indicated that even if psychotic symptomatology can be controlled by medication, once discharged, these patients continue their antisocial behavior, stop using the medication, and eventually become psychotic again. As mentioned before, these are rare cases that usually end up with permanent inpatient reclusion in specialized psychiatric services and may appear as surprisingly well adjusted in such institutions under conditions of clear and consistent environmental control. They represent the most dangerous type of patients with antisocial behavior, and the protection of family and society is the dominant concern in their management.

ANTISOCIAL PERSONALITY DISORDER

The antisocial personality disorder category represents the most frequently seen personality disorder with significant chronic antisocial behavior and the most resistant to any available present-day treatment. Antisocial personality disorder clearly presents in the two main categories mentioned above, the passive-parasitic type and the aggressive type. The corresponding clinical characteristics have been described in classical work, extending from Hervey Cleckley's (1941) *The Mask of Sanity* to Michael Stone's (2009) *The Anatomy of Evil,* with detailed description of the types and degrees of severity within a broad spectrum of psychopathology of these patients. It remains controversial as to what extent the term *psychopathy* should be applied to a particular subgroup, such as the most extremely dangerous, aggressive type of this psychopathology (Coid and Ullrich 2010). The negative prognosis for all present treatment approaches, however, covers the entire spectrum of antisocial personality disorder.

From a clinical perspective, there are two predominant characteristics of this syndrome. One is the severe narcissistic personality structure, which more than 90% of patients with antisocial personality disorder display as a dominant feature (Hare et al. 1990). A small percentage, however, present with personality features that are predominantly characterized by paranoid and schizoid traits, in the context of generally introverted habitual behavior patterns that contrast sharply with the expansive extroverted characteristics of most antisocial personalities. On the other hand, in addition to these characterological features, they evince the typical antisocial behavior of the aggressive or the passive-parasitic type. The second characteristic in patients with antisocial personality disorder, in addition to the predominant characteristics of the narcissistic personality in terms of grandiosity, entitlement, and incapacity for emotional empathy (despite sharp awareness and evaluation of other people's behavior and intentions), is a history of antisocial behavior beginning in childhood. These patients were usually given the diagnosis of conduct disorder if the early contacts with psychiatric professionals dated from childhood years. These patients typically manifest an absence of feelings of guilt and concern for the antisocial behavior in which they engage, although they may pretend to feel guilty during clinical examinations, particularly once a particular antisocial behavior has been discovered by the examining psychiatrist.

Their relationships with family members, friends, and acquaintances are clearly exploitive, and they show no capacity for an authentic emotional investment in a relationship with others from which they would obtain no benefits. Typically, this emotional indifference and callousness may even show in their behavior toward pets. Sometimes the exploitive nature of these patients' relationships may be masked by a surface pretense of interest and concern that, on further exploration, proves to be false. They show a remarkable inability to tolerate anxiety, and, indeed, situations that ordinarily would provoke anxiety may trigger antisocial or hostile behavior. These patients lack a genuine capacity for experiencing sadness and mourning. Under conditions of serious threats to their sense of well-being or autonomy they may develop strong paranoid features and engage in aggressive efforts to escape from any situation they cannot control.

Patients with antisocial personality disorder may show a potential for suicide if they feel pushed into a corner, which also relates to a general absence of fear of illness or death. Here, narcissistic grandiosity and omnipotence may combine with a total lack of concern for self once all sources of pleasure are judged to be unavailable. These patients may get involved in objectively dangerous situations, and although such dangers have an exciting effect on them, they also reveal a deep sense of invincibility.

Given these descriptions, it is not surprising that these personalities show no capacity for falling in love and an absence of tenderness in their sexual relations. Those aggressive types of antisocial personalities who are expressing their pathology mostly in sexual behavior may carry out dangerous forms of sadistic sexual attacks.

Remarkably, these personalities do not learn from experience despite grievous negative consequences and may repeat failing behavior again and again. By the same token, they can be very effective in planning criminal actions, without concern about the long-term effects of their present behavior that, unavoidably, will lead to their discovery or failure. They convey the impression that they have no sense of time, of future, or of long-range planning beyond the immediate action in which they are engaged. This peculiarity is what brings about the surprising failure of social survival in individuals who often appear as extremely savvy in planning for antisocial actions. Patients with passive-parasitic features who carry out major fraudulent operations should have been able to predict, one assumes, their eventual exposure, but they cannot think ahead over that time span.

These patients also show a characteristic incapacity to identify with the moral values of other human beings. They do not have the capacity for an emotional investment in a therapeutic relationship. When they get involved in a psychotherapeutic endeavor, manipulativeness, pathological lying, and flimsy rationalizations of irresponsibility typically characterize their behavior. They have an impressive capacity to present themselves in very different ways according to what they perceive to be the expectations of the other person with whom they interact. They have been called "holographic" because of surprising and, for the diagnostician, confusing shifts in their presentation and behavior.

Because of the lack of capacity to respond to psychotherapeutic treatment in patients with antisocial personality disorder, it is extremely important to carry out a careful differential diagnostic assessment with the following syndromes, all of which have better prognosis with psychotherapeutic interventions. I shall stress the relevant differentiating features in brief descriptions of these various syndromes.

SYNDROME OF MALIGNANT NARCISSISM

I have described this syndrome in earlier work (Kernberg 1984, 1992), and it is now quite generally accepted (Bender 2014; M.H. Stone, "The Dark Side of Narcissism: Antisocial Personality Psychopathy and Malignant Narcissism," unpublished manuscript, 2016) to represent an intermediate area between antisocial personality proper and narcissistic personality disorder with antisocial behavior. The syndrome of malignant narcissism is characterized by the typical narcissistic personality structure in addition to significant paranoid characterological features, ego-syntonic aggression against others and/or self, *and* antisocial behavior. These patients present the characteristics of severe identity diffusion and usually have significant failure in their capacity for work or profession, for intimacy in their sexual life, and for maintaining ordinary social relations. They often tend to be confused with regressed patients presenting a borderline personality disorder, but the combination of the dominant features of a narcissistic personality, the paranoid tendencies, and marked aggression in combination with antisocial behavior permits the specific diagnosis of the syndrome.

These patients also differ from individuals with antisocial personality proper in that they still have the capacity for some nonexplotive investment in others—in maintaining a nonexploitive sexual relationship, for example—and they still may show a capability for some idealization of a more normal way of living to which they aspire and the capacity for guilt feelings under circumstances when they become aware of their responsibility in hurting a person who is important to them. In other words, they still possess an "island" of a potentially ideal, good relationship that has appeal to them. This makes a psychotherapeutic relationship possible, and if the treatment provides an adequate, firm frame that protects the patient, the environment, and the treatment itself from destructive acting out, these patients may prove to be psychotherapeutically treatable. A history of significant relationships, a capacity for love, the ability to take good care of a pet, and the willingness to be honest with another about their violent, chaotic, aggressive behavior provides an element of authentic humanity. These favorable prognostic indicators stand in sharp contrast to the permanent distance and emotional unavailability of the antisocial personality proper and signify a much better outcome.

These patients differ from patients with antisocial personality disorder in their capacity to tolerate severe anxiety and depressive reactions. Ego-syntonic aggression may be directed against others in the form of provocative violent behavior, destruction of property, arrogant and controlling interactions, or angry temper tantrums, but these patients do not show the dangerousness of the aggressive behavior of antisocial personality disorder nor the pervasive conscious exploitation of significant others.

The severity of the pathology of these patients is reflected in the high frequency of inpatient treatments they require. Malignant narcissists constitute the outer limit of patients who respond to psychodynamic psychotherapies, particularly transference-focused psychotherapy (TFP). Their treatments usually require strict limits on their activities, and patients with overwhelming antisocial features, deceptiveness, and/or grave chronic self-mutilations may require supportive technical approaches.

NARCISSISTIC PERSONALITY DISORDER WITH ANTISOCIAL FEATURES

Narcissistic personality disorder with antisocial features has a better prognosis and is open to the general psychotherapeutic treatment approaches for pathological narcissism (Kernberg 2014). Antisocial behavior is a prognostically negative factor, but treatment is not necessarily impossible. These are usually patients with passive-parasitic antisocial behavior, often geared to gratifying a specific narcissistic need such as stealing objects that they need for their professional endeavors without having the funds to acquire them in a legal way. Others may engage in aggressive antisocial behavior as leaders or members of criminal groups but with a definite capacity for loyalty and commitment to some ideal. These patients are able to be involved in nonexploitive behavior with significant others despite their typical narcissistic difficulty in establishing love relations in depth. They may evince authentic interests and ideals beyond their own survival. Antisocial behavior has a specific function in sustaining these patients' narcissistic grandiosity but is typically restricted to a particular area rather than involving all their social interactions. One university professor in the arts would steal rare books with reproductions of paintings as his only antisocial behavior. Their treatment, in short, is psychotherapeutic, which also corresponds to all the less severe modalities of antisocial behavior that follow, with increasingly positive prognosis as we go down the list. Depending on various individual features, some of these patients may obtain maximal benefit with unmodified, standard psychoanalysis.

OTHER BORDERLINE PERSONALITY ORGANIZATION DISORDERS WITH ANTISOCIAL FEATURES

Here, I am referring to antisocial behavior in patients with severe personality disorders, all of which are characterized by the syndrome of identity diffusion—that is, they evince a lack of integration of the concept of self and lack of integration of the concept of significant others, but without the dominance of a narcissistic personality structure. This group includes, among others, antisocial behavior in a borderline, schizoid, paranoid, or an infantile or histrionic personality disorder. From a psychodynamic viewpoint, the antisocial behavior usually is closely connected to a dynamic feature of their personality.

For example, in the case of paranoid personality disorders, dishonest behaviors may be intended to damage a perceived enemy or to manipulate social situations in order to take revenge, and the antisocial behavior may be rationalized to the extent of "fitting" into a generally preserved ethical orientation. In infantile or histrionic personality disorders, chronic lying (including pseudologia fantastica) may serve to create an embellishment of one's life in an attempt to generate unusual interest on the part of others. In this connection, however, the tendency toward chronic lying may by itself constitute a severe limitation to the engagement in a psychotherapeutic relationship and may, in the end, defeat the therapeutic efforts.

In general, all the patients of this group have the potential, once their major splitting operations and projective identifications can be explored and resolved in the treatment situation, to experience authentic guilt and concern over their aggression and reach the depressive position in working through their antisocial behavior. Although at this point there are no specific empirical research findings indicating which patients of this group may benefit more from a psychodynamic or from a cognitive-behavioral approach, it seems reasonable to conclude that the more the symptoms are specific to antisocial behaviors and/or other circumscribed symptoms, cognitive-behavioral approaches would be a first priority. If, however, the severe personality disorder affects patients' functioning in the major areas of life tasks—that is, in work and profession, in love and sex, or in their general social functioning—a psychoanalytic psychotherapy such as TFP is the first choice.

NEUROTIC PERSONALITY ORGANIZATION WITH ANTISOCIAL FEATURES

This category is the only one that was specifically clarified by Freud in his concept of "criminals out of unconscious guilt" (Freud 1916/1957). These are, indeed, patients with neurotic personality organization—that is, with normal identity and antisocial behavior. This group would include obsessive-compulsive, depressive-masochistic, and hysterical personality disorders. The antisocial behavior may present a bizarre quality in the sense that it is usually expressed in such ways that it leads to discovery and punishment or self-punishment. For example, a physician with an obsessive-compulsive personality stole chocolates and other sweets in the cafeteria of the hospital where he worked, which led to an embarrassing discovery. In another example, a respected biology researcher falsified data of an experiment and repeated this experiment several times to nullify the false results that she had reported. In the course of psychotherapeutic treatment, the acting out of unconscious guilt feelings over a particular psychological complex may become quite obvious and permits resolution of the syndrome. These patients have very good prognosis with psychoanalysis and psychoanalytic psychotherapies, and the question is whether treatment can be made available before they seriously risk their social, intimate, or work situation.

ANTISOCIAL BEHAVIOR IN ADOLESCENT ADJUSTMENT DISORDERS

I am referring here to antisocial behavior during adolescent development of anxiety and/or depressive disorders, in the context of dominant unconscious conflicts that get acted out in their social behavior, in their intimate relations, at home, or at school. Emotional crises and related impulsive behavior may present with provocative features, as temper tantrums, and, in certain social conditions, with occasional antisocial behavior. These adolescents usually present isolated episodes of dishonesty, physical attack, participation in invasion of property, or stealing, clearly in the context of severe emotional turmoil and generalized conflicts in their social life.

Here, if the diagnostic evaluation of the adolescent reveals an identity *crisis* (in contrast to a severe personality disorder with identity diffusion), the prognosis is excellent. Identity crises can be differentiated from the severe manifestations of identity diffusion by the persistence, in the middle of the emotional regression, of a clearly differentiated sense of self and realistic assessment in depth of the personality of the significant others in their immediate family and social environment. Timely psychotherapeutic engagement usually clarifies the issues and permits symptom resolution. If, on the other hand, it seems that what is involved is a severe personality disorder, then one must evaluate to what extent the antisocial behavior is more than situational in the context of bad judgment or peer pressure than seemed to be the case initially and whether one of the previously described syndromes is involved. Usually, the combination of adolescent time-limited antisocial behavior in the context of emotional turmoil and impulsivity, anxiety, and depressive reaction provides the elements justifying the inclusion in the present category. It also needs to be taken into consideration that culturally fostered antisocial behavior by social subgroups in school, or a culturally tolerated adolescent behavior, may be involved, such as shoplifting of cosmetics by adolescent girls, which is quite prevalent in American culture.

DISSOCIAL SYNDROME

Dissocial syndrome was originally described in British literature related to the study of antisocial adolescent gang behavior and was included in DSM-I as a subgroup of "sociopathic personality disturbance" (American Psychiatric Association 1952). Patients with this syndrome were described as living in an abnormal moral environment but capable of strong loyalties. They usually are members of adolescent gangs engaging in antisocial activities. Here, one should differentiate the personality features of the various gang members. Frequently, gang leaders may have antisocial personalities or severe narcissistic personalities with antisocial behavior, whereas the followers show a broad spectrum of less severe personality organization or are youngsters in adolescent crises. They include youngsters with infantile or histrionic personality disorders or dependent personality disorders, as well as adolescents with severe conflicts at home who are searching for a supportive social environment that they find in the social life of the gang. Antisocial behavior in this syndrome is typically carried out in a group setting. Sometimes simply separating an adolescent from this social subculture may take care of the problem, whereas severe conflicts at home, including major psychopathology in the family environment, may constitute important factors that motivate the adolescent's reluctance to abandon the social culture of the gang. The combination of psychotherapeutic interventions with patient, family, and school may be very effective.

ANTISOCIAL BEHAVIOR WITHOUT PSYCHOPATHOLOGY

Some people steal because they are hungry and find themselves in a situation in which they believe they have no other way of obtaining the minimum they need to survive. They may be victims of a social pathology rather than individual psychopathology. It is, of course, essential in all cases to study the psychosocial environment that fosters, supports, encourages, or, to the contrary, strongly and rigidly opposes the antisocial behavior in which any patient is engaged.

Diagnostic Evaluation

The practical implications of this diagnostic spectrum are important. Prognosis and treatment indication depend on the diagnostic assessment and, particularly, the indication or contraindication for a specific psychotherapeutic engagement. As mentioned earlier, pseudopsychopathic schizophrenia is a rare entity that usually must be managed within the forensic field. For these patients, the most important clinical considerations are the extent to which the psychopharmacological treatment of psychosis will reveal a patient able to function with or without antisocial behavior, the corresponding dangerousness, and the indication for possible lifelong hospitalization.

In most cases of antisocial behavior, the most important practical diagnostic question is whether the patient presents an antisocial personality disorder proper or one of the less severe syndromes with antisocial behavior. The differential diagnosis usually is not too difficult to establish in a series of diagnostic interviews, with careful consideration of the past history of the patient, information from all possible sources regarding present and past antisocial behavior, and evaluation of shifting clinical characteristics through a sequence of interviews.

What follows are some examples that illustrate the application of this spectrum of severity of syndromes with antisocial behavior and the differential diagnosis among these various conditions.

A patient was hospitalized after killing his cousin with a shotgun, severing her head, and impaling it in the garden of the house where they lived. He was observed dancing around the impaled head and taken into custody. In the hospital, he was found to be hallucinating and delusional, diagnosed as presenting a schizophrenic illness and treated with atypical antipsychotic medication. After several weeks of treatment, he recovered ordinary reality testing and evinced no delusions, hallucinations, or abnormal behavior, but was remarkable for his total lack of guilt over the crime he had committed. After a further period of observation of several weeks, he brutally assaulted another patient after having been discovered stealing possessions of that patient. The tentative diagnosis of pseudopsychopathic schizophrenia was confirmed after months of neuroleptic treatment in the hospital, when, after a successful escape from the hospital, he stopped all medication and again developed a psychotic condition with manifestations of intense violence that led to his capture and rehospitalization.

Another patient, a young East German adult who was involved with a gang of neo-Nazis that set fire to buildings housing immigrant Turkish workers in a German city, revealed in his psychiatric examination severe narcissistic personality features, including a haughty and paranoid attitude toward personnel (rationalized in terms of his nationalistic ideology), and seemed ready to engage in battle following any minor provocation. He had initially been considered as possibly presenting an aggressive type of antisocial personality structure, but it emerged that he was involved in a yearlong love relation with a young woman, who had become pregnant and delivered a child, and this girlfriend had threatened him with ending their relationship if he did not stop his participation in the attacks on Turkish immigrants. It was this threat that led him to confess his participation in the racial assaults to the investigating authorities and to accept psychotherapeutic treatment offered to him in the context of his forensic evaluation. He was in love with this girlfriend and did not want to lose his relationship with their baby. This case illustrates the syndrome of malignant narcissism—that is, antisocial behavior in the context of a narcissistic personality, paranoid features, and ego-syntonic aggression.

Very different, again is the previously mentioned case of the university professor in the arts, who became an expert in stealing art books over many years while manifesting no other antisocial behavior and was diagnosed as having a narcissistic personality with antisocial behavior.

In contrast, a man who had paid a member of the Mafia an enormous amount to kill his father presented an extremely difficult diagnostic problem. The recipient of that money had been taken into custody for other criminal behaviors, without having carried out that murderous act. He confessed the nature of this financial arrangement, which led to the imprisonment and psychiatric examination of the patient. He revealed a schizoid personality with significant paranoid features, a social withdrawal that conveyed the impression of the possibility of a psychotic process that, however, could not be confirmed. It remained unclear to what extent this was an antisocial personality disorder of the rare paranoid-schizoid personality type or a psychotic illness with antisocial features. The legal system managed his case as that of an aggressive antisocial personality disorder.

Another patient, an accountant, managed over a period of years to appropriate and spend his wife's inheritance, steal the savings of his children, and accumulate a huge debt of unpaid taxes before all of this was discovered, while proclaiming his profound love for wife and children. His history of stealing and diversion of funds reached back into his childhood. He had never shown any aggressive behavior toward others, self, or objects. He pretended to feel guilty over his behavior only at points where it had been discovered and kept his antisocial behavior secret as long as he was able to sustain his secrets. This patient presented a passive-parasitic type of antisocial personality disorder.

I have referred earlier to the physician with an obsessive-compulsive personality who stole chocolates and candy from the cafeteria of the hospital, practically assuring in the process that he would be observed and found guilty of such behavior. Psychoanalytic treatment of this patient confirmed the hypothesis of criminal behavior motivated by unconscious guilt, and several years of treatment liberated him completely from this psychopathology.

It needs to be kept in mind that isolated acts of antisocial behavior, even severely aggressive acts including murder, may be symptoms of other pathology or specific disorganized mental states. Murder as an act of jealousy or the suicide and murder that occasionally complicate psychotic regressions in major depression are examples. It is the repeated enactment of antisocial behavior, the chronicity of it, that alerts the diagnostician to the differential diagnoses that I have spelled out.

In all cases detailed, the mental status examination constitutes the most important basis for the differential diagnosis. We do not yet have specific biological markers or neuropsychological or projective test batteries that would provide the corresponding differential diagnosis. Clinical test batteries may be helpful auxiliary diagnostic tools in some circumstances, but the diagnosis in the end rests on clinical psychiatric evaluation.

The method of structural interviewing developed at the Personality Disorders Institute of the Weill Cornell Medical College Department of

Psychiatry may be particularly helpful in such diagnostic studies (Kernberg 1984), and the test batteries developed by Robert Hare (Hare et al. 1990), as well as the refined criteria of severity of antisocial syndromes developed by Michael Stone (2009), provide additional information. In cases of chronic dishonesty, the information provided by third parties—family members, school, work, the forensic system—is essential. Delicate problems evolve when patients, citing their right to confidentiality, attempt to interfere with the diagnostician's obtaining full information. The extent to which legal support should and can be obtained to permit the diagnostician to expand the patient's evaluation, the question of whether in some cases it has to be recognized that an adequate diagnostic study is not possible under the given circumstances, the setting up of observational periods and hospitalization or partial hospitalization—all require highly individualized decision making. The clinician needs to recognize that sometimes conditions for an adequate diagnostic study simply cannot be obtained, and therefore its impossibility must be acknowledged and accepted.

An important question that often arises, particularly in the case of the aggressive type of antisocial behavior, is the dangerousness of the patient's pathology. The extent to which patients still give some indications of the availability of a moral dimension influencing their behavior, the severity of paranoid features and impulsivity, the potentially lethal nature of previous aggressive outbursts, the severity of the emotional dysregulation—all contribute to the evaluation of the immediate and the long-range dangerousness of the case.

The circumstances of the initiation of the diagnostic evaluation, the possibility of manipulative exploitation of this diagnostic encounter, secondary gain from psychiatric evaluation, and treatment as contrasted to the exclusively legal, forensic system management provide further diagnostic and prognostic indicators.

It is important that countertransference reactions in the evaluation of these patients be carefully monitored. There is a danger both in naïveté and in an uncritical paranoid stance of devaluation and contempt for the patient. Some patients may be frightening, and it is important for the diagnostician to have a realistic assessment of the risks involved for himself or herself. Preventive protective action may become necessary for the diagnostician to feel safe. When questions about antisocial behavior are raised with the patient, it is important to maintain a moral but not moralistic approach to avoid a critical or punitive attitude, in contrast to a descriptive and investigative attitude, in dealing with the patient's behavior. The therapist, I repeat, cannot be naïve and must accept the fact that at times he or she will be lied to and should not be tempted to deny the patient's conscious deceptiveness by describing the patient as "confused."

Sometimes only repeated examinations over a period of several weeks, while new information is brought into the sessions confronting the patient with issues that he has avoided to mention before, permit the therapist to diagnose more sharply the absence of a moral dimension in the discourse of the patient. A patient who initially professes his or her remorse over antisocial behaviors already known to the therapist may insist that "this is all there is" regarding such antisocial features. Yet, when later independent sources of information provide the therapist information about additional important antisocial behavior, the patient may react again, professing deep guilt feelings about it and suggesting that he or she simply "forgot" to mention the new information.

Psychological tests may provide further information regarding the patient's narcissistic pathology and may help to clarify if a psychotic illness needs to be considered. However, in most cases tests do not permit the therapist to establish the differential diagnosis outlined earlier: clinical judgment and information from reliable external sources constitute the essential basis for a diagnostic conclusion.

An important feature of the diagnostic evaluation is the patient's dangerousness. This issue is relevant for the initial evaluation as well as for the assessment of the degree of supervision and control required at each stage of the patient's legal, custodial, or general psychiatric hospitalization and treatment. The key prognostic factors to be considered are, first, whether the patient definitely presents an antisocial personality disorder; second, the severity of the aggression toward self or others, as revealed by the history of illness; and third, whether there is a total absence of any moral constraints—in other words, total unavailability of any superego function—which would reinforce the dangerous potential of aggressive or delinquent behavior. In addition to these features, the patient's overall level of impulsivity, the prevalence of paranoid tendencies, the striking absence of any nonexploitive object relationship, and evidence of a severe, sadistic perversion complete the constellation of high-level dangerousness that needs to be considered in the therapeutic management and that should include appropriate protection of the patient, the therapist, the patient's immediate social environment, and society at large.

References

American Psychiatric Association: Diagnostic and Statistical Manual: Mental Disorders. Washington, DC, American Psychiatric Association, 1952, p 38

Bender DS: Therapeutic alliance, in The American Psychiatric Publishing Textbook of Personality Disorders, 2nd Edition. Edited by Oldham JM, Skodol AE, Bender DS. Washington, DC, American Psychiatric Publishing, 2014, pp 189–216

Bender L: The concept of pseudopsychopathic schizophrenia in adolescents. Am J Orthopsychiatry 29:491–512, 1959 13798781

Cleckley HM: The Mask of Sanity. St Louis, MO, CV Mosby, 1941

Coid J, Ullrich S: Antisocial personality disorder is on a continuum with psychopathy. Compr Psychiatry 51(4):426–433, 2010 20579518

Durst R, Jabotinsky-Rubin K, Fliman M: Pseudopsychopathic schizophrenia—a neglected diagnostic entity with legal implications. Med Law 16(3):487–498, 1997 9409132

Freud S: Criminals from a sense of guilt (1916), in Standard Edition of the Complete Psychological Works of Sigmund Freud, Vol 14. Translated and edited by Strachey J. London, Hogarth Press, 1957, pp 332–333

Hare RD, Harpur TJ, Hakstian AR: The Revised Psychopathy Checklist: reliability and factor structure. Psychol Assess 2(3):338–341, 1990

Holmesland P, Astrup C: Pseudoneurotic and pseudopsychopathic schizophrenia: a follow-up. Neuropsychobiology 12(2–3):101–105, 1984 6527748

Kernberg OF: Severe Personality Disorders: Psychotherapeutic Strategies. New Haven, CT, Yale University Press, 1984

Kernberg OF: Aggression in Personality Disorders and Perversion. New Haven, CT, Yale University Press, 1992

Kernberg OF: An overview of the treatment of severe narcissistic pathology. Int J Psychoanal 95(5):865–888, 2014 24902768

Stone MH: The Anatomy of Evil. Amherst, NY, Prometheus Books, 2009

PART IV

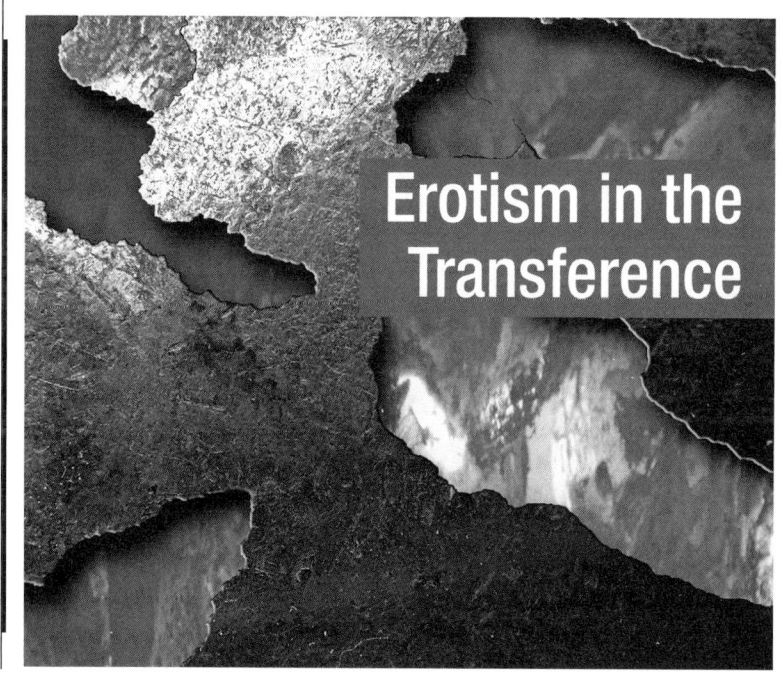

Erotism in the Transference

CHAPTER 12

Erotic Transference and Countertransference in Patients With Severe Personality Disorders

Part I: The Evaluation of Sexual Pathology

What follows is an overview of our experiences in diagnosing and treating patients with severe personality disorders and related significant conflicts in their sexual life at the Weill Cornell Medical College Personality Disorders Institute. This overview includes patients treated using transference-focused psychotherapy (TFP) and standard psychoanalysis but also includes those treated with a more supportive approach.

This chapter was originally presented as a paper at the Third International Conference of the International Society of Transference-Focused Psychotherapy, Parma, Italy, October 13–15, 2014. I wish to thank my colleagues and the patients whom we have attempted to help for their contributions to this chapter.

A First Major Obstacle

We have been impressed by the emerging contradiction between our emphasis on the need to thoroughly explore love and sex, work and profession, social life, and creativity as important sources of satisfaction with life—as well as sources of inhibitions, conflicts, and pathology in the lives of our patients—and the reluctance that psychoanalysts and psychoanalytic psychotherapists frequently show when it comes to the exploration and management of these domains, especially sexual problems. From beginning therapists to seasoned psychoanalysts, we have found a remarkable reluctance to explore the details of patients' sexual experiences, fantasies, and interactions and the erotic elements of transference and countertransference as they become apparent from the very first encounter with a patient. Part of this reluctance may be related to cultural conventionalities, but part also seems to relate to a puzzling decrease of interest in erotic life within psychoanalytic literature. Leading psychoanalytic theoreticians, such as André Green (2010), have expressed astonishment over the neglect of infantile sexuality. Ruth Stein (2008) wondered to what extent eroticism was being neglected in the middle of contemporary controversies between drive theory and object relations theory. The centrality of infantile sexuality seems to have become an orphan in the midst of this debate. The fact that strong cultural taboos remain regarding infantile sexuality seems obvious. Empirical research on the observation of the erotic behavior of infants and children has practically disappeared, with scant research dollars available for this line of inquiry.

In our work, it is evident that erotic elements play an important role in the initial evaluation of patients. Therapists do get an immediate sense of the degree of erotic attractiveness, inhibition, or repulsion evoked by patients—the extent to which aggressive erotic display and seductiveness, rigid inhibition, and significant dissociation between love and tenderness, on the one hand, and erotic desire and excitement, on the other, is an important aspect of the patient's difficulties. By the same token, therapists' correspondent countertransference reactions may indicate an important conflictual area to explore in the treatment. Patients may be erotically attractive or repulsive, and frequently seem to be so totally asexual that the thought about this subject does not occur to the therapist.

In theory, therapists—and especially analysts—are aware of the importance of systematically exploring patients' sexual fantasies and activities, preferences and inhibitions, and the role that erotic feelings and behavior have as part of their relationships, both in intimate relationships of sexual love and in their demeanor within the social context. A certain degree of erotic tension is always part of what emotionally characterizes group behavior in social networks. Very often, despite an initial history that reveals significant sexual difficulties, a dissociation of sexual material from other areas of the patient's experience may develop, contributing to making his or her actual erotic behavior "disappear" from the discourse.

For example, one patient consulted a senior psychoanalyst for a significant inhibition in her sexual response. She was able to achieve mild excitement after sexual penetration, followed by a gradual disappearance of her erotic response during intercourse, and then total incapacity to reach orgasm in any kind of sexual interaction with her partner. Interestingly enough, this symptom disappeared from the subject matter of the analytic sessions and had not been taken up at all during the next 3 years of standard psychoanalytic treatment, in which very important oedipal conflicts and competitiveness had been explored in depth. Patient and therapist may establish "bastions" of silence (Baranger and Baranger 1969)—unconscious collusion to avoid sexual matters. Often, sexual behavior may be referred to in such general terms that any real information is lost. "We had a very good sexual experience last night. It was great, very different from other times." That seems like the beginning of an explorative dialogue, but, in fact, no further exploration occurs.

This practical problem is matched by subtle shifts in the focus on dominant psychological conflicts within a psychodynamic approach. In recent times, new knowledge regarding early attachment, and of the psychopathological consequences of insecure attachment and its central role in the development of object relations, has, appropriately, been at the center of attention of psychoanalytic thinking regarding early development. However, these advances have been accompanied by a significant neglect of the erotic element of early development. Contemporary knowledge of the neurobiology of affects centers around the development of major affect systems with specific central nervous system structures, neurotransmitters, and hormonal components. These specific primary affect systems include the attachment system itself, the erotic affect system, and the play-bonding system—all of which imply positive, pleasurable, affiliative motivation—and the fight-flight and the separation-panic system as negative, aversive motivational systems. These primary affect systems may be viewed in the context of a general affective "seeking" system that motivates a general, positive exploration of the environment and provides reinforcement to the activation of other systems stimulated by environmental interaction. It is as if the concern with the development of secure or insecure attachment has displaced the attention to the other positive affect systems, particularly the erotic aspects of the infant–

mother relationship. Clinically, the focus on the immediate positive and negative affective relations of couples, and of the transference itself, tends to be formulated in terms of an enmeshed, avoidant, or secure attachment, and the erotic domain remains in the shadows.

Primary dependence linked to the attachment system appears as the only major positive motivational source of the mother–infant relationship and reflects a frequent reluctance to consider *eroticism* and *aggression* as intimately involved in motivational systems operating jointly with attachment in the earliest internalization of object relations. The contribution of mother's erotic response to her baby in evoking the infant's capacity for erotic response at a primary unconscious level, as well as the unconscious induction of that capability in her interactions with the baby, is theoretically accepted, such as in Laplanche's (1970/1976, 1987/1989, 1999) work, but this contribution tends to be neglected clinically. Ruth Stein (2008) refers to the importance of this primary erotic induction and its role in originating a mysterious, exciting, oceanic experience that will mark a sharp differentiation from the experience of ordinary normal living, determining a lifelong tension between reality-oriented, rational self experience and the passionate expansion of the sense of self as a limitless subjectivity.

Independently from psychoanalytic explorations, Bataille (1957) concluded in his study of eroticism that human experience was marked by a sharp isolation between experiences controlled by the sense of time and space and objectivity, and other existential ones, with a sense of infiniteness, subjectivity, and transgression of ordinary limits and boundaries in contrast to the adaptive boundaries in the stabilized experience of reality. Sexual and religious ecstasies represent such experiential conditions. One may translate these two realms of emotional experience as a function of adaptation to social reality, on the one hand, and the tolerance of emotional freedom for a full and limitless exploration of subjectivity, on the other. They represent a duality that provides interest and liveliness to daily experience. The elimination of the passionate world would reduce life to a dull, constricted realistic functionalism, whereas an exclusive immersion in the subjective world of passion would become self-destructive and cause the loss of boundaries in relation to reality, including extreme self-destructiveness as the result of the search for total, unlimited pleasure.

A Mature Capacity for Successful Love

What can we expect as the ideal of a mature capacity for sexual love, as expressed by an integration of eroticism and tenderness, idealization and responsibility, enjoyment and passion? By *ideal*, we do not imply unrealistic goals with the implication that patients should live up to them, but a frame of what might be optimally possible in order to highlight the greatest difficulties to achieve such a condition. What are the most severe limitations determining the distance that separates the patient from the rich life that he or she might have? We are not talking about an ideal of "normality," but a theoretical outline that facilitates the diagnosis of problematic issues that restrict the capacity to love. To begin with, such an outline should include a sharp focus on the capacity to experience sexual pleasure proper, to establish object relations in depth, and to establish one's own and joined value systems in the relationship within a couple. An optimal way to evaluate the capacity for maturity in loving is to evaluate a patient who is involved in a love relationship or has been in a love relationship that can be explored as such.

SEXUAL FREEDOM

We would expect a patient to be able not only to achieve sexual arousal, excitement, and orgasm in ordinary sexual intercourse, but to enjoy the freedom of experimenting with aspects of polymorphous infantile sexuality, voyeuristic, exhibitionistic, masochistic, sadistic, fetishistic, heterosexual, and homosexual fantasies and activities—at least in ways in which these motivations and corresponding activity can be expressed in the context of free, intense, passionate, and playful sexual relations that would tolerate all these elements of sexual experience under the organizing principle of genital intimacy.

This capability would be expressed within the relationship of a couple, in the context of feelings of love—that is, an appreciation of the personality of the partner together with gratitude for the intimacy, the expression of tenderness and idealization of the person as well as the body of one's partner. It also would show in the intensity of sexual interest, the frequency of intercourse, the frequent enactment of the arousal→excitement→orgasm→relaxation cycle, and the capacity of total freedom from shame in the intimate relation of the couple. Full sexual freedom is not too infrequent in many patients, but what we do see frequently is the total dissociation of sexual freedom from the primary love relationship, in which aspects of dissociated conflicts around preoedipal and oedipal aggression dominate; thus, sexual freedom has to be examined in the context of the capability for an object relation in depth with the object of sexual desire. Can sexual freedom and love be maintained in a relationship with one's partner, or will they become necessarily kept apart as a result of unconscious conflicts?

OBJECT RELATION IN DEPTH

An *object relation in depth* means the capacity for passionate love; a tolerance for ambivalence, in the sense that any frustrations or disappointments that generate rage may be expressed without threatening the basic loving commitment; the interest in the personality of the partner; the concern for the other's enjoyment of daily life together; and happiness with the stability of the relationship. In such an intimate object relation, there would not be room for "power" games, and there would be a sense of fair distribution of work responsibilities and mutual help, the capacity to enjoy closeness as well as tolerating separateness. The unavoidable presence of oedipal conflicts—with their triangulation fears and triangulation revenge, the jealousy arising from the fear that somebody else will be more attractive to one's partner than oneself, the temptation to establish a parallel relationship with another as a revengeful reversal of the infantile triangular experience of being excluded—should be tolerable, without such fantasies taking over and controlling the behavior of the individual (Kernberg 1995). All of this is involved in and reflects the tolerance for ambivalence and would indicate the achievement of the capacity for a love relationship in depth.

Of course, a clear sexual identity that implies a stable, predominant selection of a heterosexual or homosexual partner, a harmonious acceptance of behaviors in consonance with one's core sexual identity, and the intense idealization of another who fulfills the search of one's oedipal ideal are also involved in the capacity for sexual passion. So, emotional intensity of love, admiration of the personality of the other, and intensity of erotic desire come together in the capacity to initiate a relation by falling in love, and transforming falling in love into the stable development of a consolidated love relation as indications of the capacity for object relations in depth. The wish to become a couple also reflects an unconscious identification with an ideal image of a parental couple, daring to identify with its role or establish a better relationship than that of one's own parental couple.

THE COUPLE'S JOINED VALUE SYSTEM

The establishment of a joined value system with the person one loves does not just refer simply to a sense of commonality or harmony with respect to political, religious, or other ideological commitments, but also refers to a basic agreement regarding joint moral principles involved in the couple's profound respect for each other's ideas and interests. It includes ongoing wishes to learn from the other and share one's own thinking; and the wish to protect the couple from threatening invasion by the remnants of old unresolved conflicts with their families of origin, the disappointments and resentments, guilt and revenge; and the availability of forgiveness cemented in basic trust. Henry Dicks (1967) has stressed that practically all couples carry with them aspects of unresolved conflicts from childhood with their respective parental images that tend to be unconsciously reactivated in the present. The members of the couple tend to reactivate the past in their present relationship in an unconscious effort to work through and resolve old conflicts, and this temptation may blow up in episodes of "private madness," determining irrational behavior and crises that a couple should be able to tolerate and resolve without an accumulation of resentment.

The objective then is to explore in great detail the sexual configurations of patients' lives at the time of the initial diagnostic evaluation and then to keep track of these issues throughout the treatment in the context of the activation of transference/countertransference enactments.

General Preconditions for the Therapist

To penetrate a patient's intimate sexual world is a complex and delicate aspect of the exploration of the patient's pathology. The therapist's personal freedom from unresolved sexual conflicts becomes an important aspect of his or her capacity to register the complexity of the patient's sexual life. We assume that psychoanalytic training frees candidates from major blind spots and that the therapist's own sexual difficulties should have been explored and resolved. In practice, however, at the Personality Disorders Institute at Cornell, we have found in careful supervisory work with experienced psychoanalysts, as well as with beginning or relatively young therapists, that countertransferences to patients' sexual experiences constitute an important potential limitation to the therapist's freedom for full exploration of this complex area, and that some general characteristics of the therapist's personality may represent important compensating factors that permit the analyst to be open to patients' problems beyond limitations in the therapist's personal sexual life. We have found that it helps if the therapist has a full personal love life, including a fully satisfied sexual life with a degree of freedom of sexual fantasy, play, and exploration in the context of a gratifying, stable love relationship. These conditions help the therapist to be alert to the patient's limitations in this area and to be able to explore them without undue inhibition or emotional distance. It also is helpful when the therapist feels comfortable with the awareness of his or her and others' reaction to the erotic component of all social interactions, the awareness of sexual "vibes" emitted by or absent in others and himself or herself in social situations. Sometimes, a striking intensity of conscious or unconscious seductive "irradiation" and different degrees of erotic response by the therapist may be evoked by patients, with or without the therapist's being disturbed by them, potentially broadening the therapist's understanding of the patient's sexual conflicts.

Ideally, the therapist should relate to the dialectic referred to in Bataille's (1957) approach to psychic experience—that is, the freedom of shifting between times of reality-based, objective work focused consistently on dealing with daily life tasks, challenges, and interactions, and times when, under controlled circumstances, it is possible to "let go," to submerge oneself in an intense, passionate sexual encounter, in the ecstatic reaction to a work of art, in an experience of friendship, in a state of religious ecstasy, or even in the unpredictable intoxication related to drugs. This statement could be misunderstood as proposing some built-in "psychoticism" in the therapist's personality, which is certainly not the intention or the clarification of this point. It is a matter of being open to ecstatic experiences: sexual, artistic, religious.

In the description a patient gives about his or her sexual life in the initial encounter as part of the diagnostic evaluation of patients with severe personality disorders, we have found it helpful to be open and alert to the availability or the foreclosure of any erotic aspect of the emotional atmosphere that evolves between the therapist and the patient. It is helpful when the therapist has the capacity to transcend the conventional internal restrictions on such a freedom to explore the erotic dimension in the relation with the patient in the therapist's fantasy, given the patient's gender, age, and pathology.

Given his or her internal freedom, the therapist will be better able to explore fully the patient's sexuality during the treatment. The barrier to homosexual identification that may evolve between a homosexual patient and a heterosexual psychotherapist determines one particular difficulty in the exploration of the patient's sexual life. The therapist should acquire the freedom to identify fully with the vicissitudes of the sexual life and experience of all patients, including the case of homosexual therapists exploring the sexual life of heterosexual patients. In theory, we take this for granted, but practical experience frequently reveals potential limitations, inhibitions, and uncertainties in the therapist's capacity to identify with patients' erotic experiences. Obviously, the therapist's capacity for empathy with different sexual experiences is relevant in the evaluation of patients with organized perversions.

With cases of serious sexual inhibitions and the restriction of organized perversions, primitive sexual countertransferences may emerge during the treatment that the therapist may have difficulty tolerating and must analyze regarding their relation to the patient's projective processes. It is important that the therapist tolerate primitivity in his or her own sexual fantasy life. A consequence of the degree of sexual freedom the therapist possesses regarding his or her sexual life and fantasy is the capacity to confront the patient fearlessly with his or her difficulties and to explore the patient's sexual fantasies and experiences in depth without a seductive attitude or a superego-derived critical one. This necessarily includes being able to confront the patient with painful aspects of sexualized transferences with concern for the patient and the trust that the patient will be able to capture this attitude of the therapist.

Diagnostic Evaluation

What follows are some further thoughts regarding the diagnostic evaluation. I have described elsewhere the structural interview as a method that is particularly helpful in the evaluation of patients with severe personality disorders (Kernberg 1984), and I shall limit my comments to focus on the evaluation of the patient's sexual life within the context of that interview. It is important to obtain detailed information about the patient's love life and his or her sexual experiences. The old-fashioned concern that detailed history taking would interfere with the development of the transference and the assumption that the important issues in the patient's sexuality and love life would emerge naturally during the treatment, rather than artificially distorted in a focused exploration, has proved false in our clinical experience. Detailed initial evaluation permits arriving at a better diagnosis and treatment indication, and it provides an important source of information that will become relevant in orienting the therapist at later points in the treatment, even more so as the patient's life situation changes in the context of the treatment, with new understanding, elaboration, and working through of the patient's past.

We are interested in the extent to which there is a true capacity for commitment in the patient's love relations, capacity for full enjoyment of the sexual aspects of the relationship, and the commonality of aspirations, goals, and value systems of the couple. If the patient is significantly involved with a partner, we explore the patient's awareness of the personality of that person as part of the structural interview revealing the patient's capacity for object relationships.

The exploration of the patient's sexual life includes exploring the nature of his or her sexual behavior, the capacity for sexual interest or arousal, the freedom to approach a love object sexually, the increase of sexual excitement before and during intercourse, the capacity to reach orgasm, the frequency of sexual interactions and orgasm, the freedom to employ fantasy and play in his or her sexual activities, the freedom from undue shame and guilt over sexual intimacy, and the extent to which his or her internal freedom is reflected in the capacity to respond positively and openly to this inquiry. The frequency of the patient's sexual activity (both interactional and masturbatory), the degree of satisfaction, and the nature of his or her sexual fantasies are important as well as the frequency and the nature of dreams with sexual content. Masturbatory fantasies, particularly frequently repeated specific scenarios, are an important window into dominant conflicts in the patient's sexual life: the unconscious conflicts condensed in such stable scenarios gradually may be clarified during psychoanalytic treatment.

The therapist's countertransference disposition will provide parallel information as an assessment, as well as a response to the patient: whether the patient is attractive or not; whether the patient seems to be emitting sexual "vibes" or not; whether the patient is reacting in a paranoid, inhibited, rejecting, seductive, or provocative way; and whether the patient is presenting himself or herself, by means of demeanor, clothes, or attitude, as a person who would make an attractive impression on others, or a seductive one, or a disgusting one, or a suspicious one. Age and gender of the patient may influence the direction and sequence of questions. An important countertransference element may be the therapist's reluctance to fully explore the sexual behavior of patients with a great difference in age: adolescents being seen by older therapists, and older patients being seen by young and relatively inexperienced therapists, typically illustrate sources of therapist's inhibitions.

On the basis of this inquiry, it should be possible to assess the patient's degree of sexual freedom, including the extent to which his or her sexuality is inhibited by guilt or shame reactions, is used in a proper context, is used in teasing or seductive ways, or is characterized by a harmonious integration into the patient's thinking, behaviors, and fantasies. At the same time, while we gain information about the quality of the patient's object relations from descriptions of sexual partners, we are alert to indications of severe identity diffusion. The extent to which the patient's capacity for love, emotional intimacy, and passionate commitment is integrated with sexual desire and freedom—or the extent to which there is a severe dissociation between the capacity to love on the one hand, and for sexual excitement and erotic interest on the other—can be diagnosed in this context. There are patients with full development of an intense and varied sexual activity who evince a traumatic or narcissistic limitation in their capacity for object relations, and impulsive sexual encounters replace the capacity to establish love relationships, whereas other patients reveal a capacity for object relations in depth in the context of significant inhibition of their sexual freedom. The extent to which polymorphous infantile sexual components are integrated into the adult patient's sexual life, or the extent to which the patient is restricted to one particular infantile sexual trend (in the case of perversions), needs to be connected with the freedom or restriction of the object relations that the patient is able to establish.

An important element that emerges during this inquiry is the nature of the patient's superego functioning and the extent to which there is excessively severe superego pressure expressed in exaggerated experiences of guilt and shame. Alternatively, in cases of severe impulsivity and chaos in the expression of sexual impulses, one issue may be the extent to which failure or deficiency in superego functioning is involved in the aggressive use of sexual excitement, seductiveness, and need to control, dominate, and exploit others. We are interested in the patient's capacity for concern, responsibility, honesty, and consistency in his or her respect and treatment of sexual partners in contrast with sadistic dominance, irresponsibility, and exploitation. Patients who are involved in an intimate love relationship at the time of their evaluation facilitate the exploration of these major areas of the relationship of the couple.

Sexual Conflicts at the Level of Neurotic Personality Organization

In a highly simplified way, one might differentiate an overall level of unconscious conflicts at a neurotic level of personality organization from one at a borderline level of personality organization in terms of the predominance of advanced oedipal conflicts within the neurotic range of pathology versus the predominance of unconscious conflicts related to preoedipal aggression condensed with archaic oedipal conflicts in borderline personality organization. Predominance of advanced oedipal conflicts is reflected in unconscious guilt over oedipal sexual impulses and characterologically structured self-affirmative and self-defeating behaviors reflecting such unconscious guilt. The unconscious search for triangular relations as an expression of oedipal conflicts is frequently enacted, particularly with direct and reverse triangulations: a tendency to be fixated in self-defeating, frustrating love affairs, and an unconscious intolerance of potentially happy love relations. Being abandoned by one's love object's choosing a rival or one's unhappy love for somebody committed to somebody else represents *direct triangulation*. *Reverse triangulation* may be reflected in infidelity, simultaneous love relations with two partners, or the revengeful abandoning of a love object. Frequently, oedipal guilt is reflected in various degrees of sexual inhibition, dissociation between idealized love relations accompanied by sexual inhibition on the one hand, and sexual freedom in relationships that are frustrating or devoid of emotional intimacy on the other. Masochistic sexual promiscuity, represented by a series of unhappy love relations, needs to be differentiated from narcissistic sexual promiscuity, which is an endless sequence of temporary idealizations and rapidly following devaluations that destroy all relationships within a limited period, or else stable but superficial object relations accompanied by dissociated sexual promiscuity.

A hallmark of the neurotic level of sexual conflicts is the capacity for establishing object relations in depth, the tolerance of ambivalence in love relations with deep and stable commitments, and the capacity for interest in and availability in depth to a love life with another person with whom a deep mutuality of understanding can be established. In contrast, in borderline personality organization, the predominance of splitting mechanisms and related primitive defensive operations, particularly projective identification, is reflected in chaotic relationships and the incapacity to appreciate in a realistic and deep way both the partner's personality and his or her own. This basic situation is further complicated in the case of narcissistic pathology, in which lack of the capacity of investment in love relations is reflected in a typical, chronic dissociation of sexual interests from shallow emotional relations and, under extreme circumstances, a practically complete replacement of any sexual intimacy by almost mechanical sexual encounters, "Internet sexuality," or a total sexual inhibition reflecting the loss of any sexual interest.

Intensive, long-term psychoanalytic psychotherapy or psychoanalysis represents a symbolic replica of the oedipal situation, an ongoing intimate relationship that fosters the patient's development of sexual desire with a person—the therapist—with whom an intimate relationship develops, of particularly sexual openness on the part of the patient, while total implicit prohibition of any sexual involvement replicates the inhibition of the original oedipal scenario. The difference between the original oedipal situation and the treatment situation is the possibility of full exploration of oedipal desires: their frustrations and related conflicts, the development and exploration of disappointment reactions, resentment because of the unavoidable nonavailability of the oedipal object, and eventually the sublimatory resolution of the conflict within the openness to and search for alternative, realistic gratification of intimate sexual love and commitment in external reality.

A lack of resolution of oedipal conflicts at a level of neurotic personality organization is most typically expressed in the pathological reaction to experienced rejection or abandonment by a love object that reinforces the neurotic desire and passionate love toward unavailable objects. This may become a major resistance in the transferences of neurotic patients with masochistic personality structure, replicating in the treatment their temptation for the search for impossible, unavailable love relations in external life. Defensive, aggressive deterioration of love relations with clearly available but unconsciously guilt-provoking oedipal objects is replicated in transference developments of hostility and competitiveness as defenses against underlying erotic impulses. Typically, however, all these conflicts develop in the context of a capacity of a relationship in depth, and aggressive oedipal competitiveness, revengefulness, or defensive reactions against dependency and against intimate involvement are expressed in the context of such a potential for an object relation with depth and commitment.

In contrast, under conditions of borderline personality organization, the activation of aggressive impulses reflects a condensation of conflicts of oedipal and preoedipal nature, with predominance of preoedipal aggression, primitive aggressive impulses, and defenses against related, frustrated early dependent needs, and the predominance of sadomasochistic over loving experiences from earliest life on. Here, all dependency is charged with mistrust and resentment, and the need for omnipotent control and revenge, in replacement of the capacity to enjoy realistically available dependency. The need to deny all dependency upon a hated and envied parental object complicates these dynamics further in the case of narcissistic pathology.

The following case illustrates the nature of the conflict that facilitates the differential diagnosis between a relatively high-level, neurotic structure and the particular condensation of conflicts typical for borderline personality organization.

> The patient was a woman in her middle 40s, who was involved in a long-term relationship with a man who loved her and was disposed to marry her but was hesitant to follow through because of violent attacks of jealousy that the patient expressed regarding any other women whom they would pass on the street and her boyfriend would look at. Such situations would trigger intense rage and violent verbal, and at times physical, attacks on her boyfriend. She would also have occasional rage attacks with other people who frustrated her wishes, but the most intense, repetitive, and destructive attacks were on her boyfriend. These attacks were

triggered by whatever reason that would justify her suspecting him of his being interested in another woman and suspecting him of being dishonest with her by having secrets, including suspicions whenever he arrived later than they had arranged to meet. After each of these rage attacks she realized that they were inappropriate, "crazy," and affecting her relationship with him, but she was totally unable to control herself.

Her mother was a dominant and intrusive woman who encouraged the patient never to trust any man and not to commit herself to any relationship in depth, while apparently being quite permissive regarding transitory sexual affairs in which the patient would engage. The patient's father, a withdrawn, passive man, lived in a chronically resentful relationship with his dominant wife, letting her run the household while keeping to his own business, and he avoided getting involved with the problems his daughter had in her love relations.

In the transference, this patient presented an ambivalently dependent relationship with the therapist, to whom she would complain about her tribulations, begging him to help her with her rage attacks but systematically ignoring his efforts to help her understand the deeper reasons for her behavior. It had become very clear in the context of TFP, two sessions per week, over 1.5 years, that she treated the therapist as if he were a replica of her distant, uninterested, and weak father, identifying herself unconsciously with her dominant mother in her depreciative attitude toward the therapist and in enacting her mother's suspicion, distrust, and hatred of men during her rage attacks against the boyfriend. She was both submitting to mother and, having incorporated mother into her superego as a primitive internalized persecutor, identifying pathologically with her mother during those crises. At a deeper level, it became clear that she did not dare to compete with her mother and feared the establishment of a better relationship with her boyfriend and a potentially better marriage with him than what her parents had achieved. At a point when the relationship between her and her boyfriend seemed to improve and they decided to jointly operate a business they had created and that proved quite successful, she could not resist the temptation to bring her mother into the business. Her mother then rapidly attempted to take over the control of the business and clearly fostered whatever conflict she could trigger in the relationship between her daughter and her boyfriend. The patient became highly critical of her mother, being angry and resentful at times, though in a clearly dissociated way, but also submissive and engaging her mother even more. She clearly was fostering her mother's invasive intrusion into the relationship with her boyfriend, with enormous difficulty in realizing and confronting the contradictory nature of these opposite trends of interactions with her mother. At the same time, she showed that same contradiction in her behavior with the therapist, oscillating between pleading dependency and submissiveness, and opposition and dismissal, which also characterized the conflictual behavior with her boyfriend.

This case, obviously simplified in this presentation to highlight the essential conflict and related defenses, illustrates a strong predominance of oedipal conflicts, but with an infiltration of a more primitive relationship with a needed and unavailable, but also angry and controlling, mother, revealing an insecure attachment and a deep incapacity to trust. Her defensive repertoire included both the repression of oedipal impulses toward father and of deep guilt feelings toward mother, and the more primitive splitting mechanisms that facilitated the activation of contradictory behavior regarding dependency and rejection, and the projection of her own hostile impulses onto her boyfriend through her accusations of cheating and disloyalty.

In the transference, it became necessary to analyze both her identification with and submission to a primitive hostile and controlling mother, and the sacrifice of a gratifying love relationship in the context of which her erotic sexuality could be satisfied. She was able to have intense, "wild" sex with her boyfriend when their relationship was about to end, but she showed a remarkable inhibition in her capacity for sexual response at times when their relationship was a very good one and she was happy and gratified with his love of her. The activation of the dyadic relationship with her mother, in which she was alternately projecting her self representation onto the therapist while identifying with mother and, at other times, perceiving the therapist as a hostile mother who was trying to brainwash her into subservience while she experienced a helpless self representation in relating to mother, required a lengthy, repetitive analytic working through. This process evolved into the development of both guilt feelings and a more ego-syntonic erotic transference to the therapist, a gradual overcoming of her oedipal guilt, and the direct expression of her hatred of her mother that she had never dared to experience.

This treatment involved repetitive confrontation of her aggression against her boyfriend, her destructive denial of the transference analysis, the denial of the external reality reflected by her collusion with mother's invasive and destructive behavior toward the couple, and the reenactment of these difficulties with the therapist in the course of repetitive role reversals in the transference.

Erotic developments in the countertransference signal the extent to which the patient's erotic conflicts are being repressed, suppressed, denied, projected, or acted out. In the case of predominant repression of erotic impulses, erotic reactions in the countertransference may be minimal or absent, except for transference reasons of the therapist, if this patient presents some particularly exciting features for him or her. If the erotic reactions of the patient are overtly denied but expressed in a dissociated way in bodily appearance or expression, or in the clothing and expressive attitudes in the sessions, erotic countertransference may provide an important indication of the activation of such erotic conflicts in the transference and may lead to their interpretive approach. If the patient is suppressing concrete fears over sexual seduction on the part of the therapist, in the context of projection of his or her sexual impulses onto the therapist, erotic countertransference may be low or absent; however, if the patient is struggling with conscious sexual desires in the transference, the suppression of that information may nevertheless correspond to very intense erotic countertransference reactions. The dissociation of erotic impulses from the expression of emotional tenderness and dependency in the transference again may reduce significantly any erotic countertransference. Finally, with direct acting out of erotic transferences in the treatment situation, the therapist may respond with a positive erotic countertransference if the patient's reaction is not dominated by aggressive implications. In the case of the use of seductiveness to disarm or control the therapist or to destroy the treatment situation, the therapist not only may have no erotic counterreaction to the patient but may experience anxiety over the experienced aggressive implication of suddenly, or not so suddenly, expressed surface sexual behavior. In the case of the treatment of patients with severe personality disorders, the frequent tendency to acting out makes this an important issue to be managed and requires from the therapist an open confrontation of the patient's sexual behavior in the session, without punitive or seductive implications, maintaining a firm but respectful attitude in exploring the patient's behavior.

As mentioned earlier, the typical characteristics of neurotic structures include the capability for full-fledged development of emotional commitments reflected in the capacity for a tender loving relationship with a significant other, in the context of some degree of sexual inhibition. Sexual inhibition, in turn, may present as a direct sexual symptom such as some degree or type of impotence in men or inhibition of sexual desire, excitement, or orgasm in women (which in turn may require different treatment strategies in terms of the possibility of using sex therapy as an auxiliary treatment in the milder cases). Neurotic structure may also present as splitting between sexual freedom in relationships that lack intimacy, on the one hand, and sexual inhibition in the context of a deep love relationship on the other. As a general rule, both in patients with sexual inhibition and a split between sexuality and tenderness and in patients with sexual perversion, it is the working through of oedipal conflicts in the transference relationship that results in fundamental therapeutic effects. This constitutes a crucial difference with more severe personality disorders, in which the disturbances in the patient's identity and related primitive object relations require an extended, complex working through of the consideration of archaic oedipal conflicts with preoedipal aggression.

Perhaps masochistic scenarios and the expression of masochistic character pathology in the transference represent the most typical expression of sexual difficulties at a neurotic level of organization. In relatively simple cases, patients may have suppressed erotic feelings for the therapist that clearly become evident in the nonverbal manifestations of the patient's communications to the therapist and may involve intense erotic countertransferences that may inhibit the therapist from confronting the patient's transferences because of the fear of its seductive effects, or the fear of the patient's experiencing such a confrontation as an aggressive rejection or condemning intervention.

As an illustration, a female patient in her late 20s sought consultation because of severe difficulties in her relations with men. Her boyfriends, for unknown reasons, rejected or abandoned her after what initially seemed like a very positive relationship, in what turned out to be the enactment of a masochistic pattern of behavior on her part. Unconsciously, she would provoke them to reject her. She presented herself in the sessions in a very typical manner. She was always dressed in gray clothing, unattractively put together, with a clear neglect of the way she dressed and presented herself, a hairdo that would seem to conflict with her facial features, cigarette ashes on her dress, and only one highly significant erotized aspect; her dresses always showed deep décolletage, and a significant portion of her breast was exposed and was experienced disturbingly as exciting by her male therapist. In exploring her strong fears of criticism by him, this element of her presentation was never taken up in the session. She had to interrupt her treatment because of an important fellowship in a different country. After leaving, she wrote him an extended letter, in which she told him how very attracted she had been to him from very early on and how intensely she suffered by the fact that she could see him so frequently, feel so close to him, and yet be so terribly frustrated by him. Obviously, here, the full expression and working through of the masochistic love relation in the transference was missed. The therapist had not been able to elaborate the information given by his countertransference and to interpret the correspondent transference situation.

More frequently, a different masochistic scenario may prevail. Patients come to treatment and reveal a present, highly unsatisfactory relationship. For example, a woman mentioned how her boyfriend treated her as a slave, ignored her wishes in "dragging her along," and was more attentive to his computer than to her. After having sexual intercourse with her and spending the night, he then would organize his daily life with total neglect and lack of consideration of her. It seemed like a caricature of a sadomasochistic relationship, which the patient complained about bitterly without making any move to confront him or to end the relationship. In the transference, the therapist was at first experienced as very helpful in listening to her and empathizing with her suffering, but eventually the therapist was experienced as an "enemy" who was trying to destroy her relationship with her boyfriend, who "was all she had." The transference became hostile and aggressive, and the therapist interpreted how the patient would have to continue depending on a "bad" object while having to reject and distort what she was being offered from a "good" object. The systematic exploration of this negative transference, and of the development of negative therapeutic reactions related to unconscious guilt over being helped, gradually permitted the patient to become aware of the deep anxieties related to her sexual relationship with her boyfriend. Unconsciously, she had the fantasy that if a relationship with a man really were a satisfactory one, she would lose her relations with her parents, and, at a deeper level, she was submitting to and identified with a sadistic parental pair, which could be explored in the transference.

Often such a masochistic scenario is obscured by regressively dependent transference reactions that stimulate "rescue fantasies" in the therapist. In a regressive mode, the patient misinterprets any minor frustration from the therapist as a major rejection, develops inordinate demands, and unconsciously replicates in the transference the frustrating relationship with the boyfriend. This may be accompanied by the abandonment of the bad relationship but in a self-defeating way tends to isolate the patient further and activates this negative relation in the transference. Masochistic scenarios sometimes may tempt therapists to be seduced into excessively supportive attitudes, to the extreme of breaking ordinary treatment structures in providing the patient with the love that supposedly he or she can expect from no one except the therapist.

References

Baranger W, Baranger M: Problemas del Campo Psicoanalitico. Buenos Aires, Argentina, Kargieman, 1969
Bataille G: L'Erotisme. Paris, Minuit, 1957
Dicks HV: Marital Tensions. New York, Basic Books, 1967
Green A: Illusions et Désillusions du Travail Psychoanalytique. Paris, Odile Jacob, 2010

Kernberg OF: Severe Personality Disorders: Psychotherapeutic Strategies. New Haven, CT, Yale University Press, 1984, pp 3–51

Kernberg OF: Love Relations: Normality and Pathology. New Haven, CT, Yale University Press, 1995

Laplanche J: Life and Death in Psychoanalysis (1970). New York, Johns Hopkins University Press, 1976

Laplanche J: New Foundations for Psychoanalysis (1987). Oxford, UK, Basil Blackwell, 1989

Laplanche J: Essays on Otherness. New York, Routledge, 1999

Stein R: The otherness of sexuality: excess. J Am Psychoanal Assoc 56(1):43–71, 2008 18430702

CHAPTER 13

Erotic Transference and Countertransference in Patients With Severe Personality Disorders

Part II: Therapeutic Developments

Transference and Countertransference Developments With Borderline Patients

As mentioned in Chapter 12, the transference developments regarding the sexual life of borderline patients are characterized by dynamics that center on a condensation of oedipal and preoedipal issues, with prominence of preoedipal aggression. There is more frequent and sometimes dramatic acting out, so that the general technique of structuralization of

---

This chapter was originally presented as a paper at the Third International Conference of the International Society of Transference-Focused Psychotherapy, Parma, Italy, October 13–15, 2014.

the treatment to protect the treatment, the patient, and the therapist from dangerous destructiveness becomes relevant here. The dominant transference reveals the immaturity or severely damaged nature of internalized object relations, reflected in the incapacity of these patients to achieve a satisfactory love relationship. Their relationships are notable for split expressions of love and aggression leading to volatility, conflict, and chaos, with a poor object choice and an unrealistic evaluation of the partner. Given the patient's difficulty in assessing realistically the commitment of a partner to him or her, the patient may choose a partner with limited capacity, and so there are many reasons that patients like these are prone to enter into unsatisfactory relationships. At the same time, an apparent sexual freedom and enjoyment of the sexual relation with the partner, a greater erotic freedom as compared with what evolves in neurotic structures, is actually a favorable prognostic indicator. The most extremely ill borderline patients may evince a primary inhibition of all aspects of sexuality, all capacity for erotic engagement, with an incapacity to enjoy skin eroticism, incapacity to masturbate, absence of sexual arousal, and incapacity for sexual excitement and orgasm. These are patients with more severely negative prognosis, and they present special complications in the treatment situations. Extreme sexual inhibition to the extent of absence of all sexuality is not secondary to repression, as is the case with neurotic structures, but derives from lack of stimulation of the primary erotic affect system. Erotic affect activation tends to be drowned by the predominance of severely negative, aggressively determined interactions with primary objects. In contrast, patients with a chaotic sexual life and sexual promiscuity, who do enjoy sexual enjoyment and do evince a general erotic capability, have a much better prognosis for treatment.

A frequent presentation of borderline patients is a condensation of erotic wishes and fears and conflicts around primitive dependency, typically shown in erotic behavior geared to gratifying dependent needs in the context of deep feelings of distrust or even despair of the possibility that anybody may be interested in them except in the context of sexual desire and excitement. Here, apparent sexual freedom may be a desperate measure to maintain a love relationship otherwise threatened by the intense splitting of idealized moments and periods of aggressive explosions. Even in cases in which this is not the primary motivation for a surge of sexual intimacy, love relations with their erotic component may be expressed with such demands for continuous, absolute dedication to the patient that a hostile intention of taking control and possession of the sexual partner becomes destructive and drives the partner away, leaving the patient feeling rejected, abandoned, and confused.

Sexual promiscuity of borderline patients, particularly those with infantile or histrionic personality structures, must be differentiated from narcissistic promiscuity. This becomes quite evident in the incapacity of any intense loving engagement on the part of narcissistic personalities, as their grandiose needs lead to transitory infatuations followed by rapid devaluation of their love objects. Patients with infantile or borderline personality have a much greater capacity for lasting, if also conflictual, engagements.

Borderline patients may present some degree of superego deterioration, such as irresponsibility or lack of concern for self and partner, but still show the capacity for guilt feelings in the context of their awareness of this aggressive acting out and mistreatment of their partner.

Sexually traumatized patients who begin treatment with a phobic reaction to the possibility of exploring past traumatic experiences out of a fear of sexual retraumatization present a particular challenge. These patients may aggressively refuse to talk about past traumatizations, develop defensive affect storms in the context of paranoid reactions to the therapist, and implicitly reproduce a situation of sexual traumatization in the transference. It is important to differentiate these cases from cases of posttraumatic stress disorders in which there has been a relatively recent severe sexual traumatization (a few months to 3 years before the initial evaluation) but no indication of major personality disorder. In patients with posttraumatic stress disorder without the complication of personality disorder, the treatment indication is a careful, gradual working through of the traumatic situation in the context of an atmosphere of safety in the therapeutic situation. This is very different from the treatment of patients with sexual traumatization, which constitutes an etiological factor for a severe personality disorder and emerges either at the beginning of the treatment or during the psychotherapy. In these latter cases, one must assume the incorporation of the traumatizing experience as part of the character structure, with the patient's unconscious, double identification with victim and perpetrator. In the transference, the patient enacts this relationship between victim and perpetrator in role reversals, so that the patient must be helped to realize the reactivation both of his or her role as victim of a sexual assault and the therapist as the perpetrator, and of the patient's unconscious identification with the perpetrator while projecting the self representation as victim onto the therapist. This internal structure needs to be analyzed in the transference and resolved. There is a risk to treating a patient under such circumstances exclusively as a victim of sexual trauma, in that the unconscious identification with the perpetrator and the related intense activation of aggression in the transference are dissociated or repressed, leaving the patient in the victim stance, and reprojecting the perpetrator role prevents full resolution of the sexual trauma and causes continued difficulties in the patient's sexual life.

Borderline patients present a wide range of sexual behavior that includes polymorphous infantile features; the freedom of fantasy; play and enjoyment in action of sadistic, masochistic, voyeuristic, exhibitionistic, and fetishistic features; and alternate heterosexual or homosexual identification in their erotic life. This implies a prognostically positive feature insofar as these patients, when their internalized object relations can be worked through, and as split-off or primitive part object relations become mature object relations (integration of positive and negative features), develop the capacity for realistic depth, interest, concern, and reciprocity in their relationships. They then are able to integrate the polymorphous sexual activity under the overall expression of their sexual involvement into a full, passionate relationship. The resolution of chaotic sexual behavior, therefore, lies in the transference resolution of the character pathology rather than in the specific analysis of the unconscious significance of each of these partial sexual trends.

In contrast, in cases of well-established perversion (paraphilia)—that is, when the capacity for sexual excitement and orgasm is restricted to the linkage with a particular polymorphous infantile feature—it is important that this particular perverse sexual relationship be activated, explored, and resolved in the transference, which permits the resolution of the perversion proper. Very often such patients, in the early stages of treatment, devalue ordinary sexual relations in the light of a total immersion in the idealization of their perversion. It is useless to attempt to "dissuade" the patient from this restricted idealization. Activation and resolution in the transference of this particular behavior provides the key to change. This requires the therapist's openness to fully experience in his or her countertransference the empathy with the patient's polymorphous perverse experiences as part of the analysis in the transference of the perverse scenario. This means internal freedom of the therapist to empathize, for example, with sadistic, masochistic, or exhibitionistic impulses of the patient, and be part of the disposition to tolerance of primitive regressions in the countertransference.

For example, I once treated a woman who would cut herself all over her body, becoming excited by the appearance of blood. At one point in the treatment, I developed disgusted and excited feelings from the sudden memory of a film I had recently seen that showed a sadistic murderer cutting the throat of a woman at the moment when she was reaching orgasm. I dismissed this memory as disgusting and shocking, and only became aware a few weeks later that this countertransference development corresponded to fantasies of this patient that I should shoot her. She felt that if I were to kill her, she would remain in my mind forever, and she would die happy with the idea that her existence would remain linked with my entire life.

Borderline patients' strong tendency to act out the transference may create problems in the management of the treatment. For example, a patient may attempt to attack the therapist sexually, such as one of our female patients who tried to kiss her male therapist and to tear off his shirt. While the therapist had to keep her physically at a distance without engaging in a physical fight or an aggressive counteraction in his verbal behavior, he was also able to stop this session while keeping himself in what still may be described as a respectful and neutral, though controlling, demeanor. Another patient, who had been involved in a sexual relationship with a previous therapist and had a long history of masochistic relations with men, appeared in one session without any underwear, spreading her legs in an exhibitionistic acting out and had to be confronted with the fact that the treatment had to be carried out while preserving ordinary, socially appropriate boundaries.

Gender, age, and the nature of the pathology influence the clinical characteristics of the activation of erotic transferences. Female patients develop more easily full-fledged erotic transferences with male therapists, repeating, in a way, the social gradient of traditional patriarchal culture, the relationship of a dependent woman with a controlling powerful man. Male patients in treatment with female therapists have greater difficulty in expressing their sexual feelings fully toward their idealized therapist, enacting the problem of the little boy who is not able to gratify the sexual implications of their idealized mother figure. Here, the acting out of sexual conflict in the form of displacement of erotic behavior to other people is more frequent and needs to be considered in the transference analysis. Male therapists generally tend to have greater difficulty with the sexualized transference of homosexual patients if the therapist is heterosexual, while heterosexual women therapists better tolerate sexual transferences of homosexual women that, usually, are condensed with strong oral-dependent features. Older male therapists may have greater problems with adolescent girls' sexual activation in the transference than older women therapists, and, as we shall see, the situation changes completely in the case of narcissistic pathology, in which a different way of dealing with erotic transferences and activation of sexual conflicts in general dominates the scene.

As mentioned in Chapter 12, therapists' erotic countertransference disposition to patients' activation and intensity of erotic impulses in the transference and the correspondent countertransference fantasies are important diagnostic indicators and therapeutic tools. The sexual freedom and maturity—the capacity for passionate love of the therapist—become important therapeutic elements in the treatment. More experienced analysts and psychoanalytic psychotherapists tend to become accustomed to and more tolerant and capable of managing their countertransference reactions. There evolves an element of learning from experience that is enriched by the fact that the treatment of patients and the analytic exploration of their sexual life bring about the possibility of new life experiences that go beyond those of the ordinary sexual life of analyst and therapist. To treat this pathology opens up the broad spectrum of human sexuality and has a growth potential for the therapist. By the same token, patients' acting out, fostered by the very treatment of cases in which significant inhibition had limited the patients' potential of creatively dealing with the conflicts of their sexual life, also may become a source of new life experience for them. Sometimes, the boundary between an important positive new life experience and the acting out of the transference is difficult to establish.

Love Relations of Narcissistic Personality Structures

The most prominent problem of narcissistic personality disorder is the incapacity to love (Kernberg 1995). This deficit is regulated by means of promiscuous sexual conquests, characterized by a never-ending cycle of transitory infatuations followed by rapid disappointments and devaluation. Traditionally, we see this pattern more prominently in male narcissists. The cultural double morality in patriarchal social structures that fosters men's sexual freedom, while restricting women to virtuous domesticity, is an important reason for this different expression of narcissistic pathology. Historically, women's narcissistic pathology has been expressed much more in other areas of family life. However, with the development of the women's rights movement, and the gradual equalization of social functions, sexual freedom, and workforce participation, this sexual pattern has become more frequent in women. Similar cultural influences affect other personality disorders as well, and the dominant cultural conventionalisms influence character formation and pathological personality traits. Thus, for example, while masochistic love relations are more frequent in women than in men, masochistic sexual perversion (paraphilia) is more frequent in men, and characterologically, men's submitting themselves to chronically frustrating and suffering situations in the context of work and profession is more frequent than parallel masochistic tendencies in women.

Frequently, the severity of the narcissistic patient's incapacity for stable object relations leads to casual sexual encounters and sexual excitement and gratification as his or her only open channel to involvement with others. There are patients with stable couple relations, from a conventional viewpoint, sometimes in a joint interest with a narcissistic partner who is comfortable with this arrangement but without real emotional involvement and generally with little sexual involvement as well. The increased frequency of "Internet sex" and ready access to pornography may gratify the experience of sexual excitement and provide the material for masturbatory gratification while avoiding the need to be "dependent" on any human relationship that would be experienced as a restrictive limitation of personal freedom. With some frequency, narcissistic personalities present a constellation of reverse triangulation—that is, a stabilization of their love life by having two or more partners in parallel over an extended period, an arrangement that protects them from total commitment to one person and from a sense of being restricted. It provides them with a sense of control over these relationships and, at the same time, constitutes revenge against the oedipal traumatization of having been the excluded child of the relationship between the parents. Thus, the unconscious motivational conflict typical of borderline organization—that is, a condensation of oedipal and preoedipal features under the dominance of early aggression—is replicated in this relatively frequent triangular pattern, which may provide an apparent stability to a couple within the limitations given by such an arrangement.

The development of perversions in narcissistic personality structures is potentially more serious and dangerous than the development of perversions under conditions of nonnarcissistic borderline and neurotic conditions. Here, the intense sadistic impulses that may constitute an important aspect of narcissistic personalities, related to inordinate envy as a dominant psychodynamic of the development of the pathological grandiose self, may be expressed as dangerous sadistic perversions that are not controlled sufficiently by adequate superego features, and that under the most severe circumstances, in cases of malignant narcissism, determine objective dangers for partners in sadomasochistic involvements.

In this connection, it needs to be kept in mind that patients with pathological narcissism function along a broad spectrum of severity: from very highly functioning patients with good surface impulse control and stability in the capacity for work and in ordinary social life, in whom the narcissistic pathology is expressed only in problems of sexual intimacy, to the other extreme, patients with a total breakdown of the capacity for work and profession, social life, and any object relationship involved in their sex life (see Chapter 9, "An Overview of the Treatment of Severe Narcissistic Pathology," of this book). More than anything else, the severity of the narcissistic pathology determines the prognosis for the specific problems in these patients' love life. There are narcissistic patients who present significant inhibition of their capacity for sexual excitement, intercourse, and orgasm, related to unconscious distrust and projected aggression interfering with the engagement with potential partners. Narcissistic men may present various syndromes of premature and retarded ejaculation, and narcissistic women may experience various degrees of sexual inhibition. However, in women as well in men, the most frequent situation is the maintenance of the capacity for sexual excitement and orgasm in the context of a severe limitation of the capacity for an object relationship in depth—that is, an incapacity for love and for passionate engagement. The most extreme cases of pathological narcissism, which present a total deterioration of superego functions in their social interactions, often involve a completely uncontrolled "sexual freedom" and the possibility of life-threatening sexual perversions. One of our patients with an antisocial personality structure reached excitement and orgasm in masturbating while throwing bricks from rooftops on women walking below on the street.

In diagnostic interviews, patients with narcissistic personalities typically reveal their incapacity to love, admitting that they have never fallen in love and have only had experiences of brief infatuations. The exploration of their unconscious dynamics reveals intense conflicts around envy and devaluation, also expressed in conscious reactions of envy, excessive competitiveness, and devaluation of others that may disturb their sexual life. For example, with some frequency they may be concerned about who is obtaining more pleasure in sexual intercourse: they themselves or their partner? They feel resentful if their partner seems to obtain more pleasure or be a more effective lover than they are. These patients cannot tolerate being very dependent on a love object, because dependency signifies a humiliating inferiority. Under the control of a pathological grandiose self, their security and well-being depends on maintaining a sense of superiority and freedom from envy by being able to devalue what others are or have. Their inability to depend on anyone goes hand in hand with the incapacity to let anybody else depend on them: they cannot tolerate that a partner depends on them, because to depend on them means that the other person is inferior, which pulls them down, and which in addition is felt to be an exploitation of them. They project their own tendency to greedy exploitation onto the partner and perceive any dependency on them as a dangerous restriction and exploitation. The partner should not be inferior to them—that would pull them down—but the partner cannot be superior, either, because that would generate their envy. The partner must be equal to them in some way and yet submissive to their omnipotent control. To keep a potential partner at that level creates an implicit strain on the developing relationship that militates against the initial infatuation and leads to the gradual deterioration of any intimate relationship.

In the transference, these problems are replicated in narcissistic patients' incapacity to depend on the therapist or analyst. They convey the impression of an apparent lack of transference developments by keeping the therapeutic relationship coldly objective and uninvolved. By the same token, however, they provide most important evidence for the development of a severe narcissistic transference relationship. These patients may present a fragile idealization of the therapeutic relationship as a "learning experience" that they wish to incorporate to resolve their difficulties by themselves. At bottom, their incapacity to depend on the analyst is expressed in their attempt to appropriate for themselves the analyst's knowledge and make it theirs but without having to acknowledge any dependency or gratitude. The interpretations they receive are easily dismissed or are absorbed as part of a "learning process" that leads to no further deepening of what they have received and no further initiation of self-exploration in the light of the analyst's interpretation. The unconscious envy of the analyst is also reflected in a particular negative therapeutic reaction. Precisely at points when these patients feel that they have been helped significantly, they feel worse: a paradoxical development that protects them from experiencing envy of the analyst's capacity to help them. In general, narcissistic patients have much greater difficulty in acknowledging their envy of the therapist than in acknowledging their envious reactions prevalent in all other relationships.

Narcissistic patients' sexual seductiveness evinces a quality of possessiveness and control. They attempt to take possession of a potential love object they experience as exciting and desirable, with an initial idealization of the sexual object; but, once they feel the new partner really loves them and wishes to give himself or herself totally over to them, these patients' internal devaluation of what they admired, desired, and envied destroys the attractiveness of what they first wanted to acquire. At a deeply unconscious level, narcissistic personalities envy the other gender and want to acquire all the capabilities and possessions of both genders. This may be the underlying dynamic of some homosexual narcissistic patients, and there also are other cases of narcissistic pathology that are particularly centered on the need to deny the envy of the other gender. At severe levels of narcissistic pathology, the aggressive possessiveness and devaluation of partners may take the form of openly sadistic behavior, an ongoing effort to devalue and control the freedom of behavior of the other that is quite frequent in cases of malignant narcissism.

One patient, with deep envy of his wife, who was successfully developing her profession and social standing and who he felt was overshadowing him, suggested to her an open marriage. He used their participation in group sex to induce her to have simultaneous sexual relations with five men while he watched her, and in the process devalued her completely as "a piece of meat." This led to the end of the marriage in the context of brutal divorce proceedings. In many cases, the repetitive cycles of temporary idealization and rapid devaluation of partners decrease over the years, and, in contrast to the enjoyable playboy or playgirl attitude in their 20s and 30s, an erosion of this pattern may set in, with boredom and indifference in their 40s and 50s. This development may lead to a total breakdown and loss in the interest of sexual intimacy, and a practical abandonment of all efforts to establish some form of sexual intimacy with a partner.

In the treatment of narcissistic personalities, the first obstacle, of course, is the analysis and resolution of the pathological grandiose self, which should be deconstructed into its component internalized real and ideal self and object representations, gradually leading to the emergence of the underlying borderline structure, the severely split idealized and persecutory object relations that reflect more directly the condensation of oedipal and preoedipal conflicts. Typically, in favorably evolving cases, the analysis of the narcissistic transferences occupies a major period of the total analysis or psychoanalytic psychotherapy, and it is only in the context of the transference analysis that their concrete sexual fantasies and conflicts may be understood and resolved.

A frequent development, although not exclusive to narcissistic pathology, is the *syndrome of perversity*—that is, the unconscious transformation of something good and valuable the patient receives in the treatment into an aggressive acting out against others. It is one more expression of unconscious envy that parallels the development of the psychotherapeutic process, one more form of negative therapeutic reaction, and it may lead to intense negative countertransference reactions. Obviously, it is one more manifestation of the conflicts around unconscious envy that need to be worked through in the treatment.

Total Apparent Obliteration of Sexuality

I refer here to cases of total absence of sexual activity, fantasy, and relations, possibly affecting a patient's social life to the extent that there may be no social life at all. There are different cases involved here requiring a careful differential diagnosis. First, there is a syndrome that includes the most severe cases of borderline personality organization, but without a narcissistic personality proper, in which a primary, total inhibition of all erotic potential has taken place. It is the case of such severely temperamentally negative predisposition, and overwhelmingly negative affect activation in the context of a traumatizing environment, that the erotization of the body surface and the erotically stimulating aspects of normal attachment have not taken place (Laplanche 1970/1976). Negative, particularly aggressive affects, override the possibility of primary erotic stimulation. It is only in the context of the treatment, with the activation of chaotic relations with others, self-mutilating behavior, sadomasochistic relations, the breakdown of social relations, and the absence of the capacity for intimacy, that the typical condensation of oedipal and preoedipal problems of borderline patients may be worked through in the transference of these patients. This gradually permits the emergence of the erotic impulses that were practically obliterated in the first few years of life. In these patients, after a long period, primitive sadomasochistic sexual fantasies may emerge in the sessions that provide important views of archaic idealized and persecutory early relations with related sexual implications of bodily penetration, incorporation, and destruction.

I referred earlier to a patient who developed the intense erotic fantasy of wanting to be shot and killed by me in order to be fused with me by means of my guilt feelings for the rest of my life. Another patient, in an advanced stage of her treatment, fantasized that she was lying naked in a stadium, as part of a convent, with the entire stadium filled with nuns surrounding her, while Mother Superior penetrated her at center stage with a huge metallic penis. The nuns, while watching, would get sexually excited, and that, in turn, would excite her sexually. This fantasy facilitated the patient's reaching orgasm through masturbation for the first time in her life. Still another patient developed, in the course of her treatment, the capacity to masturbate while she rested on a bed covered with a rubber sheet. She would urinate while masturbating and be able to achieve orgasm with a fantasy she was being bathed by her father, who was touching her genitals while lovingly bathing her. At an advanced stage of treatment, with an emergence of sexual fantasies in the context of such sadomasochistic scenarios, the full exploration in the transference of the patient's sexual life becomes very important and potentially may bring fundamental change.

There are some patients with total inhibition of erotic responsiveness in which the addition of sex therapy by a psychodynamically savvy therapist collaborating with the analyst or psychoanalytic psychotherapist of the case may be able to bring about significant change. It needs to be stressed that this refers to extremely severe cases in which the patient has total nonrepressive inhibition of his or her erotic potential, and it is generally undertaken in the latter stages of the psychotherapy treatment.

A second type of patient with practically total loss of the capacity for erotic response is the patient with narcissistic personality who, after many years of sexual promiscuity, has lost his or her capacity for temporary infatuations and sexual involvements and whose sexual life gradually has become practically extinguished. Here, the analysis of the narcissistic personality structure should reactivate the patient's erotic potential in terms of the capacity for sexual arousal, excitement, and orgasm.

A third case is that of the "dead mother" syndrome, patients with a severely narcissistic personality structure in which the dismantling of all internalized object relations, including the concept of self, has become so dominant that their internal capability for emotional relationships seems to be erased. Originally described by André Green (1993), these patients have a history of severe chronic depression in the mother in their first few months or years of life, an unconscious identification with such a mother experienced as a dead image, and the wish to maintain or reestablish the relationship with such a mother by accompanying her in that emotionally dead union. Consciously, these patients are characterized by a remarkable lack of interest in life. Life becomes a burden, given their total lack of motivation. On the surface, their capacity for ordinary social object relations seems to be appropriate, but basically their relationships are extremely distant and empty: all the aggression has been vested in the destruction of their internal life. Some of these patients can be helped to reconstruct their earliest conflicts related to a deeply frustrating mother. They may be able to reactivate their rage at having been ignored and abandoned in the transference: if that stage of treatment can be reached, the prognosis improves. Other cases simply end in a profound sense of frustration and disappointment by both patient and therapist because of the impossibility of activating a regressive transference relationship.

Under all these circumstances, in cases of obliteration of sexuality of the kind mentioned, there may develop an absence of erotic elements in the therapist's countertransference as well, a tendency to abandon all thoughts and feelings of erotic implications relating to that patient. The therapist should be alert to the problem of total absence of any erotic feature to his or her reaction to the patient and make use of it to explore with the patient the correspondent deficit in his or her life as a major issue to be resolved, if possible. This is as important as the patient's relationship to work and profession and to friendship and social life. In such cases, it is essential to maintain alertness to any, even the vaguest, manifestation of an erotic activation that potentially may emerge. Again, this emergence may only occur in the context of the activation of severely sadomasochistic features that already represent an advantage in this situation. In other cases, patients may evince a potential for an erotic component in their reaction to art or other cultural manifestations that evoke in them a sense of diffuse, longed-for opening of a space and of "letting oneself go." Here, the basic dilemma of life, the oscillation between the rational and the ecstatic aspects of existence—referred to initially in context to the contributions of Bataille (1957; see Chapter 12, "Erotic Transference and Countertransference in Patients With Severe Presonality Disorders, Part I")—becomes relevant.

References

Bataille G: L'Erotisme. Paris, Minuit, 1957
Green A: On Private Madness. Madison, CT, International Universities Press, 1993
Kernberg OF: Love Relations: Normality and Pathology. New Haven, CT, Yale University Press, 1995, pp 143–162
Laplanche J: Life and Death in Psychoanalysis (1970). New York, Johns Hopkins University Press, 1976

PART V

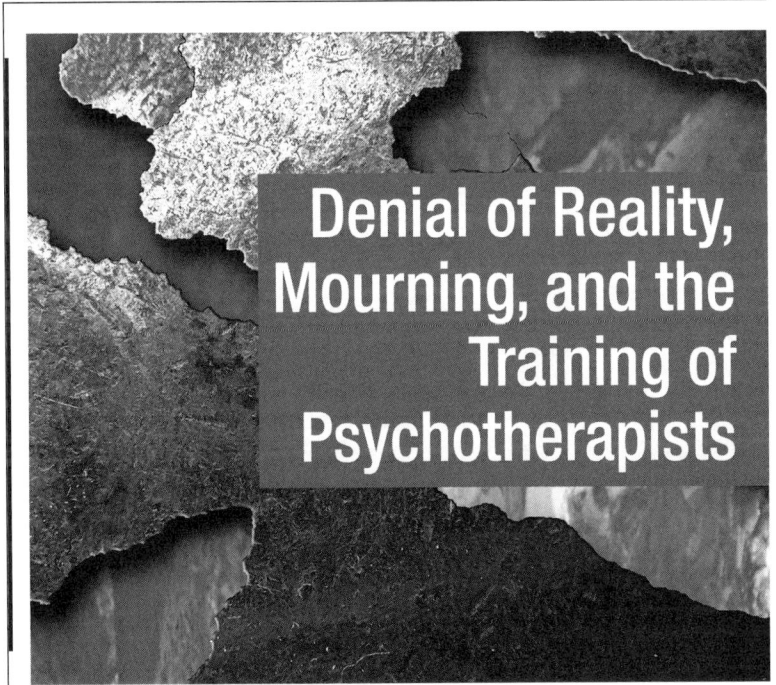

Denial of Reality, Mourning, and the Training of Psychotherapists

CHAPTER 14

The Denial of Reality

What follows is the exploration of a frequent complication in the psychoanalytic psychotherapy of severe personality disorders, and one that we also encounter at times of significant regression in the psychoanalysis of patients with that level of severity of illness. While the analyst is attentive to the patient's free association and the display of unconscious defensive operations and impulses in the patient's fantasies and associations, a parallel, incongruent, or bizarre element of the external reality emerges in the patient's discourse that points to potentially severe developments in his or her external life, which the patient seems to be ignoring or mentioning so casually that their importance easily may escape the attention of the therapist.

The analysis of the "total transference" includes the expression of the transference both in the developments in the session and in the parallel developments in the patient's external life, sometimes clearly in the form of acting out or else in somatization. Here, however, it is only the therapist's putting together in his or her own mind those fragmented, bizarre, or ignored aspects of reality that appear so puzzling and that would not

---

This chapter was originally presented as a paper at the Biannual Congress of the German Society for Personality Disorders, Munich, Germany, July 10, 2016.

become part of the information that the therapist receives directly from the patient if the therapist did not use his or her common sense in reformulating to himself or herself an aspect of the patient's external reality beyond the patient's apparent capacity to grasp it at that point. To put it differently, one aspect of the transference is acted out in such a way that an effective denial on the part of the patient requires an unusual effort of the analyst to understand something almost imperceptible within that reported external reality. The therapist's common sense, at times, may leave him or her with new, unanswered questions about apparently strange aspects of that reality. Only direct inquiry of the patient about these aspects may permit the therapist to put together a totally denied, highly significant process that has been developing outside the sessions.

The ordinary interest of the analyst in listening to free association is to penetrate deeper layers of the patient's mind, to establish contact with unconscious conflicts enacted in the here and now. In contrast, in these unusual, strange occurrences referred to, the therapist's inquiry must include a clarification of aspects of the patient's external life that ends up uncovering issues effectively eliminated from the patient's awareness by his or her denial of reality.

Let me present a few examples of these kind of developments:

> A female patient in her early thirties was a research scientist in a highly prestigious, complex research organization, where she headed a research team that was part of a larger project. Long-standing conflicts with authority figures, related to profound ambivalence toward an admired but feared authoritarian father, affected her relationship to men. Idealizing and submitting to powerful men first and then ending up in a rebellious rejection of such men was a central focus in the analysis of the transference. Her relationship with men had ended with a painful breakup on several occasions, in what, at bottom, was a masochistic intolerance of a good sexual relationship.
>
> In the middle of a tumultuous relationship with what seemed to be a very nice partner, she mentioned to the therapist her anger with the mistreatment, as she saw it, of a member of her team by the financial office of the research institution. She had expressed her protest over this financial problem to her project leader, but without obtaining a satisfactory response. Over several weeks, she occasionally mentioned her discussion of this situation with coworkers on her team, who, it seemed, agreed with her and expressed their general resentment at the bureaucratic rigidities of her institution. The dominant affective situation in the transference involved her fantasies that the therapist would naturally always sympathize with the views of the patient's boyfriend rather than with her, "the typical alliance of men in power."
>
> The occasional ironic or angry references to her research institution at first did not draw the attention of the therapist, who was used to her

The Denial of Reality

protests over social injustices. At one point, the patient mentioned, rather casually, that she had decided to ask for an appointment with the director of the research institution, and at a later session she announced with a triumphant tone that she had obtained that appointment for a near, future date. It needs to be stressed that all the relevant comments in the sessions were rather isolated bits of information, expressed in the current of free associations without an apparent internal continuity of these thought processes.

The therapist experienced a sudden sense of alarm as he was reviewing her latest session with the announcement of the appointment with the director. Was that a typical acting out of the patient's rebellious protest against authoritarian powers, with a profound, unconscious masochistic implication? The therapist now raised the question with the patient as to what her intentions were and what process had led her to appeal to the ultimate authority of that large institution. In the following sessions, the therapist found out that, indeed, the patient was going to present a major complaint about faulty procedures in the financial management of her project, implying irresponsible neglect of this situation by the project director, the director of the overall program of which this project was a component, and the director of the division in which this entire development had taken place. The therapist asked the patient if she had discussed the situation with each of these superiors, whether she had expressed her dissatisfaction to them, and whether she had informed them of the next steps she was planning to take. She had not.

This led the therapist to become very concerned about the patient's forthcoming interview with the director of the research institution: the patient had bypassed three levels of authority in planning to address her protest to the highest level of the organization, and this might involve a serious risk for her future in that very hierarchical workplace. She was a very promising but junior member of the staff and was still uncertain about the possibility of a permanent position. The total situation now could be explored in the context of her pattern of rebellious protest as an expression of deeper masochistic urges, in turn linked to unconscious prohibition against a happy sexual relationship with a desirable man, an oedipal conflict.

Another example involves the psychoanalytic treatment of a patient with a severe narcissistic personality disorder who had obtained a position in a very exclusive high school specializing in the education of outstanding and unusually gifted adolescents. This school had very high expectations of their faculty, and all new teachers were hired on a 1-year "mutual acquaintance" basis—that is, in a provisional situation that might lead to a permanent position or to the end of this teaching assignment after the probation year. The patient was a very gifted, charismatic teacher, fully aware of his capacity to activate adolescents enthusiastically and certain of his desirability for the school. After making a very positive impression on everybody, he felt secure in the job and expressed his subtle but definite arrogance and depreciative attitude toward authorities and colleagues in occasional humoristic remarks and unconsidered attitudes that led to a few incidents, which he referred to in his free associations as amusing illustrations of his superiority. The analyst became concerned whether this might threaten the patient's position at the school. The patient calmly dismissed the analyst's concern, with an attitude of possessing much greater experience of the school system than the analyst. The analyst interpreted the projection onto him of the patient's own repressed and dissociated feeling of inferiority and concern over failure but did not trust his overall assessment of the dangerous situation in which his patient was finding himself. He actually missed the full clarification of incidents that, from a viewpoint of common social intelligence, should have alerted him and the patient of dangerous consequences following some of these negative interactions at the school. Toward the end of the year, the patient was notified that his contract was not going to be renewed, which shocked and depressed him. It emerged only now how unusually favorable and privileged the conditions of this job were that the patient, most probably, would not be able to replicate elsewhere. Here the patient's omnipotent control blocked the analyst's full experience of his own concern and the realistic assessment of the patient's social situation.

A third example is apparently simpler but illustrates a lack of common sense by the analyst about the information from a patient working in an organization for social welfare that she was quitting her job because she was "bored." The patient had been in analysis a relatively brief period, and the analyst knew that she had held an important position in that place of work over many years. Her categorical statement in one session that she had decided to leave this job because of "boredom" caught him by surprise, but he felt it prudent not to question the patient about the reasons that would lead her to leave the job at this point after so many years, and it was not clear to him what role transference developments might play in this decision. It did not occur to him to ask her what she meant by saying that she was bored (i.e., Bored by what? How did this boredom show? How come now when for many years the job was not boring?). The analyst felt he should not raise all these questions, because he felt that, in general, raising direct questions to patients should be avoided in analysis and that, particularly in this case of a woman who he felt was highly sensitive to any criticism, it would be experienced as a critical stance toward her decision.

Several months later, she announced that she had taken another job in an institution dealing with underprivileged families and that she hoped it would be a less stressful job than the one in the previous organization where she had worked. A few weeks later, she complained that people were talking about her and that, unfortunately, the same thing was repeating itself in her new job as had happened in the previous organization, where everybody talked about her behind her back, which had proved intolerable. Now the nature of the "boredom" became clearer—namely, a strong paranoid reaction toward coworkers, particularly female coworkers, and the direct linkage to paranoid developments in the transference became evident. This example may seem rather trivial in the sense that the exploration of what may have been considered an acting out by her sudden decision to resign from the other job did not take place. However, it is linked to the other examples by the lack of use of common sense in interpreting the situation and by not confronting the patient with a denial of reality implied in the patient's behavior and recognized in the analyst's countertransference.

In general, what these cases have in common is a distortion of reality usually totally ignored by the patient and presented in such suddenly rationalized or fragmented ways that it is difficult for the therapist to capture it. Often this goes hand in hand with the splitting off of aspects of reality that are recognized at times, or in theory, but are disconnected totally from the emotional life of the patient at other times. For example, one patient, a man with a severe narcissistic personality structure, who had reached an agreement with his wife to have an "open marriage" at a time when this was a culturally fashionable aspect of "liberation" in some social circles, seemingly enjoyed his own sexual promiscuity while theoretically granting the same rights to his wife. Emotionally, however, he was convinced she would never become interested in another man and that his attractiveness would override any such temptation on her part. She, however, also initiated an extramarital relationship that developed into an intense love relation. The patient was shocked: he had ignored her indignant reaction to his proposal that she interpreted as a devastating lack of commitment to their marriage and that triggered her questioning their relationship. The combination of his grandiosity, the devaluation of his wife, and the denial of the reality of her emotional reactions, all of which became clear enough throughout time in the discourse of the patient, led to his traumatic experience of her decision to end the marriage.

Sometimes little "tidbits" of information in a patient's discourse seem strange and irrelevant enough not to draw the analyst's attention to them. They should be considered as possible indications of an aspect of reality that is being denied by the patient and presented as part of a broader picture reflecting the patient's defensive organization regarding his or her reality. Frequently, such denial tends to cover chronic self-destructive behavior that may accumulate throughout time and finally emerge as an unexpected traumatic situation or even a catastrophe. Only a retrospective review of all the information provides the data that clearly indicate a logical progression of developments in external reality. Sometimes an essential aspect of reality is suppressed, an apparently minor link in a chain is underlined, and the total picture is recovered only much later, sometimes too late.

The implication of what I have described is that in some severe cases of psychopathology, free association may be distorted unconsciously at the service of the denial of external reality, and the analyst's task may be to interpret that denial of reality as an affectively dominant subject in the sessions. However, to interpret the denial of reality requires the analyst to formulate in his or her own mind a vision beyond the patient's presentation of it, a construction of reality that permits the therapist to clarify its significance and reveal important mechanisms of denial at work in the patient's communications. It means having to pay attention to the patient's reality through the patient's communication of it beyond the patient's awareness and understanding, and being prepared to explore the meaningful blindness of it as part of the patient's defensive operations. If denial of reality is accompanied by significant acting out outside the sessions that draws attention by itself to what is going on in the patient's external life, the task, paradoxically, becomes easier. But when no major acting out seems to be occurring, and there are only relatively small, apparently unimportant happenings that seem strangely interspersed with other material in the patient's free associations, the task becomes much more difficult. These forms of denial are frequent in cases of patients with borderline personality organization in which splitting mechanisms are dominant and point to the defensive use of free association against the awareness of external and not only internal reality of the patient.

The psychoanalyst's interpretive interventions under such circumstances present a particular difficulty. As the case material mentioned already illustrates, the clarification of what has been masked or subtly distorted in the patient's communication, the confrontation of implications of the information that the patient is denying, and the interpretation in depth of the total situation that the patient has created may appear to be an "intrusion" into the patient's external life. The analyst may appear as taking a stand that is outside technical neutrality, and it even may appear to reflect countertransference acting out. In fact, in practice, in our experience at the Personality Disorders Institute at Weill Cornell Medical College, we have observed these concerns as a major difficulty of therapists working analytically with severely ill patients. In an effort to maintain a technically neutral stance, and to avoid acting out of countertransference reactions to patients' denial of significant aspects of their reality, analysts and therapists are reluctant to intervene by interpreting the denial of reality.

The following is an important differentiation to keep in mind: the difference between a supportive or re-educative stance that may reflect an analyst's behavior enacting countertransference problems, on the one

The Denial of Reality

hand, and the need to clarify systematically an external reality to interpret its motivated denial on the part of the patient, on the other. The difficulty of this differentiation may result from the lack of understanding of technical neutrality as interventions that are made from a position outside the internal conflicts of the patient—that is, they are supposed to be neutral regarding the dynamic forces in mutual conflict in the patient's mind. Forceful, even, at times, categorical statements that clarify a reality may be technically neutral, whereas at other times, very carefully and thoughtfully pronounced interpretations that take sides in the patient's internal struggles are not. Sometimes the analyst may feel reluctant to raise a set of related questions to clarify an obscure aspect of a situation, as if that represented an intrusion into the patient's reality, an acting out of the analyst' curiosity or his or her own interests, and, once again, an abandonment of technical neutrality.

It is a common assumption within analytic circles that the more an analyst can avoid raising direct questions, by means of thought-provoking interpretations of the relevant issues, the purer or more elegant is the analytic technique. Further, the assumption holds that much raising of questions reflects lack of technical skills, such as the trivial but so frequently heard question, "and how did you feel about that?" (Busch 2014).

The denial of reality may represent one element of a broader splitting of reality into opposite segments of experience, reflecting massive projective identification of the intrapsychic conflict onto the perception of the outer world. However, when the process is gross enough to become manifest as the counter position of an idealized and a persecutory aspect of experience, the splitting operations are clear enough to lend themselves to interpretive interventions. The subtler aspects of denial of reality discussed here usually serve long-range masking efforts, particularly severely self-destructive ends, and the lack of their perception may seriously affect the patient's life. In very severe cases, the analyst has a special function in addition to his or her attention to verbal behavior, nonverbal behavior, countertransference, and the subtle aspects of the analytic fields. Now the therapist also has the task of "scanning" the patient's environment, reproducing in his or her mind an external world that may be distorted as a function of the patient's defensive needs and unconscious acting out. This usually is a silent, quite obvious, aspect of analytic listening to patients with better-functioning ego and an integrated world of representations of significant others, patients within the neurotic level of structural organization, where analytic assessment of the psychosocial reality of the patient's life can be taken for granted. Therefore, this is a problem that emerges relatively seldom in standard analysis of neurotic patients. It becomes predominant only in the pathology of severe borderline and narcissistic pathology and may require active attention on the analyst's part.

An active attention to the reality of a patient's life may seem to run counter to the principle of interpreting "without memory or desire" (Bion 1967). Perhaps this is the place to clarify once again that to interpret without memory or desire does not imply blindness to the history of the patient's life and problems and to the nature of his or her external world. It means entering each session with a true openness, to be impressed and guided by the predominant affective issues now dominating the total therapeutic situation. However, during that evocative situation, with the activation of the patient's unconscious reality and conflicts, relevant "memory and desire" also emerge in the therapist's countertransferences as material to be understood, analytically worked through, and interpretively used.

A penetrating, systematic history taking and analytic exploration of the patient's present reality at the beginning of the treatment, his or her reality in work and profession, love and sex, social life, and creativity, and the dominant conflicts in all those areas give fundamental initial information that at a certain moment of the treatment will prove helpful as it emerges in the awareness of the analyst's mind during the sessions. Psychoanalysts traditionally have been well prepared to have such a potential vision of the patient's infancy and childhood in their mind, but we have learned that this must be extended to a full awareness of the patient's present reality—its intricacies, potentials, and dangers—because it is in that present reality that the patient's unconscious conflicts and the transference are going to be played out. This knowledge facilitates the therapist's alertness and awareness of the denial of reality we are exploring.

The interventions geared to clarify an obscure and denied segment of the patient's reality may create the danger of effectively interfering with free associations, transforming them or reducing them temporarily to a therapeutic "dialogue" that in turn may be used for defensive purposes by the patient. Some argumentative interchanges that evolve during analytic sessions between patient and analyst not only indicate transference and countertransference acting out, but also may gratify the ongoing defensive effort by the patient to avoid the regressive experience of confronting deeper levels of unconscious conflicts in the transference. This is a risk increased by excessive questioning by the analyst, which orients the patient's thinking defensively into the reality aspects of that obscure area of reality the analyst is interested in clarifying. Thus, the interpretation of the denial of reality must be applied sparingly and directed to areas of severe potential self-destructiveness by the patient in the interest of protecting the patient and the treatment.

The analyst's view of the totality of the patient's present life also acquires particular importance in cases in which a major life problem has become so chronically structured into the patient's daily life, so routinely expressed with secondary defensive rationalizations that keep the total situation stable, that the analyst becomes blinded against the ongoing awareness of that problem. For example, difficulties may evolve with patients who present chronic distancing from their spouse or sexual partner, who find compromise solutions to life together that are practically comfortable for them both, within an unconscious collusion to bury any emotional intimacy, suppress their sexual life, or deny profound differences in overall values, interests, and ethical commitments.

Patients may come to treatment because of their sense of dissatisfaction with their life and in the initial evaluation clearly convey particular areas that are inhibited or paralyzed by unconscious conflicts. Throughout treatment this becomes covered again by a pattern of customs and routine. They may thus induce an unconscious collusion between patient and analyst not to explore the corresponding problems. This may be considered one example of the bastions of unconscious collusions in treatment described by Baranger and Baranger (1966). Acute conflicts, symptoms, and traumatic developments in a patient's life may obscure these underlying long-term problems initially mentioned in the patient's evaluation and then going underground. The analyst should be able to maintain an internal overview of the patient's life, particularly from the perspective of what would be an optimal life situation for this particular patient that he or she has not been able to achieve—because of which he or she is suffering—possibly without clearly being aware of what he or she is missing.

The careful scrutiny of the patient's external life situation in the course of the treatment brings up not only problems related to the denial of reality but the entire course of the patient's changing relationship to work and profession, love and sex, social life, and creativity. It often raises in the therapist's mind the question "Are there more or alternative or better ways this patient could enrich his or her life experience?" Obviously, countertransference reactions, guilt feelings, and rescue fantasies of the therapist may play a role, as does projective counter-identification with the patient's own dissociated or guilty wishes to expand his or her life experience. However, the effect of social and political constraints also may play a role in a patient's life, restricting the patient's horizon, while the therapist may be aware of open roads of inquiry the patient is ignoring.

I treated a 27-year-old African American woman from one of the poorest neighborhoods of New York City with transference-focused psychotherapy. She presented an infantile-histrionic personality disorder, with drug abuse, sexual promiscuity, and irresponsibility in work situations connected with serious interpersonal problems. She lived with her mother and six siblings in a rundown apartment. Her father had abandoned the family when she was 4 years old, and the present home atmosphere was totally chaotic. Despite this, the patient had been able to graduate from high school with consistently high grades, a fact to which nobody in her family seemed to have paid any attention. They lived in extreme poverty. At one point in the treatment, it occurred to me that, given her success in high school and her financial situation, she might be eligible for a college scholarship, which would significantly improve her long-range employment possibilities. I raised that issue in the middle of our exploration of important masochistic features in her relationship with men, her self-devaluing and impulse-driven lifestyle. She obtained that scholarship and ended up studying and graduating from a local college, securing a growth-facilitating position in a local industry, and entering an educated middle-class social community. Her life situation improved greatly, and her opportunities for finding adequate men increased in parallel to her growing capacity for establishing object relations in depth.

The therapist's position of technical neutrality may be compromised by such an intervention, but it should be possible to explore and interpret the consequences of such a temporary shift. Questions geared to clarify something the therapist does not understand, and which the patient is avoiding to clarify, reflect the authentic, task-oriented curiosity of the therapist that is part of his or her diagnostic and therapeutic function. A genuine interest in the patient's well-being as the obvious objective of the treatment to help the patient improve his or her life experience and condition is an important, objectively required aspect of the analytic work. And so is the active exploration, in the analyst's mind, of the patient's entire present life situation, the denial of aspects of reality that need to be interpreted, and the unrealized life potential that the patient may be missing, even without an unconscious blinding about his or her potential. An actively engaged analyst may still be a technically neutral one.

The therapist's creativity in imagining a better life for patients with severe personality disorders who unconsciously are so involved in enacting self-destructive tendencies in their life situations is an important function in the ongoing evaluation of external reality. During the very early diagnostic evaluation of a patient's difficulties, it helps to be able to imagine oneself in the patient's situation, in his or her skin and concrete life circumstances. What would we do in such a situation, to "get out from under," to break through the barriers of self-restricting psychopathology? Such imaginary scenarios may expand the horizon of the therapeutic objectives beyond the expectations of the patient and protect the therapist's stance against contamination by the patient's self-destructive tendencies during the treatment. Such a disposition on the part of the therapist is totally compatible with a position of technical neutrality.

In short, denial of reality includes both denial of potential self-destructive acting out and blinding toward potentially healthy opportunities for growth and development. Technical neutrality facilitates full transference development and transference interpretation and, in turn, is protected by consistent countertransference analysis. The combination of these technical instruments permits the diagnosis and interpretative resolution of the denial of reality, a development particularly important in cases of severe personality disorders. Technical neutrality may be challenged but can be maintained under these conditions.

A patient may have sacrificed a creative talent and, over time, it turns out that this was a useless, unnecessary sacrifice and is related to his or her self-destructive tendencies. The patient may not, or no longer, be aware of this sacrifice; however, it still affects him. A woman may consult for treatment because of sexual inhibition but over the years rationalize this inhibition as being a reasonable result of many years of living together with her spouse and the loss of the romantic aspects of the couple's relationship, reinforced by a husband's loss of sexual interest under conditions of lack of response by her over an extended period. A patient may start his analysis with an expressed wish to resolve a problem, then not refer to it over many months, unconsciously managing the analyst's attention to stay away from the problem as well. It is perhaps particularly under conditions of apparent trivialization of free association, at times when nothing seems to be going on in the sessions over a period of time, or when the nature of the patient's discourse turns stubbornly to the external realities of daily life, that periods of countertransference reactions may evolve in which the analyst is distracted and matters unrelated to the patient intrude in his or her mind, when in fact he or she may be responding to what is now active in the intersubjective field rather than in the verbal interaction focused on free association. At such points it may be helpful for the analyst to activate, in his or her own mind, the total patient situation: What important issues are affecting this patient's life and are not being taken up in the sessions? Is there any discrepancy between the apparent tranquility and affective superficiality of the patient's communications at this time, the analyst's countertransference contamination by this atmosphere, and the split-off, ongoing presence of a major unresolved problem?

This is a different situation from the more specifically focused denial of reality we were exploring before. Now it is the total life situation of the patient that becomes the focus of the analyst's concern, and the question can be raised: What is the relationship between that major unresolved chronic issue and the present "triviality" in the sessions? Simply raising these questions in the analyst's mind often changes the nature of the intersubjective field, increases the analyst's awareness of how, in subtle ways, a neglected subject is emerging in transference and countertransference thoughts and fantasies. This may become the affectively dominant subject of the sessions as it gets connected with other aspects of transference/countertransference development. It represents another expansion, I suggest, of Betty Joseph's (1985) concept of the "total transference," which includes mental realities not directly expressed in the sessions but painfully recovered by the analysis of the total relationship between the treatment at this point and the patient's external life.

Interpretive interventions that bring this issue into the content of the therapeutic hours may be experienced by the patient as a traumatic intrusion and disturbance of his or her present equilibrium. It is important that such interventions clearly correspond to important problems in the patient's life, whose resolution may improve his or her effectiveness and well-being, and do not represent the analyst's own ideological assumptions of perfect life arrangements artificially imposed on the patient's present equilibrium.

The comments about denial of reality and the analyst's concern about the total reality of the patient's life point to the delicate balance between the analyst's interests in helping the patient achieve a better life experience and his or her respect for the equilibrium that the patient has established for himself or herself. It may become a conflict between commitment and discretion, and should not be an acting out of *furor sanandi*. It points, however, to an implicit analytic task of helping the patient to improve his or her life beyond the resolution of the symptoms and difficulties that brought him or her into treatment. Often this expanded goal cannot be achieved, but the very fact that sometimes it can points to the therapeutic potential of this analytic approach.

The technical modification proposed in this chapter within the overall technical approach of transference-focused psychotherapy involves an actively focused questioning about strange or bizarre bits of information that may reflect silent or masked severe acting out of a patient's self-destructive tendencies. Unconsciously, the patient may attempt to prevent the therapist from becoming aware of the preparation or expression of dangerous self-destructive behavior on his or her part. That is what is involved in the need to clarify, confront, and interpret the denial of reality. In addition, self-imposed limitations the patient establishes or enacts regarding his or her expectations, aspirations, and goals in life constitute a broader, subtler, but eminently important expression of self-defeating tendencies that the therapist should raise questions about when relevant. That also is implicit in the denial of reality.

Conclusion

The questioning and confronting interventions discussed in this chapter may be considered to present advantages and disadvantages. Among the disadvantages, one may cite the potential interference with free association and the temporary transformation of the therapeutic work into a dialogue between patient and therapist, and this may be exploited as a defensive maneuver on the part of the patient. Raising questions also may reveal intentionality on the part of the therapist, reducing the position of technical neutrality. In the same context, raising questions may facilitate acting out of countertransference disposition. All of these are negatives.

On the positive side, raising questions in the context referred to earlier expands the field of investigation to acting out of transference developments in external reality, even beyond the field signaled by Betty Joseph. Raising a focused question about an area in which severe self-destructive behavior is being enacted may gain time and protect the patient from acting out that would result in serious damage. Raising questions about patients' self-restrictive and self-limiting life objectives may contribute to expanding and enriching patients' lives. At the end, this approach is harmonious with the overall transference-focused psychotherapy approach that proposes "impatience" in every session and consistent patience over the long run.

References

Baranger W, Baranger M: Insight and the analytic situation, in Psychoanalysis in the Americas. Edited by Litman R. New York, International Universities Press, 1966, pp 56–72

Bion WR: Notes on memory and desire. Psychoanalytic Forum 2:272–273, 279–290, 1967

Busch F: Creating a Psychoanalytic Mind: A Psychoanalytic Method and Theory. London, Routledge, 2014, pp 78–87

Joseph B: Transference—the total situation. Int J Psychoanal 66:447–454, 1985

CHAPTER 15

The Long-Term Effects of the Mourning Process

In an earlier paper (Kernberg 2010), I pointed to some aspects of the mourning process that in my view had not been considered sufficiently in the literature. I proposed that mourning is a permanent process, with profound impact on the structures of the mind, on object relations in general, and on the capacity for deepening the understanding of subjective experiences of self and others. I suggested that the mourning process culminates in the consolidation of a permanent relationship with the lost object while still internalizing some aspect of the object's characteristics as part of the self experience. This development points to the double process of identification: the incorporation of aspects of the lost object into the self and the setting up of a permanent dyadic relation of a representation of self with the representation of the lost object. This development within the ego coincides with new developments within the ego ideal, modifying superego functions in general, in the context of the internalization of

---

This chapter was originally presented as a paper at the Winter Meeting of the American Psychoanalytic Association, January 20, 2013; this chapter was originally published as Kernberg OF: "The Long-Term Effects of the Mourning Process," in *Grief and Its Transcendence: Memory, Identity, Creativity*. Edited by Tutter A, Wurmser L. London, Routledge, 2016, pp. 89–94. Copyright © 2016 Routledge/Taylor & Francis Group. Adapted with permission.

the life project of the lost object—the identification within one's own ego ideal with what the lost object would have wished to achieve in life, and what the person whose death is mourned would have said or done, reacted to or felt, expected himself or herself to achieve, and hoped for the mourner to achieve. The organization of internalized value systems, the integration of the mature superego, is thus modified and enriched.

Still, the mourning process would continue as repeated pain over the loss, with the lost object becoming a permanent painful "absent presence," and connected with this experience, the reactivation of guilt feelings over not having fully appreciated the lost object during life and guilt feelings over having failed the loved one while they were alive. The more ambivalent the past relation with the object, the more painful are such guilt feelings, to the extent that pathological mourning may be characterized by significant pathology. In this latter case, the despair over the impossibility to repair real or fantasied guilt is reflected in depressive symptomatology, resulting in the possibility of suicidal wishes as the expression of the wish to expiate deep guilt feelings. Implicit dynamics may involve fantasies that self-elimination would permit the good parts of the self to survive, with the simultaneous destruction of all the bad parts of the self reflecting the negative feelings, including hatred of the lost object and the related unconscious introjection of the hated part of the object as part of the self. Under extreme circumstances, the despair over the permanent nature of the loss coincides with the condemnation symbolized by the words inscribed over Dante's entrance to the Inferno, "Abandon all hope, ye who enter here."

But the purpose of this chapter is to describe the process of mourning under the optimal conditions in which ambivalence had not been so marked or extreme, and where mourning processes reactivate what Freud (1917[1915])) and Melanie Klein (1940) described as the normal mourning processes and, in Melanie Klein's contribution, as the reactivation and reworking through of the depressive position as the central process of such mourning.

Approximately 5 years after my initial contacts with the persons I described in my earlier contribution (Kernberg 2010)—who had lost a spouse after decades of living together, and who had remarried, and whom I had been able to interview extensively—I revisited them with the question of what further changes may have taken place in them throughout those 5 years. (I was able to contact a majority of them, in addition to further reviewing patients' material and my own experience, having undergone similar vicissitudes in my own life.)

To begin, essentially the same processes that I summarized as the main observations communicated in my previous work continued to be present. Again, during these interviews, mourning reactions became reactivated, together with information provided regarding experiences similar to those they had reported in the original interview 5 years prior, perhaps somewhat attenuated in some cases, but nonetheless, an intense, lively upsurge of reactivation of mourning under sudden emergences of past experiences triggered by present-day life situations. In addition, however, new elements emerged that had not been so clearly observable before.

First, I found a generally changed attitude of these persons toward the potential of serious illness and death. There was a decrease of the anxiety that one might expect would be elicited by the development of symptoms of a potentially serious illness or death, both their own and those close to them. This decreased fear of death and dying at times surprised the subjects of my inquiry themselves. They made comments such as "If he was able to go through this, I shall be able to do it," a sense of being accompanied by the beloved person who had died in the imagining of one's own process of dying, and fantasies of the possible reencounter with the dead person after one's own death even in persons without any religious inclination or convictions in that regard. The sense of death as a reencounter acquired an important function of dealing with one's own death, particularly if the conviction of being loved by one's departed partner was very powerful. From an analytic perspective, this may be rooted in both oedipal and preoedipal experiences as the assurance of the permanence of the love of the internalized mother imago. For those who had religious convictions about life after death and who had remarried, fantasies and questions emerged about what would happen to them with the competing love of two persons, the past and the present spouse. This same issue was explored by C.S. Lewis in his dramatic autobiographical essay "A Grief Observed" (Lewis 1961), in which he solved that painful question for himself in the assumption that in the love of God all other conflicts could be reconciled. From a dynamic viewpoint, one may speculate about the projection of oedipal triangulations into the fantasied world after death and the corresponding efforts of defensive denial or sublimatory resolution of conflicts around direct and reverse triangulation (Kernberg 2012).

It impressed me that a more general attitude of tolerance of conflicts seemed characteristic of all the persons interviewed, accompanied by a greater degree of understanding of the viewpoints of others with whom they had experienced themselves in a serious conflict, and an increased capability for forgiveness toward others who had disappointed them or treated them with hostility. This greater degree of tolerance seemed to go hand in hand with greater tolerance for the ambivalence of human relations in general, an increased curiosity in the experiences and motivations of other persons, and the sense of greater understanding and greater freedom to be of help to other persons who were undergoing a mourning process. While some of these changes might be attributed to the general emotional maturation and deepening of self-reflection as an expression of the developmental process of essentially normal individuals, the intensity of this process in the subjects I reinterviewed seemed to them clearly related to the ongoing subtle process of long-term mourning for a lost object.

This greater degree of tolerance may extend to the fantasies about the lost object. For example, in situations of unresolved, significant guilt feelings, the mourned-for object may also be experienced as more tolerant and forgiving toward the surviving partner. The fantasy of a desired reencounter upon the survivor's own death now may include this more benign and forgiving lost object. The opposite may evolve in cases of *pathological mourning:* as part of depressive symptomatology, the person may experience the frightening fantasy that he or she will be rejected on such an encounter in the afterlife, resulting in an expansion of a panicky sense of abandonment.

Returning to the interviews, one other experience shared by practically all persons was the increase of thoughts and reflection regarding other losses in their lives, a review of what originally might have been almost peripheral, barely noticed processes of mourning regarding persons other than close and intimately related relatives and friends, but, of course, particularly so regarding one's own mourned parents, children, or siblings. Revisiting past mourning processes tended to be accompanied by the emergence of the lost love objects from the past, particularly one's parents, in the manifest content of dreams, very often in the context of scenes of early childhood or adolescence in which the dreamer is both a child and the present adult relating to a live image of the lost object. Old conflicts were relived in combination with the expression of new insights regarding these conflicts in the very interaction dreamed about, so that vivid repetition of the past in the context of present-day reflections about it were condensed into the dream experience. Vivid dreams involving dramatically realistic new experiences with the lost partner were quite frequent and were naturally followed by a painful awakening.

One subject told me that he felt that he lived in two worlds: one of daily reality, in which he felt immersed in the reality of his present human world, and one of his dreams, in which his deceased wife would appear as naturally linked to his present experiences, relating to his present network of close relationships—a scenario that would appear as perfectly realistic during his dreams.

A greater sensitivity to the nuances of present-day intimate relations and friendships seemed to evolve in parallel to the processes referred to this point: a combination of understanding in greater depth and appreciation of the importance of intimate relations and the mutuality of friendship. Octavio Paz's statement that "friendships are the leaves of the tree of life," mentioned by one of my subjects, was reflected in concrete experiences of the enrichment of his daily life.

Although the acceleration of the experience of time is a generalized human experience as part of the aging process, this very process seems accentuated in persons who are grieving losses of persons with whom they shared an intimate relationship over many years. The normal contrast between childhood and early adulthood, when external reality seems stable while the individual experiences himself or herself in a period of rapid change, and later life, in which the experience of changes in external reality points to the transience of existence, seems to be reinforced as a consequence of a severe loss, inducing a higher sensitivity to change, to the ephemerality of experience. That, in turn, deepened the intensity and value of relationships, and of the complex nature of one's own and others' personalities. It also deepened, at least in some of the persons whom I reinterviewed, the experience of art and the search for permanent values in the ethical as well as the aesthetic sphere. One person referred to Dali's famous sculpture "Horse Saddled With Time," in which one of Dali's blanket-like, soft surface clocks embraces the back of a harried, tense, and frightened-looking running horse, as a reflection of the transitoriness of experience. Another person stated succinctly that the relationship with those one loved was the only stable reality in a world of constant change. Obviously, personal conflicts, anxieties, and challenges determine the vast variety of reactions to the passage of time, but the very intensity of the awareness of this passage seemed related to the long-term processes of mourning.

In contrast to the heightened awareness of the transitory nature of experiences as well as aspects of external reality, several individuals I interviewed referred to the unexpected reactions they experienced toward objects concretely related to their mourned partner. An object that was dear to the lost person—a piece of jewelry, a painting, a song, an object of art or literature closely related to the lost person's interest—would intensify its meaningfulness and impact, triggering brief but deep mourning reactions. These seemed to be memory "rocks" in an ever-changing sea of reality. Most subjects were surprised by the intensity of sudden mourning reactions upon encountering of one of these objects. One person mentioned the drawing of an angel by Paul Klee, produced during the late stage of his illness, that his deceased wife had given him a few months before her death. On the wall of his office, it functioned as a bridge to an immediate contact with her, the memory of their conversations about Klee's art and life, and as a silent communion between them.

For psychoanalysts and psychoanalytic psychotherapists, the personal experience of a profound mourning process may increase their capacity to respond to their patient's mourning process. It may increase their understanding that patients need an open space and the therapist's capacity to fully tolerate, understand, and accompany the patient in his or her suffering, without premature reassurance or foreclosure of the process. The optimal way to help patients at this juncture is to permit them to share fully with the therapist their experience of the lost object, the very presence of this absent object in the content of the therapeutic hours. This involves the lost object becoming alive in the emotional experience of both participants, an increasing reality of the permanence of the lost object in the mental life of the patient as the memory becomes a shared reality in the therapeutic encounter. Therapists' sensitivity to patients' intolerance of the mourning process may increase their facilitating the diagnosis of paranoid regressions—the patient's blaming others for the death, and reacting with rage and wishes for revenge—and of pathological mourning reactions—severe, unrealistic guilt feelings and self-blame with depressive symptomatology and potentially suicidal impulses. The analytic resolution of these manifestations of intolerance of normal mourning may help the patient tolerate and elaborate the normal mourning process. Perhaps the greatest therapeutic challenge, under such circumstances, is the dominance of denial of mourning processes as an aspect of narcissistic pathology. The patient's apparent indifference to what from the outside appears as a dramatic loss may trigger strong negative countertransference reactions. The analyst's deep awareness that, together with the unconscious devaluation of the lost object, the patient is also impoverishing his or her own internal life may increase the analyst's tolerance and working through of this countertransference reaction. This radical indifference, of course, should not be confused with defensive hypomanic reaction to intolerable mourning, a denial of depression seemingly easier to integrate and work through.

In conclusion, if all true learning is essentially painful, the learning derived from the long-term effects of mourning processes probably is among the most painful contribution to learning in depth about intimate human relationships and their contribution to the richness of life. The underlying mechanisms involve the internalization of a highly significant object relation into both ego and superego structures in the context of the prevalence of love over hatred; the tolerance of the depressive position in contrast to the regressive defenses of narcissistic and paranoid structures or the condition of pathological mourning; and the corresponding capacity of working through of the depressive position, and of reinstating and deepening the relation with internalized good objects in the structure of one's mind.

References

Freud S: Mourning and melancholia (1917[1915]), in Standard Edition of the Complete Psychological Works of Sigmund Freud, Vol 14. Translated and edited by Strachey J. London, Hogarth Press, 1957, pp 237–260

Kernberg O: Some observations on the process of mourning. Int J Psychoanal 91(3):601–619, 2010 20590930

Kernberg OF: The Inseparable Nature of Love and Aggression: Clinical and Theoretical Perspectives. Washington, DC, American Psychiatric Publishing, 2012, pp 263–264

Klein M: Mourning and its relation to manic-depressive states. Int J Psychoanal 21:125–153, 1940

Lewis CS: A Grief Observed. San Francisco, CA, HarperCollins, 1961

CHAPTER 16

A Proposal for Innovation in Psychoanalytic Education

In this chapter, I propose that psychoanalytic education needs to advance into two apparently contradictory but essentially linked and indispensably complementary directions:

1. A clear, precise, scientifically based body of theory that reflects its specific contribution to psychological science and its applications, a true science of the dynamic unconscious, in contrast to "ecumenical" tolerance of unproven parallel or contradictory belief systems. This scientific approach also should apply to a system of therapeutic technical interventions that is sharp, precise, and comprehensive and can be scientifically subjected to empirical testing.
2. An honest, open, unashamedly subjective and existential exploration of emotional reactions and interactions in the treatment situation, what may be called a romantic attitude to what is actually alive—

This chapter was originally presented as a paper at the International Psychoanalytic Conference in Reykjavik, Iceland, October 9, 2014.

or dead—in the therapeutic encounter, within that technical frame. This discussion will illustrate steps in the direction of these objectives.

Renovation of the Structure of Psychoanalytic Education

I believe that the educational stagnation and underlying authoritarian structure of psychoanalytic education derive largely from the present-day training analysis system as a major source of inhibition of the educational process. In earlier work (Kernberg 2006a, 2007), I explored how the defensive conservatism regarding changes in our educational methodology, the dogmatic approach to the conceptual aspects of theory and technique, and the unresolvable, unanalyzable idealization of the training analyst as a combination of excellent clinician, ideal supervisor and seminar leader, and administrative leader of the institution are intimately linked. The protective segregation of psychoanalytic institutes from their scientific and academic counterparts, the restriction of the teaching faculty that excludes scholars in related disciplines from participating in the central educational venture, the infantilization of the candidates whose idealization of their training analysts cannot be fully resolved, the distrust of alternative ideas and schools of thought that differ from the dominant approach of any particular institute—all are major symptoms of the training analysis system and have been quite extensively analyzed and documented in recent contributions.

I propose that realistic quality control of the graduate psychoanalyst be assured by the development of a psychoanalytic specialty board that is similar to board-certified specialties in psychiatry. Such a board would offer certification in psychoanalysis to all graduates after a certain number of years of experience (probably somewhere around 5 years), which would provide the possibility for the graduate to have added one more "generation" of advanced or completed psychoanalyses since his or her graduation. Although we desperately need research on objective criteria for competence in carrying out psychoanalytic treatment, in practice it should be possible to assess the competence of all graduates. As part of the development of methods of selection of training analysts in recent years, we have gained empirical experience in evaluating their acquisition of technical expertise in carrying out psychoanalytic treatment. That experience, combined with the relative ease with which their theoretical knowledge may be evaluated, should allow the assessment of competence if and when seriously attempted. Körner (2002) has stated convincingly that psychoanalytic competence can be evaluated in terms of theoretical knowledge, technical expertise, and a psychoanalytic attitude. To develop instruments of theoretical knowledge should not offer major difficulties; also, there exists empirical evidence that the level of technical experience in psychoanalytic psychotherapy can be assessed (Mullen et al. 2002). Additionally, regarding a psychoanalytic attitude, Tuckett (2005) has suggested convincingly a method for evaluating the analyst's attitude in terms of his or her intuitive understanding of the patient's material, the analyst's capacity to develop a corresponding formulation in his or her mind, and the analyst's capacity to communicate it in appropriate interventions. This proposed method dovetails with the current practice of evaluating candidates for training analysis status by having the candidate present selected sessions from his or her analytic work and be prepared to discuss the patient's dynamics and his or her understanding and interventions in this context.

The expectation that during the, say, 5 years of experience beyond graduation the candidate for certification has carried out sufficient analytic work could be realistically broadened with alternative pathways to achieving clinical competence. These pathways include psychoanalytic treatments proper as well as experience in psychoanalytic psychotherapies, psychoanalytically influenced publications, and research concerns that demonstrate that the graduate has continued to use his or her psychoanalytic education to develop further his or her knowledge and depth in the understanding of unconscious conflicts, as well as their motivational impact on personality and psychological functioning, and has applied this knowledge in psychoanalytically based treatments.

Again, while acknowledging how little we have advanced in operationalizing criteria of analytic competence so that arbitrariness in the corresponding decision-making process cannot be fully eliminated, realistically the combination of knowledge, technical sophistication, and analytic attitude, combined with the nature of interests developed during the time span after graduation, should make it possible to confirm the expertise of the psychoanalyst to justify certification, and with it, the authorization to analyze candidates as well.

The supervisory function, in this proposed model, would be completely disconnected from the certification of the clinician in psychoanalysis. Talented supervisors would be recognized for their capabilities from their candidate years on, in terms of their creative and clarifying function in group seminars, which could be assessed further in the appointment of assistant supervisors at the time of graduation. Supervisors may also be selected from other sources such as colleagues recognized for their supervisory functions in study groups of the society, or for appreciated supervisory functions of psychoanalytic psychotherapy in departments of clinical psychology or psychiatry.

The stress on the evaluation of the scholarly productivity and research of psychoanalytic institutes leads to a related issue: the relationship between psychoanalytic institutes and the university. I have explored this issue in more detail elsewhere (Kernberg 2011), and I only wish to summarize here some major conclusions. I believe that the research function and scholarship in psychoanalytic education are essential to the survival of psychoanalysis as a profession and a science. In the long run, they will increase the need and objective pressures on psychoanalytic institutes to realign themselves within university settings. Various alternative models for such a relationship already exist, including a psychoanalytic institute within departments of psychiatry or clinical psychology, or a psychoanalytic institute as part of a psychoanalytic "center"—with various branches or structures throughout the university, or as an independent university institute in close liaison with several university colleges (Ferrari 2009; J. Körner, personal communication, 2009; Levy 2009). In any case, these various models of integration or rapprochement would facilitate research by combining the professional and clinical resources of psychoanalytic institutes with the research expertise and financial resources of university structures, thus fostering joint research projects related to or representing psychoanalytic theory, technique, and applications.

By the same token, such a relationship would break down the intellectual isolation of psychoanalytic institutes, permit the appointment of distinguished university professors as institute seminar leaders and scholars in residence, and open the executive structure of the psychoanalytic institute to scholars and research methodologists who may not have undergone psychoanalytic training, but who are strongly interested in psychoanalysis as a science. Theoretical, clinical, and applied seminars within psychoanalytic institutes thus could lead to depth and excitement of interdisciplinary studies, further increased by opening institute seminars to university faculty and students, so that only highly specialized seminars in psychoanalytic technique would be reserved for psychoanalytic candidates (and, it is hoped, at some point, to high-level trainees in psychoanalytic psychotherapy as well).

Another significant change in the proposed model of psychoanalytic education is that the analysts of candidates would no longer automatically occupy a position in the organizational structure and leadership function of the institute. The proposed model conceives the executive leadership of the institute as constituted by representatives from the supervisory body, seminar leaders, the research body, and representatives from the student body. The entire faculty would be involved in the selection of the director of the institute. The director of the institute would have the authority to appoint the various committees' leadership and would be responsible to the faculty, the psychoanalytic society, and/or the university setting within which the psychoanalytic institute may function. While variable arrangements may develop between the executive committee of the institute and the faculty at large, this model stresses the "functional"—in addition to the "democratic"—selection of supervisors, research faculty, seminar leaders, and student body representatives as the members of the executive committee of the psychoanalytic institute.

The seminar leaders in turn would be appointed separately from the certification process. Theoretical, clinical, research, and applied psychoanalytic subjects should be taught by recognized experts in the field, including non-analysts interested in psychoanalytic theory as it applies to related disciplines and experts in research methodology.

I have mentioned at several points the participation in the institute's academic life of a research faculty, both analysts and non-analysts, throughout the educational activities and the organizational structure of the institute. A specific department of research within each psychoanalytic institute is a highly desirable goal and should not be difficult to achieve once the fundamental importance of the development of new knowledge is recognized as an essential component of psychoanalytic education. Research faculty represented across the entire committee structure of the institute, including the executive committee, without consideration of whether the research experts are psychoanalysts, should provide support to seminar leaders in raising important questions of research interest and inviting and facilitating candidates and faculty to participate in specific research projects, provide research consultation and counseling to candidates, carry out a mentoring function for specifically research interested candidates, and present specialized seminars as electives on research methodology (Kernberg 2006b).

The proposed model also implies the selection of academically interested and motivated candidates and the fostering of their academic careers simultaneously with their psychoanalytic education. This represents a sharp contrast to the past tendency of many institutes to foster an almost exclusive dedication to psychoanalytic training and practice proper, with the idealization of "training analyst" as the only desirable career ladder inspiring the psychoanalytic candidate.

One other major but presently underdeveloped function of psychoanalytic institutes would implement teaching and research on the application of psychoanalytic theory and technique to a broad spectrum of derived psychotherapeutic approaches: individual, couple, family, and group psychotherapies based on psychoanalytic principles—in short, the development of a broad spectrum of psychotherapeutic modalities and expertise that increases the relevance of psychoanalysis for the mental health professions. A natural outgrowth of this effort would be to study the effectiveness of different treatment modalities and their indications and contraindications, thus eroding the present-day contradiction between psychoanalytic training geared almost exclusively to teaching the technique of standard psychoanalysis, while in their dominant daily practice psychoanalysts employ precisely the psychoanalytic psychotherapies that are not taught, or given only cursory attention, and are generally undervalued in traditional psychoanalytic education.

A Contemporary Approach to Psychoanalytic Theory

I propose that a clear outline of classical psychoanalytic theory, as reflected in the final theoretical view of Freud, should be taught together with the contemporary modifications, questions, and controversies that have been raised regarding all aspects of these theoretical formulations. This includes the contemporary controversies among the ego psychological approach and the Kleinian, British Independent, relationist, and Lacanian schools. This exploration would include consideration of the theory of the mental apparatus; its motivation, structure, and development; the nature of unconscious processes; the topographic theory; and the spectrum of defensive mechanisms. This review would reevaluate the structural theory; the drive theory; the oedipal complex and the nature of the id, particularly with relation to infantile sexuality; and the role of aggression. Study of the structure and functions of the ego should include considerations of identity and the theory of the self as well as the role of the superego in normality and pathology.

What I wish to stress is that all these areas of the educational task would have to include the alternative, complementary, or questioning approaches that have been developed in the boundary sciences, with an ongoing exploration of the psychoanalytic theory from the viewpoint of neurobiological developments, evolutionary psychology, developmental psychology, experimental psychology, social psychology, and current knowledge in sociology and cultural anthropology that relates to various assumptions of psychoanalytic theory. Obviously, much of this needs to be taught by specialists who may not be available within the realm of a psychoanalytic faculty, therefore experts in these fields should be recruited to contribute their specific knowledge. In short, psychoanalytic theory needs to be examined in the context of the developments of modern science in other related fields.

Let me illustrate this approach with one example: the contemporary analysis of Freud's dual drive theory, in and of itself controversial within psychoanalytic approaches. Drive theory raises questions regarding the relations between this theory and the evolving contemporary knowledge of motivational systems in neurobiology. Specifically, the discoveries regarding the *neurobiological* origin, structure, and functioning of affects as primary motivational systems, and the early interactions among *genetic* dispositions, brain structures, and environmental influences from the beginning of life on (Kernberg 2012). Affective neuroscience, in short, must be explored in the context of the analysis of the theory of drives. Obviously, in clinical studies of mental mechanisms, particularly the relationship between impulsive and defensive pressures, affect-driven desires and opposite mechanisms tending to control, suppress, or repress them have been subjected to psychoanalytic studies. For example, we have empirical investigation of the mechanism of projective identification, relating it to the exploration of affective communication, by Rainer Krause and others. The study of early cognitive and affective interactions and their relations to primitive defensive operations, particularly in the study of attachment, is another example of parallel and sometimes even combined research from a psychoanalytic, behavioral, and neurobiological perspective. Development and psychopathology are vast areas where psychoanalytic clinical observation and theory may be enriched, contrasted, and developed in interaction with related sciences.

A central, unifying concept of all psychoanalytic approaches is the theory of the dynamic unconscious and its influence on conscious life. The empirical evidence of the operations of the dynamic unconscious appears to be sufficiently powerful to signal a key function of psychoanalytic theory within the general contemporary research on different states of consciousness and the relationship between declarative and procedural memory. In short, general psychoanalytic theory, theory of development, and theory of psychopathology need to be correlated with related contemporary scientific approaches. Regarding psychopathology, obviously, psychoanalytic theories of depression must be related to the new knowledge regarding neurobiology of depression, and psychoanalytic theory of character pathology with the developing knowledge regarding neurobiological and psychosocial influences in the development of personality disorders. Again, psychoanalysis may have fundamental contributions to make to other sciences that have not been exploited and only expressed in hypotheses or assumptions that, under the present circumstances, have not been taken seriously by other scientific fields because of the lack of empirical and interdisciplinary research initiated by psychoanalytic educational institutions and a neglect of investment in research.

Psychoanalytic Technique and Its Application

The lack of teaching and awareness of psychoanalytic technique and its application to the derivative forms of psychoanalytically derived psychotherapies represents, I believe, a major failure of psychoanalytic education. It is significant, and dramatic, that to this day there does not exist any comprehensive text on psychoanalytic technique! Insofar as competence in psychoanalytic technique is assumed to represent the objective criteria for graduation and advancement within one's institute, it is not surprising that this process has been sufficiently mystified to leave open a vast area of uncertainty and vagueness regarding the criteria used to assess this competence, and to enshrine, within the "training analyst" system, the tremendous subjectivity in these evaluations.

I believe that we have sufficient evidence of the basic commonality of technical psychoanalytic principles of various schools to justify a clear, common, basic psychoanalytic technique and to define how different psychoanalytic approaches vary in their use of core techniques. I will not go into details about the analysis of this problem in this chapter, but I believe that interpretation, transference analysis, technical neutrality, and countertransference analysis compose the basic components of the technical psychoanalytic approach and that the combined use of these four techniques are then applied to other aspects of the psychoanalytic situation such as character analysis; dream analysis; analysis of acting out, enactment, repetition compulsion, and working through; and the analysis of termination (see Chapter 4, "The Basic Components of Psychoanalytic Technique and Derived Psychoanalytic Psychotherapies" and Chapter 6, "The Spectrum of Psychoanalytic Techniques," of this book). The preconditions for carrying out this technical approach in the treatment of patients are given by the instructions of free association for the patient and the evenly suspended attention of the analyst. Clear definition of those four basic techniques permit one to define their specific modifications by alternative psychoanalytic approaches. In this field, we do have significant empirical evidence on effectiveness, stemming largely not only from research in psychoanalytic psychotherapies that have been employing these techniques with specified modifications, but also from empirical clinical research on psychoanalysis proper and on comparison between psychoanalysis and psychoanalytic psychotherapy. Evidence is accumulating that is relevant for the educational processes involved in teaching psychoanalytic technique in psychoanalytic institutes. It is discouraging how little this empirical evidence has been used in psychoanalytic education.

The use of contemporary educational techniques, combined with computer-based analyses of content of psychoanalytic sessions and the direct study of therapeutic interactions by audio and video recording (strenuously objected to by psychoanalytic educational institutions until a few years ago), has not proved to be detrimental to the analytic process. The specific effects of interpretation, in contrast to supportive psychodynamic psychoanalytic approaches, have been clearly demonstrated. The systematic analysis of transference has been shown to be an important therapeutic tool in the treatment of severe personality disorders, whereas until about 30 years ago, psychoanalytic assumptions of the various schools, with the exception of the Kleinian school, were that analytic approaches to such very severe cases were risky and mostly contraindicated. We now have evidence for indications and contraindications of various psychoanalytical psychotherapies for severe personality disorders.

It is realistic and feasible now to develop precise techniques for psychoanalytic psychotherapy and supportive forms of therapy based on psychoanalytic understanding and principles. Our training institutes have been reluctant to teach these approaches in an effort to preserve a "pure culture" of psychoanalytic technique proper against all the evidence of the possibility of differentiating these approaches, and the possible expansion of the application of psychoanalytic principles for a vast number of conditions in which psychoanalysis is not possible or not indicated. This has led to the development of *psychotherapy* institutes specializing in these particular techniques, in competition with pure psychoanalytic cultures, and with a social chaos in this field that also contributes to the loss of prestige of the profession that we have been witnessing.

Preservation and Enrichment of the Subjective, Intersubjective, and Existential Approaches to Psychoanalytic Treatment

The major obstacle to synergy between psychoanalysis and other scientific endeavors stems from the assumption that each psychoanalytic situation is a unique relationship between two individuals and therefore does not lend itself to objective scientific measurement. There is a naïve assumption that the analyst listening with evenly suspended attention, or with an effort to enter each session "without memory or desire" and open to reverie on the patient's material, will provide the essential and exclusive precondition on which psychoanalytic understanding and interpretation are based. I believe that this assumption is a bias derived from a lack of understanding of what a clear and precise technical approach means. The intuitive sense of what is going on between patient and therapist is obviously the basis of all understanding and analytic work. The content of free association, the patient's verbal communication and affect expression, the nonverbal manifestation of his or her behavior, and the affective tonality of this communication all influence the analyst and constitute the basis for his or her intuitive understanding. The combination of verbal communication, nonverbal communication, and countertransference constitutes the raw material on which interpretation and transference analysis are based. The analysis of countertransference is the source of important information, and the analyst's intervention from a point of technical neutrality—not implying indifference or distancing but rather a concerned objectivity—opens the field for the expression of a specific emotional experience that the patient introduces in the analytic encounter. Openness to this experience by the analyst is not in contradiction to a clear understanding of how this knowledge is to be captured and used or how the analyst's understanding can be transformed into new understanding and communicated to the patient. All recent technical analytic approaches, as has been pointed out by Fred Busch (2014), have evolved into giving primary attention to the enacted object relationship in the transference in the here and now, and to transformation of the material intuitively captured by the analyst into representational consciousness by the patient that reflects what previously could not be experienced and reflected on. I believe that the main controversy regarding "What is the correct interpretation?" usually relates to the genetic element of what is enacted, and here clearly theory influences analytic technique and should be spelled out and subjected to empirical investigation. I am referring to whether conflicts stem from a preverbal period of development or from archaic or advanced oedipal levels of development and dominance. With an optimal understanding of the unconscious processes that are developing in the here-and-now interaction, the question of genetic origins can be clarified throughout time. My point is that open, intuitive awareness of the present psychoanalytic situation within one's theoretical orientation not only is essential but can be closely studied. Theoretical differences should not be an impediment to the study of clinical and applied psychoanalysis. Theory counts, regarding the scientific nature of the psychoanalytic theory of personality, development, psychopathology, and treatment, and its scientific evaluation, as well as evaluation of the techniques of therapeutic intervention and their theoretical basis, will determine the future of the profession as well as of the theory itself.

References

Busch F: Creating a Psychoanalytic Mind: A Psychoanalytic Method and Theory. London, Routledge, 2014

Ferrari H: IUSAM-APdeBA: a higher education institute for psychoanalytic training. Int J Psychoanal 90(5):1139–1154, 2009 19821859

Kernberg OF: The coming changes in psychoanalytic education: part I. Int J Psychoanal 87(Pt 6):1649–1673, 2006a 17130087

Kernberg OF: The pressing need to increase research in and on psychoanalysis. Int J Psychoanal 87(Pt 4):919–926, 2006b 16877244

Kernberg OF: The coming changes in psychoanalytic education: Part II. Int J Psychoanal 88(Pt 1):183–202, 2007 17244574

Kernberg OF: Psychoanalysis and the university: a difficult relationship. Int J Psychoanal 92(3):609–622, 2011 21702747

Kernberg O: The Inseparable Nature of Love and Aggression: Clinical and Theoretical Perspectives. Washington, DC, American Psychiatric Publishing, 2012

Körner J: The didactics of psychoanalytic education. Int J Psychoanal 83(Pt 6): 1395–1405, 2002 12521538

Levy ST: Psychoanalytic education then and now. J Am Psychoanal Assoc 57(6):1295–1309, 2009 20068242

Mullen LS, Rieder RO, Glick RA, et al: Testing psychodynamic psychotherapy skills among psychiatric residents: the psychodynamic psychotherapy competency test. Am J Psychiatry 161(9):1658–1664, 2004 15337657

Tuckett D: Does anything go? Towards a framework for the more transparent assessment of psychoanalytic competence. Int J Psychoanal 86(Pt 1):31–49, 2005 15859220

Index

Abstinence, and technical neutrality, 60
Abstraction, and components of personality, 13, 14
Acting out
  borderline patients and, 239
  countertransference and, 63
  denial of reality and, 256
  enactment as distinct from, 82, 92
  psychoanalytic techniques and, 88–91
  technical neutrality and, 61
  transference analysis and, 59
  transference-focused psychotherapy and, 109, 117
Adjustment disorders, and antisocial behavior in adolescents, 204–205
Adolescents, and adolescence
  antisocial behavior in adjustment disorders of, 204–205
  internalized set of ethical principles and, 13
  supportive psychotherapy and, 143, 145
Advanced oedipal state of development, 12
Affective dominance
  character analysis and, 84

importance of as psychoanalytic technique, 83, 83, 84
  tactics of transference-focused psychotherapy and, 108, 147–148
Affective reactivity, and temperament, 5–6, 32
Affective system
  character traits and, 8
  neurobiology of, 32–34
Age. *See also* Adolescents; Children
  activation of erotic transferences and, 239
  evaluation of sexual behavior and difference in between patient and therapist, 224
Aggression
  narcissism and, 154–155
  supportive psychotherapy and control of, 140
  syndrome of arrogance and, 164
Aggressive type, of antisocial behavior, 197, 199, 208
Alcoholism, and antisocial behavior, 177
Analytic listening, 82
Anatomy of Evil, The (Stone 2009), 199
Anonymity, and technical neutrality, 60

Anorexia, and transference-focused psychotherapy, 124. *See also* Eating disorders
Antisocial behavior. *See also* Antisocial personality disorder
  acting out and, 90
  in adolescent adjustment disorders, 204–205
  aggressive and passive-parasitic types of, 197, 199, 208
  borderline personality organization and, 14, 203–204
  definition of, 197
  differential diagnosis of, 206–210
  narcissistic personality disorder and, 173–177, 202–203
  neurotic personality organization and, 204
  pseudopsychopathic schizophrenia and, 198–199
  superego integration and, 14
  supportive psychotherapy and, 141, 143
  syndrome of malignant narcissism and, 201–202
  transference-focused psychotherapy and, 121, 126–127
Antisocial personality disorder
  antisocial behavior and, 199–201
  differential diagnosis of, 174, 206–210
  narcissistic personality disorder and, 174
  supportive psychotherapy for, 146–147
Anxiety
  dream analysis and, 87
  somatization and, 96–97
  transference in narcissistic patients and, 193
Applebaum, Ann, 133
Arrogance, syndrome of, 156, 163–166

Assessment. *See also* Differential diagnosis; Evaluation
  of degrees of pathology in experience of self, 23
  of interpersonal functioning, 23–24
  supportive psychotherapy and, 138–139
  transference-focused psychotherapy and ongoing, 117
Attachment-separation panic system, 6
Attention, and preconditions for psychoanalytic work, 53–54
Aversive affective system, 33

Bad/feared relationships, and goals of transference-focused psychotherapy, 66
Baranger, M. and W., 97, 259
Bataille, G., 218, 222
Behavior. *See* Aggression; Antisocial behavior; Counterphobic behavior; Self-destructive behavior; Sexual behavior; Suicide
Bion, Wilfred R., 54, 86, 114, 115, 163, 178
Borderline personality disorder. *See also* Borderline personality organization
  antisocial behavior and, 203
  case illustration of interpretation in, 73–78
  defensive use of free association in, 110
  neurobiology of, 27, 41–42
  suicidal behavior and, 168
  transference-focused psychotherapy and assessment of life situation in, 118–119, 120
Borderline personality organization. *See also* Borderline personality disorder
  antisocial behavior and, 14, 203–204

Index

borderline personality disorder under conditions of, 41–42
identity diffusion and, 10
primitive defensive operations and, 137
psychoanalytic object relations theory and, 39, 42–43
sexual behavior and transference or countertransference developments in, 235–240
sexual conflicts and, 226, 227
transference-focused psychotherapy as treatment for, 43–45, 107, 111
transference analysis and, 56, 59
unresolved mourning processes and, 101
Brain structures, and affect expression, 33–34. *See also* Neurobiology
Brief psychoanalytic psychotherapy, 102
British Independent approach, and components of psychoanalytic technique, 67
Britton, Ronald, 166, 178
Busch, Fred, 282

Case illustrations
of denial of reality in narcissistic personality disorder, 252–255
of differential diagnosis of antisocial behavior, 207–208
of interpretation in borderline pathology, 73–78
of sexual conflict at level of neurotic personality organization, 227–228
Categorical system, for classification of personality disorders, 20, 26
Certification, in psychoanalysis, 274, 275
Character, as component of personality, 6–9
Character analysis, and psychoanalytic techniques, 83–86

Children, and antisocial behavior, 199. *See also* Adolescents; Development
Chronic illness, and mourning process, 267. *See also* Health care; HIV
Chronic supportive counseling, 144
Clarification, and interpretation of defenses, 55
Classification, of personality disorders in DSM-5, 10, 19–28
Cleckley, Hervey, 199
Cognitive ability, and intelligence, 14–15
Cognitive development, and empathy, 37
Cognitive differentiation, between self and other, 35
Cognitive-emotional recognition system, 37
Cognitive framing, and affect activation, 32
Cognitive learning, and narcissism, 157
Communication, and interpretation, 55. *See also* Language; Nonverbal communication
Compassion, and neurobiology, 36–37
Complementary identification, and countertransference, 62
Comprehensive Dictionary of Psychoanalysis (Akhtar 2009), 54
Concordant identification, and countertransference, 62
Conduct disorder, 199
Conflict(s)
psychoanalytic theory on struggle between impulse and defense, 52–53
sexual at level of neurotic personality organization, 225–232
technical innovations in transference-focused psychotherapy and, 113–119

Confrontation, and interpretation of defenses, 55
Contagion, and brain functions, 36
Contemptuous behavior, and syndrome of arrogance, 164–165
Contract(s). *See also* Safety
  acting out and, 90
  antisocial behavior and, 177
  supportive psychotherapy and, 139
  tactics of transference-focused psychotherapy and, 108, 120, 123–126
Control, and syndrome of arrogance, 165. *See also* Omnipotent control
Conversion reactions, and somatization, 96, 97
Core self, 35
Couch, use of for psychoanalysis, 64
Counterphobic behaviors, 7
Countertransference
  analysis of as basic component of psychoanalytic technique, 51, 53, 61–63, 280
  antisocial behavior and, 175, 209–210
  enactment and, 91
  evaluation of sexual pathology and, 222–223, 224
  narcissism and negative forms of, 188, 189, 190
  relational approach to transference analysis and, 58
  sexual behavior in borderline patients and, 235–240
  sexual conflicts and erotic developments in, 229–230
  supportive psychotherapy and, 134, 136–137, 142
  syndrome of arrogance and, 165
  technical neutrality and, 61
  techniques of transference-focused psychotherapy and, 110, 111

Crisis intervention, and supportive psychotherapy, 148
Culture, and sexual behavior in patients with personality disorders, 240

Dali, Salvador, 269
Daydreaming, and psychoanalytic field, 98
"Dead mother" syndrome, and narcissistic personality disorder, 154, 155, 171–172, 246
Death, and mourning process, 267
Deceptiveness. *See* Dishonesty
Decision making, and supportive psychotherapy, 148
Deconstruction, and dream analysis, 87
Defense(s)
  borderline personality disorder and, 43
  character traits and, 7–8
  free association and narcissistic, 181–195
  identity and identity diffusion, 9
  interpretation of, 55
  psychoanalytic object relations theory and, 39, 52–53
  psychoanalytic techniques and analysis of, 83–84
  supportive psychotherapy and, 137–138
  transference-focused psychotherapy and, 121–123
Dependency
  defenses in narcissism and, 182, 183, 184–185, 188, 192
  sexual behavior and erotic transferences in borderline patients, 236
  sexual behavior and erotic transferences in narcissistic patients, 242–243
Depersonification, of superego, 13

Depression, and somatization, 96–97. *See also* Depressive position

Depressive-masochistic personality disorder, 95, 204

Depressive position. *See also* Depression
  development of normal psychological functioning and, 39
  narcissistic patients and achievement of, 191

Detoxification, for alcohol or drug abuse, 177

Devaluation, and borderline personality disorder, 43

Development, and psychoanalytic object relations theory, 37–40

Diagnosis. *See* Assessment; Differential diagnosis; Evaluation

Dialectical behavior therapy (DBT), 170

Dicks, Henry, 221

Dictionaries, and definitions of psychoanalytic techniques, 82

Dictionary of Kleinian Thought, A (Hinshelwood 1991), 55

Dictionnaire International de la Psychanalyse (de Miholla 2002), 54

Differential diagnosis. *See also* Assessment; Evaluation
  of antisocial behavior and antisocial personality disorder, 206–210
  of antisocial personality disorder and narcissistic personality disorder, 174
  of total apparent obliteration of sexuality, 244–247

Dimensional system, for classification of personality disorders, 20, 26

Directors, of psychoanalytic institutes, 277

Direct triangulation, and sexual conflicts, 226

Dishonesty
  antisocial behavior and, 174, 176, 177, 203
  tactics of transference-focused psychotherapy and, 109, 126

Domestic violence, and antisocial behavior, 175

Dreams
  analysis of as psychoanalytic technique, 86–88
  awake life form of, 98–99
  mourning process and content of, 268
  narcissistic patients and, 191

Drive theory, contemporary analysis of, 279

Drug abuse
  antisocial behavior and, 177
  transference-focused psychotherapy and, 124

DSM-IV, and classification of personality disorders, 19–20, 21, 25–26, 27–28

DSM-5, and classification of personality disorders, 10, 19–28

Dynamic interpersonal therapy (DIT), 112–113

Dynamic unconscious, as unifying concept of psychoanalytic approaches, 279

Eating disorders, and antisocial behavior, 177. *See also* Anorexia

Edinburgh International Encyclopedia of Psychoanalysis, The (Skelton et al. 2006), 55

Education, of therapists in psychoanalysis and psychoanalytic technique, 70, 273–283. *See also* Learning

Ego. *See also* Ego identity; Id; Superego
  concept of ego ideal, 12
  concept of frailty of, 133

Ego *(continued)*
   Freudian concept of, 11
   psychoanalytic object relations theory and, 39
Ego identity, and character as component of personality, 6–9
Ego psychology, 38, 67, 112
Embodied self, 34
Emotional dysregulation, and neurobiological structures, 27. *See also* Self regulation
Empathy
   assessment of interpersonal functioning and, 23–24
   brain functions and, 36
Enactment
   acting out and, 82, 92
   countertransference and, 63
   psychoanalytic techniques and, 91–92
   transference and, 52
Envy, and negative therapeutic reaction, 95, 96
Equivalency, and development of self, 36
Erikson, Erik, 24
Ethical values, and components of personality, 11–14. *See also* Value system
Evaluation. *See also* Assessment; Differential diagnosis
   of competence in psychoanalysis, 274–275
   of sexual pathology, 223–225
Examination dreams, 87
Existential approach, to psychoanalytic treatment, 281–283
Expressive psychotherapy, 66, 68–69

Face-to-face position, and psychoanalytic psychotherapies, 64
Facial expression, and early development of self, 35–36

Family
   antisocial personality disorder and, 200
   involvement of in treatment of narcissistic personality disorder, 173, 174
   risk of suicide during psychotherapeutic treatment and, 170
   transference-focused psychotherapy and joint sessions with patient and, 125
Family history, and borderline personality disorder, 74
Fantasy, and supportive psychotherapy, 134. *See also* Rescue fantasies
Financial situation, of patient
   antisocial behavior and, 176
   discussion of in transference-focused psychotherapy, 127, 128
First Dictionary of Psychoanalysis, The (Sterba 2013), 55
Five-factor system, for classification of personality disorders, 19–20, 22–23, 25
Free association
   defensive use of by borderline patients, 110
   denial of reality and, 256
   dream analysis and, 88
   narcissistic defenses and, 159, 181–195
   as precondition for psychoanalytic work, 53, 54
   supportive psychotherapy and, 139–140
French approach, and basic components of psychoanalytic technique, 67
Frequency, of sessions
   differentiation of psychoanalysis from psychoanalytic psychotherapies, 64
   supportive psychotherapy and, 64, 139, 147

Index 291

transference-focused psychotherapy and, 64, 107, 115, 132
Freud, Sigmund, 12, 60, 154, 204, 266, 278, 279

Gating function, 36–37
Gender, and activation of erotic transferences, 239. *See also* Sexual identity
Genetics
  borderline personality disorder and, 41
  drive theory and, 279
  intelligence and, 15
German depth psychology–based psychoanalytic psychotherapy, 69, 112
Gill, M.M., 109
Goals, of treatment
  transference-focused psychotherapy and, 66, 119–120
  supportive psychotherapy and, 134, 145
Good/desired relationships, and goals of transference-focused psychotherapy, 66
Grandiose self, and narcissism, 158, 160, 161, 169, 170, 175, 176, 186, 188, 191, 193, 195, 242, 244
Gratification, derived from acting out, 91
Green, André, 90, 110, 114, 154, 168, 171, 172, 178, 216, 246
Guilt
  mourning process and reactivation of, 266
  narcissistic personality disorder and, 191, 194, 195
  negative therapeutic reactions and, 94, 95, 96

Handbuch Psychoanalytischer Grundbegriffe (Mertens 2014), 55
Hare, Robert, 209

Health care, supportive psychotherapy and problems in, 140. *See also* Chronic illness
Histrionic personality disorder. *See* Infantile-histrionic personality disorder
HIV, and transference-focused psychotherapy, 122
Homicide, and antisocial behavior, 208
Homosexuality, and sexual identity, 222, 239
Hospitalization
  pseudopsychopathic schizophrenia and, 198
  transference-focused psychotherapy as alternative to, 125
Hypochondriasis, 96–97
Hysterical personality disorder, and antisocial behavior, 204

Id. *See also* Ego
  Freudian concept of, 11
  psychoanalytic object relations theory and, 39
Identity. *See also* Ego identity; Sexual identity
  assessment of degrees of pathology in experience of self, 23
  as component of personality, 9–10, 24
Identity diffusion
  borderline personality organization and, 43
  concept of integrated self and, 24
  development of self and, 10
  integrated system of ethical values and, 13
  severe personality disorders and, 107
Identity pathology, personality disorders of, 10
Impairment, and Level of Personality Functioning Scale, 24

Impulse, conflict of with defense in psychoanalytic technique and object relations, 52–53
Impulsivity
    borderline personality disorder and, 43
    evaluation of sexual pathology and, 225
Individualization, of superego, 13
Infantile-histrionic personality disorder
    antisocial behavior and, 203
    denial of reality and, 259–260
    exclusion of from DSM-5, 22, 25
    supportive psychotherapy and, 145–146
Informed consent, for contacts with third parties, 143
Insight
    as mechanism of change in psychoanalytic treatment, 64–65
    working through and, 94
Insight-oriented psychotherapy, 66, 68–69
Intelligence, as component of personality, 14–15
Internet sex, 241
Interpersonal affective focus, in dynamic interpersonal therapy, 112
Interpersonal relationships. *See also* Family; Social history
    antisocial personality disorder and, 200
    assessment of functioning, 23–24
    outcome of treatment for narcissistic personality disorder and, 192
    supportive psychotherapy and, 140
    transference-focused psychotherapy and, 66, 113–119
Interpretation
    as basic component of psychoanalytic technique, 53, 55–57, 280
    case illustration of in borderline pathology, 73–78
    hypochondriasis and, 97
    supportive psychotherapy and, 135
    transference analysis and, 58–59
    transference-focused psychotherapy and, 109
Intersubjective approach, to psychoanalytic treatment, 281–283
Intersubjective field, 98–99, 262
Intimacy, and assessment of interpersonal functioning, 24
Intolerance of triangulation, and narcissistic personality disorder, 166–168
Intrapsychic structures
    classification of personality disorders and, 26–27
    development of personality and, 15–16
    psychoanalytic object relations theory and, 40

Jacobson, Edith, 11
Joseph, Betty, 92, 113, 262

Klein, Melanie, 39, 100, 266
Kleinian approach
    basic components of psychoanalytic technique and, 67
    enactment and, 91–92
    narcissistic pathology and, 178
    transference analysis and, 58–59
    transference-focused psychotherapy and, 113
Körner, J., 274–275
Krause, Rainer, 279

LaFarge, Lucy, 189
Language, patient's appropriation of analyst's in narcissism, 185. *See also* Communication
Language of Psychoanalysis, The (Laplanche and Pontalis 1988), 54–55

Index

Laplanche, J., 218
Latency years, and internalized value system, 13
Learning. *See also* Cognitive learning; Education
    character traits and, 8
    long-term effects of mourning process and, 270–271
Legal issues, and suicidal behavior of patients, 173
Letter of understanding, and safety contracts, 125
Level of Personality Functioning Scale, 23–24
Lewis, C.S., 267
Life situation. *See also* Interpersonal relationships; Work situation
    denial of reality in severe personality disorders and, 259, 260–262
    technical innovations in transference-focused psychotherapy and, 113–121, 122, 128
Limbic system, and affect expression, 33–34
Limit setting, and tactics of transference-focused psychotherapy, 108, 122, 177
Los Fundamentos de la Técnica Psicoanalitica (Etchegoyen 1986), 55

Mainstream approach, to interpretation, 57
Malignant narcissism, syndrome of, 154, 160, 174, 176, 201–202, 207
Mask of Sanity, The (Cleckley 1941), 199
Masochistic personality. *See also* Depressive-masochistic personality disorder; Sadomasochistic relationship; Sadomasochistic transferences
    sexual conflicts at neurotic level of organization and, 231–232
    transference-focused psychotherapy and, 122–123

MBT. *See* Mentalization-based therapy
Mentalization
    borderline personality organization and, 43, 44
    concept of, 65
    neurobiology and, 41
    transference-focused psychotherapy and increased, 66
Mentalization-based therapy (MBT)
    basic components of psychoanalytic technique and, 69
    improvement in personality functioning and, 65
    transference-focused psychotherapy compared to, 112
Mental status examination, 208
Mirror neuron systems, 36, 37
Morality, and defenses against sense of personal responsibility in transference-focused psychotherapy, 121. *See also* Ethical values; Value system
Mourning
    long-term effects of, 265–271
    termination and process of, 100–102
    working through and, 94

Narcissistic personality disorder. *See also* Malignant narcissism
    antisocial behavior and, 173–177, 202–203, 207
    case illustration of denial of reality in, 252–255
    character analysis and, 84
    classification of in DSM-5, 21–22
    "dead mother" syndrome and, 154, 155, 171–172, 246
    defensive operations and free associations in, 181–195
    denial of mourning process in, 270
    negative therapeutic reaction and, 95

Narcissistic personality disorder *(continued)*
  primitive defensive operations and, 137
  range of pathology in, 154
  sadomasochistic transferences and, 172–173
  sexual behavior and erotic transferences in, 240–244, 246
  sexual conflicts and, 226
  suicidality and self-destructiveness in, 168–171
  termination and, 100–101
  transference-focused psychotherapy and assessment of life situation in, 118–119
  transferences at fluctuating borderline level of, 160–168
  transferences at high stable level of functioning, 156–160
Narcissistic resistances, and tactics of transference-focused psychotherapy, 109
Negative narcissism, 168
Negative therapeutic reaction, and psychoanalytic techniques, 94–96
Neo-Bionian approach, to interpretation, 57
Neurobiology
  borderline personality disorder and, 41–42
  classification of personality disorders and, 26–27
  concept of personality and, 15–16, 32
  development and integration of affective systems, 32–34
  drive theory and, 279
  of empathy and compassion, 36–37
  mentalization and, 41
  self and, 34–36
Neuropsychological structures, and classification of personality disorders, 27

Neurotic personality organization
  antisocial behavior and, 204
  character analysis and, 85
  identity diffusion and, 10
  interpretation and, 73
  sexual conflicts at level of, 225–232
  termination and, 101
  transference analysis and, 56, 59–60
New Dictionary of Kleinian Thought, The (Spillius et al. 2011), 54
Nonverbal communication, and psychoanalytic psychotherapies, 64

Object constancy, 36
Object relations, and object relations theory
  aggressive internalized versus idealized in severe personality disorders, 107
  attachment-separation panic system and, 6
  character traits and, 8
  psychoanalytic theory and, 37–45, 50–53
  sexual behavior and, 220
  supportive psychotherapy and, 133
Obsessive-compulsive personality disorder, 204
Oedipal conflicts, and neurotic personality organization, 227, 229, 230
Ogden, T., 98
Omnipotent control, and narcissism, 182–183, 184–185

Paranoid personality disorder, 22, 25, 203
Paranoid-schizoid position, 39
Paranoid transferences, 174–175
Paraphilia, and erotic transferences in borderline patients, 238

Index

Passive-parasitic type, of antisocial behavior, 197, 199, 208
Pathological mourning, 268
Patient(s). *See also* Countertransference; Family history; Financial situation; Life situation; Social history; Transference; *specific personality disorders*
  effect on age difference with therapist on discussion of sexual behavior, 224
  role of in psychotherapeutic relationship, 82
  supportive psychotherapy and responsibilities of, 144–146
Paz, Octavio, 269
Persecutory affect states, and object relations, 39
Persecutory segment, of early experience, 11–12
Personality
  character and ego identity as components of, 6–9
  definition of, 3–4
  identity and identity diffusion as components of, 9–10
  integrated system of ethical values and, 11–14
  integrated view of determinants of, 4
  intelligence as component of, 14–15
  neurobiology and, 32
  psychoanalytic treatment and improvement in functioning of, 65
  temperament as component of, 5–6, 7, 32
Personality disorder not otherwise specified (NOS), 19
Personality disorders. *See also* Antisocial personality disorder; Borderline personality disorder; Borderline personality organization; Infantile-histrionic personality disorder; Narcissistic personality disorder; Obsessive-compulsive personality disorder; Paranoid personality disorder; Psychoanalysis; Schizoid personality disorder; Schizotypal personality disorder
  acting out and, 89
  antisocial behavior as aspect of, 198
  character analysis and, 84
  character traits and, 7
  classification of in DSM-5, 10, 19–28
  denial of reality as frequent complication in, 251–263
  development of transference-focused psychotherapy as specific treatment for, 49–50
  erotic transference and countertransference in patients with, 235–247
  evaluation of sexual pathology in patients with, 215–232
  indications and contraindications of supportive psychotherapy for, 146–147
  integration of internalized system of ethical values and, 13
  mourning process and, 265–271
  primitive defensive operations and, 9
  therapeutic alliance and, 86
  transference-focused psychotherapy for severe forms of, 91, 99, 106
  transference monitoring in supportive psychotherapy and, 141
Personality Disorders Institute (Weill Cornell Medical College), 5, 49–50, 106, 131, 133, 154, 192, 208, 215, 221, 256
Personal responsibility, defenses against sense of, 121–123
Perversity, syndrome of, 244

Physical abuse, and narcissistic personality disorder, 161, 164. *See also* Domestic violence
Posttraumatic stress disorder, 237
Preconditions, for psychoanalytic work, 53–54
Prohibitions, internalization of earliest, 11–12
Projective identification
   borderline personality disorder and, 43, 74
   enactment and, 91–92
   interpretation of, 74
Proto-self, 35
Pseudopsychopathic schizophrenia, and antisocial behavior, 198–199, 206, 207
Psychoanalysis, and psychoanalytic techniques. *See also* Psychoanalytic theory
   acting out and, 88–91
   character analysis and, 83–86
   definition and analysis of basic components, 54–63, 81, 82
   differentiation of psychoanalysis from psychoanalytic psychotherapies, 64–70
   dream analysis and, 86–88
   education of therapists in, 280–281
   enactment and, 91–92
   negative therapeutic reaction and, 94–96
   preconditions for, 53–54
   psychoanalytic field and, 97–99
   psychoanalytic theory in context of object relations and, 50–53
   repetition compulsion and, 92–94
   sexual conflicts at level of neurotic personality organization, 226–227
   somatization and, 96–97
   subjective, intersubjective, and existential approaches to, 281–283
   termination and, 99–102
   working through and, 94
Psychoanalytic field, and psychoanalytic techniques, 97–99
Psychoanalytic institutes, 276–278. *See also* Personality Disorders Institute
Psychoanalytic psychotherapy, and pathological mourning, 101–102. *See also* Psychoanalysis; Psychotherapy
Psychoanalytic Terms and Concepts (Auchincloss and Samberg 2012), 54
Psychoanalytic theory, contemporary approach to, 278–280. *See also* Object relations; Psychoanalysis
Psychodynamic psychotherapy, and supportive techniques, 66, 69. *See also* Supportive psychotherapy
Psychological permanence, of concept of self, 35
Psychological tests, and antisocial behavior, 210
Psychology. *See* Ego psychology; German depth psychology–based psychoanalytic psychotherapy; Psychological tests; Self psychology; Three-person psychology
Psychopathic transferences, 174–175
Psychopharmacology, and schizophrenia, 198–199, 206
Psychosis, and pseudopsychopathic schizophrenia, 198–199, 206
Psychosomatic disorders. *See* Somatization

Index

Psychotherapy, differentiation of psychoanalysis from psychoanalytic forms of, 64–70. *See also* Brief psychoanalytic psychotherapy; Expressive psychotherapy; German depth psychology–based psychoanalytic psychotherapy; Insight-oriented psychotherapy; Mentalization-based psychotherapy; Psychoanalytic psychotherapy; Psychodynamic psychotherapy; Supportive psychotherapy; Transference-focused psychotherapy
Psychotherapy institutes, 281
Psychotherapy Research Project (Menninger Foundation), 66, 133

Racker, Heinrich, 62
Reaction formations, and defensive character traits, 7
Reality
  denial of as frequent complication in severe personality disorders, 251–263
  tactics of transference-focused psychotherapy and, 108, 120–121
Reductionism, in development of theoretical fields, 4–5
Regression, and transference analysis, 59, 60
Rehabilitation, and alcohol or drug abuse, 177
Reich, Wilhelm, 84
Reinforcing adaptive defenses, concept of, 133
Rejection sensitivity, and severe childhood trauma, 42
Relational approach
  basic techniques of psychoanalytic psychotherapy and, 67–68
  countertransference and, 63
  enactment and, 91, 92
  interpretation and, 57
  psychoanalytic field and, 98
  technical neutrality and, 61
  transference analysis and, 57–58
Repetition compulsion, and psychoanalytic techniques, 92–94
Repetitive narratives, and narcissism, 184, 185, 187
Rescue fantasies, of therapists, 232
Research, and psychoanalytic institutes, 277. *See also* Translational research
Resistance analysis, 83
Reverse triangulation, and sexual conflicts, 226, 241
Rigidity, of defensive character traits, 7
Rockland, Lawrence, 133
Role responsiveness, and enactment, 91
Role reversals
  borderline personality disorder and, 44, 78
  narcissistic personality disorder and, 162
  transference-focused psychotherapy and, 107, 148
Rosenfeld, Herbert, 154, 158, 163, 178

Sadomasochistic relationship, and negative therapeutic reaction, 95–96
Sadomasochistic transferences, and narcissistic personality disorder, 172–173
Safety. *See also* Contracts
  acting out and, 90
  antisocial behavior and, 177, 209, 210
Sandler, Joseph, 91
Schizoid personality disorder, 25, 203
Schizophrenia, psychopharmacological treatment of, 198. *See also* Pseudopsychopathic schizophrenia

Schizotypal personality disorder, 23
Secondary gain, and supportive psychotherapy, 143, 146
Second chances, and contract breaches, 123–126
Seeking, and affective systems, 33
Self. *See also* Grandiose self; Self psychology
  assessment of degrees of pathology in experience of, 23
  character traits as component of personality and, 8–9
  concepts of identity and identity diffusion, 9–10
  integration or lack of integration as common factor in personality disorders, 21
  mentalization and, 41
  narcissism and, 155–156, 195
  neurobiology and, 27, 34–36
  psychoanalytic object relations theory and, 40
  subjective intrapsychic structures and concept of, 27
Self-destructive behavior. *See also* Suicide, and suicidal behavior
  denial of reality and, 255, 262–263
  narcissistic personality disorder and, 161, 168–171, 172–173
  negative therapeutic reaction and, 95, 96
  supportive psychotherapy and, 140
  transference-focused psychotherapy and, 117, 119, 125
Self-direction, and assessment of degrees of pathology in experience of self, 23
Self psychology, and technical neutrality, 61, 68
Self-regulation, and severe childhood trauma, 42. *See also* Emotional dysregulation
Seminar leaders, and education in psychoanalysis, 277

Separation reaction, and termination, 101, 102
Sessions. *See* Couch; Financial situation; Frequency
Severe personality disorders. *See* Personality disorders
Sexual abuse
  borderline personality organization and, 237
  narcissistic personality disorder and, 161, 176
Sexual identity, 220, 222
Sexuality, and sexual behavior
  antisocial personality disorder and, 200
  conflicts at level of neurotic personality organization and, 225–232
  diagnostic evaluation of pathologies in, 223–225
  ideal of mature capacity for successful love, 218–221
  narcissistic personality disorder and erotic transferences, 240–244
  obstacles to exploration of in therapy, 127–128, 216–218
  preconditions for therapist's evaluation of, 221–223
  supportive psychotherapy and, 135–136
  total apparent obliteration of in patients with severe personality disorders, 244–247
  transference or countertransference developments in borderline patients, 235–240
  transference-focused psychotherapy and, 127–128
Shame, and narcissistic personality disorder, 194–195. *See also* Shame
Social environment, and internalized value systems, 12. *See also* Life situation

Index 299

Social history, and borderline personality disorder, 74. *See also* Interpersonal relationships
Social service agencies, and supportive psychotherapy, 143–144
Somatization, 90, 96–97
Specialty board, development of psychoanalytic, 274
Splitting, and psychoanalytic object relations theory, 40
Stein, Ruth, 216, 218
Steiner, John, 161–162, 163
Stereotypes, and descriptions of persons in life of narcissistic patient, 186
Stone, Michael, 199, 209
Structural interviewing
  differential diagnosis of antisocial behavior and, 208–209
  supportive psychotherapy and, 138–139
Subjective approach, to psychoanalytic treatment, 281–283
Subservient agreeableness, and interpretation of transference, 52
Suicide, and suicidal behavior
  acting out and, 90
  antisocial personality disorder and, 200
  narcissistic personality disorder and, 161, 168–171
  repetition compulsion and, 94
  tactics of transference-focused psychotherapy and, 109, 123, 124–125
Superego. *See also* Ego
  borderline patients and deterioration of, 237
  components of personality and, 9, 11–14
  evaluation of sexual pathology and, 225
  psychoanalytic object relations theory and, 40

Supervision, and education in psychoanalysis, 275–276
Supportive psychotherapy
  acting out and, 91
  assessment and, 138–139
  contracts and, 139
  countertransference and, 136–137
  dream analysis and, 88
  establishing priorities of treatment, 139
  free association and, 139–140
  frequency of sessions, 64, 139, 147
  indications and contraindications for, 146–147
  modified interpretive approach for, 135
  newly defined strategy of treatment with, 134
  patient's responsibilities in, 144–146
  primitive defensive operations and, 137–138
  psychoanalytic techniques and, 66, 69
  repetition compulsion and, 93–94
  suicidal or parasuicidal behavior and, 170
  technical neutrality and, 136, 148
  therapeutic alliance and, 86
  therapist's relationship with external environment, 143–144
  traditional definition of and changes in, 132–133
  transference analysis and, 135–136, 141–142
  transference-focused psychotherapy compared with, 147–148

Technical neutrality
  acting out and abandonment of, 90
  as basic component of psychoanalytic technique, 51, 53, 60–61, 68, 280

Technical neutrality *(continued)*
   denial of reality and, 257, 260, 261
   supportive psychotherapy and, 136, 148
   techniques of transference-focused psychotherapy and, 110, 115, 126–127
Temperament, as component of personality, 5–6, 7, 32
Termination, and psychoanalytic techniques, 99–102
TFP. *See* Transference-focused psychotherapy
Theme, transference-focused psychotherapy and choice of, 108–109
Theory of mind, 34, 36
Therapeutic alliance, 86, 141
Therapists. *See also* Countertransference; Education; Psychoanalysis; Psychotherapy; Transference
   creativity in imaging better life situations for patients, 260–261
   personal experience of mourning process by, 270
   preconditions for evaluation of sexual pathology by, 221–223
   rescue fantasies of, 232
"Thick-skinned" and "thin-skinned" narcissists, 156, 158–160, 161–163, 182
Third parties, and supportive psychotherapy, 143
Three-person psychology, 44, 167–168
Ticho, Ernst, 119
Tiefenpsychologisch fundierte Psychotherapie (depth psychology–based psychoanalytic psychotherapy), 67, 112
Timidity, as character trait, 7
Tolerance, and mourning process, 267–268

Total transference
   acting out and, 89, 128
   denial of reality and, 262, 251–252
Trait-specified personality disorder, 22
Transference. *See also* Total transference; Transference analysis; Transference-focused psychotherapy
   acting out and, 89
   character analysis and, 85
   differences between supportive and transference-focused psychotherapies, 148
   interpretation of, 55–56
   mechanisms of change in psychoanalytic treatment and, 65
   narcissism at fluctuating borderline level and, 160–168
   narcissism at high stable level of functioning and, 156–160
   psychoanalytic technique and, 51–53
   sexual behavior in borderline patients and, 235–240
   sexual behavior in narcissistic personality structures and, 240–244
   sexual conflicts at level of neurotic personality organization and, 230, 232
   technical neutrality and, 61
Transference analysis
   acting out in context of, 90
   as basic component of psychoanalytic technique, 57–60, 280
   enactment and, 92
   narcissistic patients and, 189
   supportive psychotherapy and, 135–136, 141–142
   techniques of transference-focused psychotherapy and, 109–110

Index

Transference-focused psychotherapy (TFP)
  acting out and, 90–91
  borderline personality disorder and, 43–45, 73–78, 85
  character analysis and, 85
  dream analysis and, 88
  face-to-face position for, 64
  free associations by narcissistic patients and, 181
  frequency of sessions, 64, 107, 115, 132
  indications for, 105
  intersubjective field and, 99
  limit setting and, 177
  malignant narcissism and, 160, 174
  mechanisms of change and, 65–66
  negative therapeutic reaction and, 96
  new developments in, 113–127
  relationship of to other psychoanalytic modalities, 111–113
  repetition compulsion and, 93
  sexuality and financial situation as taboo subjects in, 127–128
  strategies of, 106–108
  suicidal or parasuicidal behavior and, 170
  supportive psychotherapy compared with, 147–148
  supportive techniques in, 133
  tactics of, 108–109
  technical neutrality and, 68, 115
  techniques of, 109–110
Translational research, 20

Trauma
  borderline personality disorder and, 42, 237–238
  intelligence and, 15
  narcissistic personality disorder and, 161, 163
  repetition compulsion and, 92–93
Trust, and development of self, 10
Tuckett, D., 275
12-step programs, 177

Universities, relationship between psychoanalytic institutes and, 276

Value system, sexual relationships and shared, 220–221. *See also* Ethical values; Morality
Verbal self, 36
Violence. *See* Domestic violence; Homicide; Physical abuse

Winnicott, D.W., 98
Work Group on Personality and Personality Disorders for DSM-5, 19–20
Working through, and psychoanalytic techniques, 82, 94
Work situation. *See also* Life situation
  supportive psychotherapy and, 137, 140
  transference-focused psychotherapy and ongoing assessment of, 118–119, 122–123

Yeomans, F.F., 108, 123